Trends in Human Hair Growth and Alopecia Research

Trends in Human Hair Growth and Alopecia Research

Edited by

D. Van Neste, J.M. Lachapelle and J.L. Antoine
Occupational Dermatology Unit, Catholic University of Louvain,
Bruxelles, Belgium

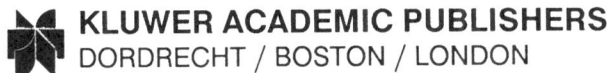
KLUWER ACADEMIC PUBLISHERS
DORDRECHT / BOSTON / LONDON

Distributors

for the United States and Canada: Kluwer Academic Publishers, PO Box 358, Accord Station, Hingham, MA 02018-0358, USA
for all other countries: Kluwer Academic Publishers Group, Distribution Center, PO Box 322, 3300 AH Dordrecht, The Netherlands

British Library Cataloguing in Publication Data

Trends in human hair growth and alopecia research
  I. Man. Hair. Growth
  I. Neste, D. Van, (Dominique)
  I. Lachapelle, J.M. III. Antoine,
J-L (Jean-Luc)
612'.799

ISBN-13: 978-94-011-7875-4   e-ISBN-13: 978-94-011-7873-0
DOI: 10.1007/978-94-011-7873-0

Published in the United Kingdom by Kluwer Academic Publishers, PO Box 55, Lancaster, UK.

Kluwer Academic Publishers BV incorporates the publishing programmes of D. Reidel, Martinus Nijhoff, Dr W. Junk and MTP Press.

Lasertypeset by Martin Lister Publishing Services, Carnforth, Lancs. England

Contents

CONTENTS

Acknowledgements

The contents of this book are based on the original contributions and presentations made at the international research symposium *The Human Hair Follicle in Biomedical Research* held at the Louvain University, Brussels, February 5–6, 1988.

Organized under the auspices of the
SRD – SOCIÉTÉ DE RECHERCHE DERMATOLOGIQUE

Local program committee:
Professor A. Kint, Rijks-Universiteit Gent, Gent, Belgium
Professor J.M. Lachapelle and Dr D. Van Neste
Université Catholique de Louvain, Brussels, Belgium

Concept and organization: Skinterface sprl, Tournai, Belgium

This International Research Symposium acknowledges financial support from the following institutions

COMMISSION FRANÇAIS DE LA CULTURE DE L'AGGLOMÉRATION DE BRUXELLES

FONDS NATIONAL DE LA RECHERCHE SCIENTIFIQUE

MINISTERE DE L'EDUCATION NATIONALE

Foreword

It is now thirty years since William Montagna and Richard Ellis edited "The Biology of Hair Growth". In his introduction, Stephen Rothman, of the University of Chicago, USA and one of the driving forces behind research on skin at the time, wrote:

"The pilary system is a perfect microcosmic structure. In this microcosmos we find birth, development, ageing and death, activity and rest, color formation and decolorification, greasiness and dryness, infection and sterilization, hypertrophy and atrophy, benign tumours and malignant ones."

He foresaw the human pilary system as a model for the study of a multitude of human diseases including ageing and cancer. It was not, however, until the seventies that the development of micro-biochemical techniques indeed allowed the use of the human hair follicle as a convenient biopsy tissue for Biomedical Research in general. Measurement of enzyme activities, and important co-factors, and culturing of cells from single follicles all became possible. In the eighties dermal papilla cells were grown in culture and this opened the way to study hair differentiation *in vitro*.

Studying hair differentiation is, in fact, studying growth regulation and it is this aspect that by far transcends the importance of studying hair growth itself. Let us not forget that metastatic prostate cancer is treated with the same drug - cyproterone acetate - that is used for the treatment of alopecia and hirsutism in women.

A breakthrough in the treatment of alopecia has recently been achieved, not so much in the sense that an effective treatment for most cases of alopecia is now available but in the sense that the approach has dramatically changed. Since Aristotle, himself balding, discovered that eunuchs did not develop baldness, treatment and research have been aimed at inhibiting androgen action in order to prevent hair loss. Minoxidil is the first drug in use for a new approach, namely the induction of local hypertrichosis without interfering in the mechanisms of androgen action.

In the coming years a series of drugs with a strong hypertrichotic effect promises to increase the effectiveness of alopecia treatment. These chemicals are potent, however, and unacceptable side-effects are to be feared in longer term use with large numbers of patients. We are therefore confronted with a major challenge both for academia and for pharmaceutical and cosmetic industries.

While the regrowth of hair may require potent drugs, their lifelong use for prevention of alopecia and for the maintenance of hair regrowth should not be necessary. There is an important task ahead in the development of effective but simple and safe treatments for the above-mentioned goal; as always in research, once that the basic understanding of a problem has been achieved, simplification is always possible.

The Commission of the European Communities has recently decided to accept research into skin diseases as one of the major opportunities in the field of "Age-Related Health Problems" research. Moreover, it was agreed that the possibility of collaboration with industry in European coordinated research actions should be investigated. This brings together a challenging scientific situation with a challenging political one.

My own personal hope is that the achievement of the above-mentioned goal to control the growth of normally differentiating hair cells will bring us closer to the understanding and control of the growth of cancer cells. May the human hair follicle continue to be a valuable model for the study of both cellular differentiation and transformation!

Fons VERMORKEN
Medical Reseach Division
Commission of the European Communities, Brussels

List of Contributors

A. Arai
Derm. Universitäsklinik
Hartmansstrasse 14
D-8520 Erlangen
West Germany

P. Bouhanna
Dermatologie
89 avenue de Villiers
F-75017 Paris
France

H. Degreef
Department de Dermatologie AZ St Pieter
Brusselsestraat 69
B-3000 Leuven
Belgium

Y. de Prost
Department of Dermatology
Hôpital Necker Enfants Malades
149 rue de Sèvres
F-75743 Paris Cédex 15
France

J. De Weert
Dermatologie Akademisch Ziekenhuis
Vrijheidslaan 20
B-9000 Gent
Belgium

D. Dhouailly
Laboratoire de Zoologie et Biolologie
Animale
Université Scientifique et Médicale de
Grenoble BP 68
F-38402 Saint Martin d'Heres Cédex
France

R. Imai
Department of Dermatology
Juntendo University School of Medicine
2-1-1 Hongo
Bunkyo-Ku
Tokyo 113
Japan

K.H. Kurz
Universitäts-Hautklinik
J. Stelzmann-Strasse 9
D-5000 Köln 41
West Germany

J. M. Lachapelle
Dermatologie UCL 3033
30 Clos Chapelle-aux-Champs
B-1200 Bruxelles
Belgium

Ch. M. Lapiere
Service de Dermatologie
Hôpital de Bavière-CHU Sart-Tilman
B-4000 Liège
Belgium

M.-C. Lenoir
CIRD
Centre Internationale de Reserche
Dermatologiques
Sophia Antipolis
F-06565 Valbonne Cédex
France

A.G. Messenger
Department of Dermatology
Royal Hallamshire Hospital
University of Sheffield
Sheffield S10 2JF
United Kingdom

X. Miller
Dermatologist
Cite Bourschterbach 27
L-9029 Warken
Luxembourg

J. Miura
Department of Dermatology
Juntendo University School of Medicine
2-1-1 Hongo
Bunkyo-ku
Tokyo 113
Japan

C. Nappe
L'Oreal-Laboratoires de Recherche
Fondamentale
1 Avenue Eugène Schueller
BP 22
F-93601 Aulnay sous Bois Cédex
France

H. Niedecken
Haut-und Poliklinik der
Rheinische Friedrich-Wilhelms-Universität
Sigmund-Freud Strasse 25
D-5300 Bonn-Venusberg
West Germany

G. Orecchia
Clinica Dermatologica
Università di Pavia
Policlinico S. Matteo
I-27100 Pavia
Italy

J.-P. Ortonne
Service Dermatologie
CHU-Hôpital Pasteur
avenue de la voie Romaine
F-06002 Nice Cédex
France

J.D.R. Peereboom-Wynia
Dermatologie-Ziekenhuis Dijkzigt
Dr Molewaterplein 40
3015 GD Rotterdam
The Netherlands

C. Pelfini
Department of Dermatology
University of Pavia
Pavia
Italy

Y. Privat
Centre Hospitalier Régional
Hôtel Dieu
Place Daviel
F-13002 Marseille
France

H. Schell
Derm. Universitätsklinik
Hartmansstrasse 14
D-8520 Erlangen
West Germany

J. Schweizer
Deutsches Krebsforschungszentrum
In Neuenheimer Feld 280
D-6900 Heidelberg 1
West Germany

G. Serre
Laboratoire de Biologie Cellulaire
CHU Toulouse-Purpan
Place du Docteur Baylac
F-31059
Toulouse Cédex
France

Ch. Sultan
Unité INSERM 58
Biochimie des Stéroides
60 rue de Navacelles
F-34100 Montpellier
France

D. Tennstedt
Dermatologie UCL 3033
30 Clos Chapelle-aux-Champs
B-1200 Bruxelles
Belgium

H. Uno
Wisconsin Regional Primate Research
Center
University of Wisconsin
1223 Capitol Court
Madison
Wisconsin 53715-1299
USA

K. Uyttendaele
Laboratory for Dermatology
Sint Lucas Kliniek
Sint Lucaslaan
B-8320 Brugge 4
Belgium

D. Van Neste
Skinterface sprl
9 rue du Sondart
B-7500 Tournai
Belgium

R. Venafra
Università di Pavia-Medimport
via Recchi 7
I-22100 Como
Italy

A. Vermorken
Research Unit for Cellular Differentiation
and Transformation
University of Nijmegen
G Grooteplein 21
NI 6500 Nijmegen
The Netherlands

Part I:
BIOLOGY AND EXPERIMENTAL MODELS

1

Embryogenesis of the hair follicle and hair cycle

J. De Weert
Department of Dermatology
State University of Ghent, Belgium

ABSTRACT

Formation of hair follicles starts *in utero* along with the first anagen stage of the first hair cycle. After the first wave of growth during the postnatal period, in human beings, each follicle has its own growth cycle that behaves independently of its neighbors, so that there is a mosaic pattern of hair replacement. Some synchronization of human hair growth occurs, however, in certain pathological conditions. After a period of continuous growth, involution of the lower part of the follicle occurs. During catagen the follicle passes in an upward migration to the telogen location. The papilla is likewise pulled upward at the end of the catagen stage. Another characteristic feature in catagen is the phenomenon of cell death by apoptosis and, after catagen, the follicle enters in telogen. This stage is only seemingly quiescent, since the germ of the new follicle is already being formed at its base. The first sign of a new anagen phase is mitotic division of the cells in the lower part of the telogen follicle. The active base of the follicle is transformed to a bulb and the entire development of a new hair with its epithelial component and connective tissue envelopes begins again in the same way as *in utero*, except for two factors: the new follicle does not originate from an epidermal bulge into the dermis, and the old dermal papilla can resume its activity.

Hair consists of compactly cemented keratinized cells and may be regarded as a holocrine secretion produced by cells formed in the base of the hair follicle. Unlike epidermal cells, the hair follicle undergoes cycles, with periods of growth and quiescence. The active growth phase is called anagen[1]. During the resting period, when the hair is retained as a 'club', the follicle is in telogen. The two periods, anagen and telogen, are linked by a transition phase or catagen. During this period, the follicles are reorganizing into an inactive quasi-embryonic state.

    This pattern of growth and rest varies from species to species. With the exception of some animals (e.g. the Merino sheep, the Angora rabbit and the

3

poodle dog in which continuous growth is maintained throughout life), molting in most mammals is more or less synchronous, the club hairs are shed at a given time of year when they are replaced by new hairs. In rodents, the growth periods occur in waves, which start on the belly and move over the flanks to the back[1]. In man, as in the guinea pig, each follicle has its own growth cycle that behaves independently of its neighbors, so that there is a mosaic pattern of hair replacement.

Some synchronization of human hair growth occurs, however, in certain physiological and pathological conditions. In pregnancy almost all hairs are in anagen and a synchronous hairfall occurs in the period of 2–3 months after the delivery[2]. In alopecia areata, the anagen follicles are precipitated into a dystrophic stage that closely resembles the catagen stage[3]. Telogen effluvium is an excessive loss of normal club hairs which occurs when anagen follicles change via normal catagen to the telogen phase too fast and too soon[4].

Knowledge of the morphology and chronology of cyclic hair changes is therefore indispensable to an understanding of the pathodynamics of various hair diseases.

Formation of the follicles, which is also the first anagen stage, starts *in utero*. In our study with albino rats of the Sprague-Dawley colony, the hair germs of the back appear on the 17th day of embryonic life. The first anlagen of the vibrissae or tactile hair follicles are seen on the 15th day. The development of the whiskers occurs earlier and faster than the formation of the follicles of the general pelage. According to Pinkus[5], the first human follicles are formed in the end of the second or in the beginning of the third month of intrauterine life, in the region of the upper lip, eyebrows and chin. Although man has no tactile follicles, the striking association of time and site of the appearance of the first follicles is an indication of human's close phylogenetic relationship to other mammals.

The first indication of the formation of a hair follicle is a crowding of cells in the basal layer of the still relatively undifferentiated bilayered epidermis. This causes a slight bulge of the epidermis: the primitive hair germ or pre-germ[5] (Figure 1). The consensus is that the epidermal change occurs before an accumulation of mesodermal cells is visible. Studies with tritiated thymidine on the rat embryo demonstrated an increase of mitosis only at the level of the epithelial cells of the early pelage-hair germs, while it was impossible to find an increase of the mitosis rate of the mesenchymal cells around and at the bottom of the growing follicle. On the other hand, mitosis was greatly increased in the mesenchymal component around the tactile sinus-hair follicle.

As tritiated thymidine is only a marker for cell division, this study does not answer the question of the possible primary inductive role of 'messengers' or proteins emanating from the mesoderm.

In the consecutive stages (hair germ, hair peg and bulbous peg stage)[6], the follicular column gradually grows into the dermis (Figure 2). The free advancing end of the peg becomes bulbous and envelops a part of the mesoder-

4

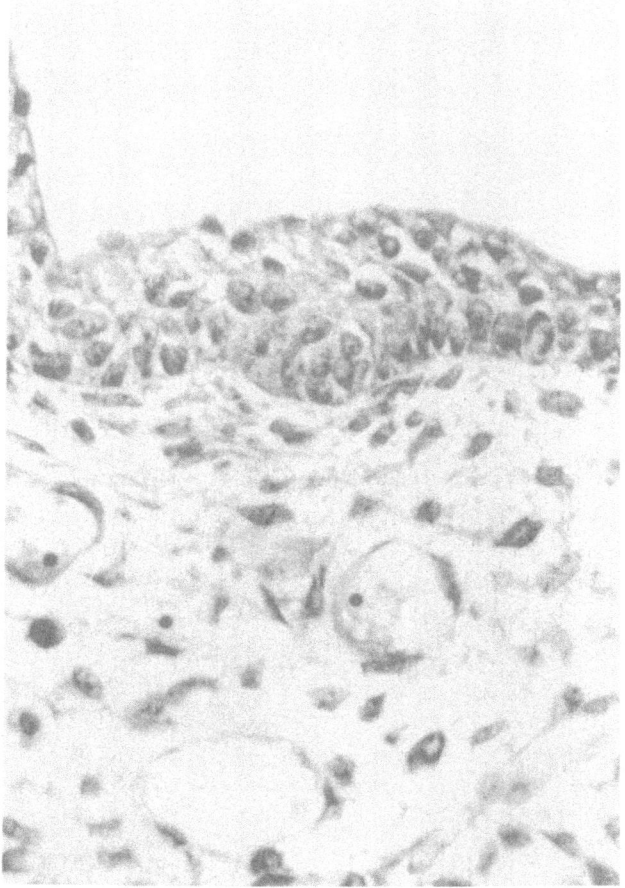

Figure 1 Primitive hair germ. (HE x 600)

mal cells gathered at the bottom of the hair germ: the dermal papilla. Simultaneously, two epithelial swellings develop at one side of the follicle (the so-called 'posterior' side). The upper bulge represents the future sebaceous gland, the lower one the site of attachment of the arrector muscle.

Once all the components of the pilosebaceous units have been established, differentiation ensues. The cells, where the first signs of differentiation are visible, are located in the outer layers of the bulb around the dermal papilla. They become fusiform and acquire eosinophilic granules: the trichohyaline granules, and will give rise to the outer layer of the inner root sheath (layer of Henle). Differentiation of the layer of Huxley and the cuticle of the inner sheath appears on a higher level, i.e. in a chronologically later phase.

At the periphery of the inner sheath are found the cells of the outer root sheath. They contain many glycogen granules, whereas in the cytoplasm to-

5

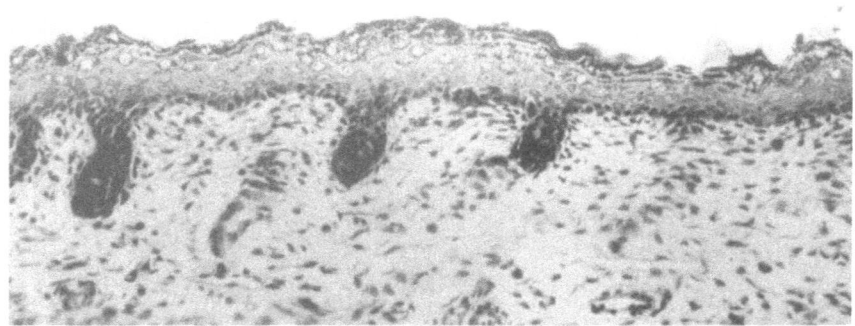

Figure 2　Hair germ, hair peg and bulbous peg (rat embryo)(HE x110)

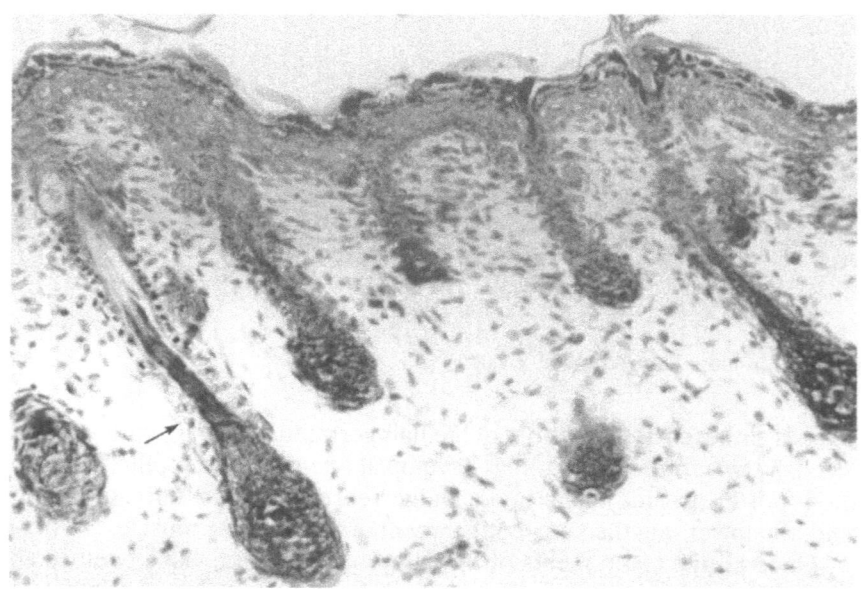

Figure 3　A group of growing follicles (rat embryo). At left differentiation of inner and outer root sheath is visible (arrow). (HE x110)

nofibrils and relatively few desmosomes are discerned (Figure 3). At the inner side of the inner root sheath cortical cells begin to differentiate. They become progressively fusiform and elongated. Filaments and bundles of filaments appear in their cytoplasm[7]. The hair cuticle originates from cuboidal cells in the upper part of the bulb. In their upward migration the long axis is initially radially oriented. Higher up, their outer edges begin to move upward, the orientation changes from horizontal to vertical, and the cells become imbricated.

At the top of the papilla, and localized in the centre of the concentric rings of cells, undifferentiated cells are found. They undergo a peculiar evolution and will form the medulla[8].

Two connective tissue elements surround the hair follicle: the basement membrane and two layers of collagenous fibres. The fibres of the inner layer are orientated parallel to the long axis of the follicle, those of the outer layer are perpendicular to it.

The fully formed anagen follicle produces for a given time a hair which is firmly fixed in the follicle. As soon as the growth phase is over (in different types of hairs this takes different lengths of time), signs of catagen appear in the follicle. The first alteration due to the catagen phase in albino rats occurs in the cells of the papilla. The fibroblasts become rounded and lie close to one another. However, the cytoplasm of the papillary cells remains unchanged, indicating that they still remain active. Cell proliferation in the matrix decreases and finally ceases. The cells in the upper part of the bulb continue to move up and to differentiate into cortex and inner root sheath.

In the evolution of catagen, the outer root sheath seems to have a special significance[9]. It remains present in the undifferentiated epithelial column and around the papilla. In its cells desmosomes, hemidesmosomes and filaments form. In addition, anchoring filaments between the basal lamina and the plasma membrane increase, indicating that cohesion between both the cells and the dermo-epithelial connection has been augmented. The synthesis of the intercellular fine fibrils and desmosome-like structures at the level of the papilla lead to the same conclusion[10]. During catagen the follicle passes in an upward migration to the telogen location. As a result of the cohesion-increasing structures, the papilla is likewise pulled upward at the end of the catagen stage[11]. At the beginning of telogen it is located against the epithelial sack, i.e. the resting matrix cells and can thus fulfil its vital role in the development of a new anagen stage.

Another characteristic feature in catagen is the phenomenon of cell death by apoptosis. Histologically, apoptotic cells are scattered single cells showing an eosinophilic staining cytoplasm with or without a pyknotic nucleus. Apoptosis in catagen was at first described by Weedon and Strutton in 1981[12]. We studied this phenomenon in the catagen follicles found at the advancing edge of patches of alopecia areata, where the catagen stage lasts for several days. Apoptosis is observed in the outer sheath cells at the level of the bulb and of the epithelial column. As the cell shrinks, the plasma membrane loosens its contact with the adjacent cell, except at the sites of the desmosome attachment. The glycogen granules accumulate into the side of the cytoplasm that is directed toward the basement membrane. Tonofilaments appear. The nucleus is released from the cytoplasm, which darkens and

7

becomes very dense. At the end of the process only small and flattened remnants of cells subsist. The presence of glycogen granules allows to identify the outer sheath origin of this cell (Figure 4).

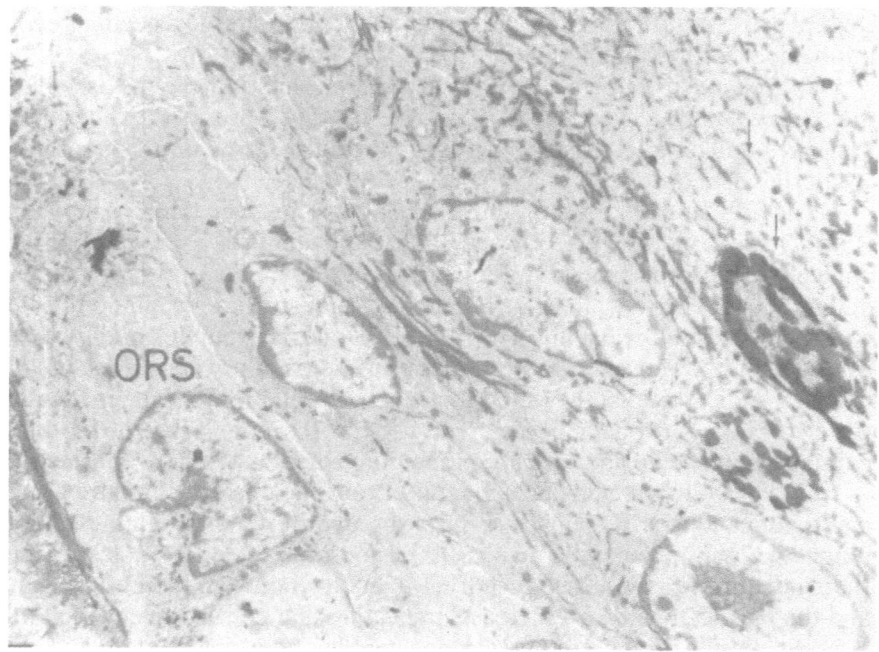

Figure 4   Formation of the club in catagen (rat). Fine fibrils and bundles of fibrils are seen (arrow). ORS = outer root sheath. (x2125)

Ultramicrographs revealed that the formation of the club is a result of cortical differentiation. Bundles of 8 nm wide are arranged in the cytoplasm (Figure 5). They increase numerically and fill the cytoplasm[13,14]. According to Pinkus[15] and Holmes[16], the lower end of the catagen hair becomes surrounded by trichilemmal keratin. At the end of catagen, or at the beginning of telogen, the club is completely structured, and is surrounded by a capsule of germ cells. The dermal papilla is reduced to a compact ball of cells located immediately below the club. The size of the whole follicle is reduced to about a half or one-third the length of the anagen follicle.

The telogen follicle is only seemingly quiescent, since the germ of the new follicle is already being formed at its base. The first sign of a new anagen phase is mitotic division of the cells in the lower part of the telogen follicle. The active base of the follicle is transformed to a bulb and the entire development of a new hair with its epithelial component and connective tissue envelopes begins again in the same way as *in utero*, except for two factors: the

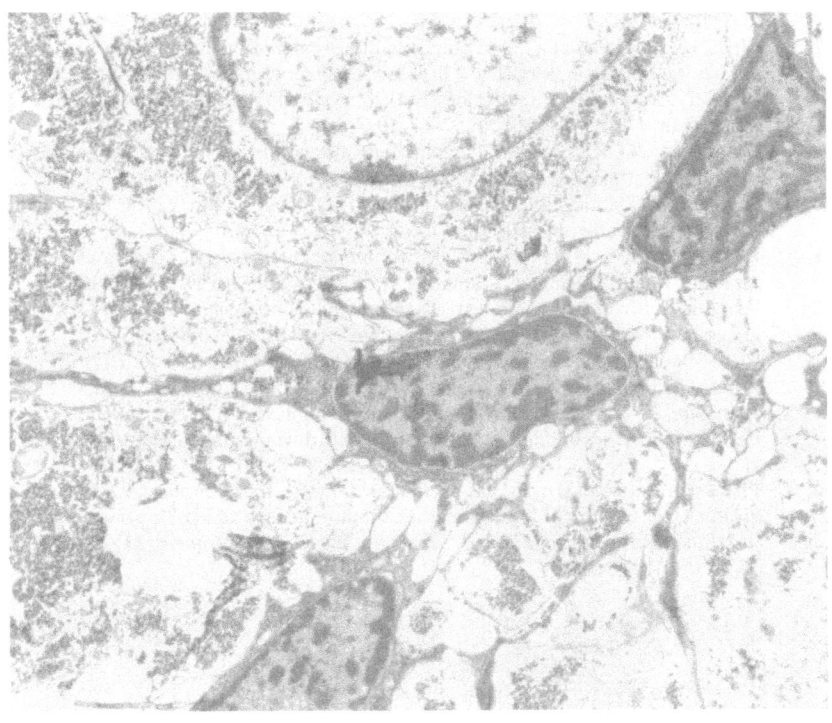

Figure 5 Ultramicrograph of apoptotic cells in the outer root sheath of an alopecia areata follicle. (x2550)

new follicle does not originate from an epidermal bulge into the dermis, and the old dermal papilla can resume its activity.

After proliferation of the epithelial cells into the dermis, the internal root sheath is formed. The top of the new hair forces its way to the surface alongside the old hair shaft. The old club hair comes out, or can persist for a long time. The growth cycle of the hair of one generation comes to an end, and growth of the hair of the next generation continues.

References

1. Dry IW. The coat of the mouse *Mus musculus*. *J Genet* **16**, 287–340, 1926
2. Lynfield YL. Effect of pregnancy on the human hair cycle. *J Invest Dermatol*, **35** , 323–327, 1960
3. Thies W. Vergleichende histologische Untersuchungen bei Alopecia areata und nar-big-atrophisierenden Alopecien. *Arch Klin Exp Derm*, **227**, 541–549, 1966
4. Kligman AM. Pathologic dynamics of human hair loss. I: Telogen effluvium. *Arch Dermatol*, **83**, 175–198, 1961
5. Pinkus F. The development of the integument. In *Manual of Human Embryology* (Keibel and Mall, eds), Vol. I, pp. 243–291. Philadelphia: Lippincott, 1910

6. Stöhr P. Entwicklungsgeschichte des menschlichen Wollhaares. *Anat Hefte Abt*, **1** (23), 1–66, 1903
7. Birbeck MS, Mercer EH. The electron microscopy of the human hair follicle. 1. Introduction and the hair cortex. *J Biophys Biochem Cytolog*, **3**, 203–214, 1957
8. Roth SI, Helwig EB. The cytology of the cuticle, the cortex and the medulla of the mouse hair. *Ultrastruct Res,* **11**, 52–67, 1964
9. Braun-Falco O, Kint A. Zur Dynamik der Katagenphase: eine experimentelle Studie an Albino Ratten. *Arch Klin Exp Dermatol*, **223**, 1–15, 1965
10. Sugiyama S, Takahashi M, Kamimura M. The ultrastructure of the hair follicles in early and late catagen. *J Ultrastruct Res*, **54**, 369–373, 1976
11. De Weert J, Kint A, Geerts ML. Morphologic changes in the proximal area of the rat's hair follicle during early catagen. *Arch Dermatol Res*, **272**, 79–92, 1982
12. Weedon D, Strutton G. Apoptosis as the mechanism of the involution of hair follicles in catagen transformation. *Acta Dermatovenereol*, **61**, 335–339, 1981
13. Roth SI. The cytology of the murine resting (telogen) hair follicle. Reprinted from: *Biology of the Skin and Hair Growth*. Proceedings of a symposium held at Canberra, Australia, 22–28 August, 1964. Eds. Sydney: Angus & Robertson, 1965
14. Parakkal PF. Morphogenesis of the hair follicle during catagen. *Z Zellforsch*, **10**, 174–186, 1970
15. Pinkus H. 'Sebaceous cysts' are trichilemmal cysts. *Arch Dermatol*, **99**, 544–555, 1969
16. Holmes EJ. Tumors of lower sheath. Common histogenesis of certain so called 'sebaceous cysts', acanthomas and 'sebaceous carcinomas'. *Cancer*, **21**, 234–248, 1968

2
Keratin expression in the human hair follicle

J Schweizer
Institute of Experimental Pathology,
German Cancer Research Center,
69 Heidelberg, Federal Republic of Germany

ABSTRACT

During the past 20 years there has been an impressive accumulation of scientific literature on the proteins which are involved in the formation and differentiation of the hair. It is clear that these studies cannot be segregated from the previous research on wool fiber proteins. Therefore a short compilation of the knowledge in this area will be presented, especially to take into account methodological aspects and difficulties associated with the biochemical analysis of hair proteins.

The first detailed description and analysis of the whole set of native hard alpha-keratins of the human hair – recently published by two different laboratories – has provided new evidence for the already widely accepted realization that these proteins represent a distinct subclass of epithelial cytokeratins which is highly conserved in mammals. They seem to be generally involved in the formation of hardened cornified structures and may therefore be regarded as molecular markers for hair/nail type differentiation.

Similar to cytokeratins, the hard alpha-keratins can be divided into two characteristic type I and type II subfamilies, each containing four individual members which are encoded by mRNAs of their own. The unambiguous identification of the whole set of proteins by gel electrophoretic methods requires sophisticated focusing conditions which have also enabled it to be shown that the different proteins undergo an increased phosphorylation during hair maturation. Reassociation studies in which collectively separated and solubilized type I and type II proteins were combined *in vitro*, revealed their capacity to assemble into 8–10 nm filaments provided, however, the reassociation conditions took into account the high cysteine content of the proteins. The presence of four protein subunits in each of the two subfamilies is indicative of the formation of an equal number of distinct keratin pairs, and preliminary immunohistochemical studies with antibodies recognizing either the basic or the acidic proteins in Western blots suggest that the oppositely charged proteins appear coordinately in the keratogenous zone of the forming hair shaft.

These new insights in the field of hard alpha-keratin composition, synthesis and localization raise a variety of new questions. It can be predicted that the strategy for the resolution of these questions will certainly involve recombinant DNA techniques to elucidate both the nucleotide and amino acid sequences of the different hard alpha-keratins and their respective mRNAs or genes. These will provide an arsenal for the generation of highly specific gene probes and antibodies which in turn will be a prerequisite to further unraveling of the complex differentiation pathways of the hair from the hair follicle germinative cells.

INTRODUCTION

The hair develops from a morphologically complex follicular structure which can be divided into three main parts: the outer root sheath, the inner root sheath and the hair itself. The outer root sheath which is continuous with the interadnexial epidermis, constitutes the outermost wall of the hair follicle and is surrounded by the connective tissue sheath. The inner root sheath consists centripetally of three concentric layers: Henle's layer, Huxley's layer and the inner root sheath cuticle. Finally the hair shaft is built up of the hair cuticle, the cortex and, depending upon species, localization and developmental stage, the medulla. The constituents of both the inner root sheath and the hair fiber arise from a germinative pool of matrix cells located in the club-shaped hair bulb which encloses the dermal papilla in a cavity at its base (for a detailed description of the hair follicle anatomy, see references 1 and 2). Similar to the differentiation of the mammalian epidermis, the terminal differentiation of the hair can be regarded as a suicide maturation pathway, during which epithelial cells produce abundant amounts of keratin, keratinize and ultimately die.

During the past 20 years there has been an impressive accumulation of scientific literature on the proteins which are involved in the formation and differentiation of the hair. It must, however, be emphasized that most of our present knowledge in this field has been a direct consequence of demands of wool research and, in comparison, considerably less information is available about the corresponding proteins in human hairs.

Recently, however, two laboratories – that of Franke, in Heidelberg, and of Sun, in New York – have independently and almost simultaneously tackled this problem and further investigated the protein composition of human hair[3,4]. These studies form the core of this review on the keratinization of human hair. It is clear, however, that these studies cannot be segregated from the previous research on wool fiber proteins. Therefore a short compilation of the knowledge in this area is necessary, especially as it takes into account various methodological aspects and difficulties associated with the biochemical analysis of hair proteins.

PROTEINS ASSOCIATED WITH WOOL FIBER DIFFERENTIATION

Previous chemical and biochemical studies have shown that the constituent proteins of wool fibers and the associated matrix material fall into three major classes, each class itself consisting of two or more subfamilies of apparently related proteins.

The designation of the three protein classes in the literature is according to a nomenclature which takes into account the particular occurrence or the preponderance of distinct amino acids (mostly cysteine) within the proteins. Following decreasing molecular weights, one distinguishes the low sulfur proteins (40–60 kDa; 1–3 mol% cysteine), the high sulfur proteins (10–25 kDa; 20–30 mol% cysteine) and the high glycine/tyrosine proteins (6–9 kDa; 20–40 mol% glycine, 12–21 mol% tyrosine; for a detailed description of the three protein classes, see references 5–7). A large body of electron microscopic and X-ray studies has also shown that the hair and wool fiber cortex contains abundant amounts of 8–10 nm alpha-helical keratin filaments which are separated from each other by an interfilamentous matrix. It is now well established that the globular high sulfur proteins and the high glycine/tyrosine proteins are involved in the formation of the interfilamentous matrix, whereas the low sulfur proteins represent the constituent proteins of the 8–10 nm filaments[5–7]. In the following, they will therefore be referred to as low sulfur keratins or preferentially 'hard alpha-keratins'. The latter classical designation was originally introduced to discriminate the alpha-keratins of the hardened cornified tissues of hair, nails and claws from the 'soft alpha-keratins' or cytokeratins from epithelia[8].

The resolution of the hard alpha-keratins of wool fibers by two-dimensional gel electrophoresis revealed two major families of proteins, each family consisting of apparently four distinct subunits. The larger and more basic proteins were designated 7a, 7b, 7c and 5; the smaller more acidic proteins were designated 8a, 8b, 8c1 and 8c2[5,6]. Subsequent amino acid sequence homology comparisons of enzymatically obtained alpha-helical fragments of distinct proteins of the two families (proteins 7c and 8c1, respectively[9,10]) have then led to the classification of wool alpha-keratins into type II proteins (comprising the more basic protein family 7a, 7b, 7c, and 5) and type I proteins (comprising the more acidic protein family 8a, 8b, 8c1 and 8c2[9–14]).

Perhaps the most important recent advance in our knowledge of hair and wool alpha-keratins is the realization that they are in many respects intimately related to the cytokeratins of keratinizing, non-keratinizing and simple epithelia[5,6]. From the structural point of view, both share a comparable X-ray diffraction pattern, arising from the alpha-helical domain in a coiled coil formation[15,16]. An antiserum raised against the protease-resistant alpha-helical domain of wool keratin was found to crossreact strongly with the keratin network of a variety of epithelia and epithelial cells[17]. Moreover, by analogy with the classification of hard alpha-keratins of wool into oppositely charged type I and type II subfamilies, all soft keratins can also be divided into an acidic subfamily, comprising mainly the smaller subunits and a basic to neutral subfamily of substantially larger subunits[33]. Again, the biochemical reason for this subdivision has been found to be due to sequence characteristics (i.e. the number and distribution of basic and acidic amino acids) of the respective alpha-helical domains[57]. Finally, preliminary sequence data from molecular cloning experiments of hard alpha-keratins show extensive homology with the corresponding data of epidermal keratins[18,19] and suggest an almost identical genomic exon–intron organization of wool component 8c1 and epidermal type I keratins[5,20,21].

It must, however, be emphasized that up to now a reliable comparison of the chemical, biochemical, physical and immunological features of hard and soft alpha-keratins is seriously hampered by a property of hard alpha-keratins which, at a first glance, seems to be only of minor importance. Indeed, earlier investigations had suggested that the hard alpha-keratins from wool and hair which are extensively crosslinked by S–S bonds and tightly associated with the matrix proteins, could apparently not be solubilized under conditions which solubilize cytokeratins, i.e. in buffers containing denaturating and reducing agents at neutral or slightly alkaline pH[22,23]. Traditionally, therefore, the methods used to solubilize hard alpha-keratins have involved either proteolytic digestion or – almost ubiquitously employed in protein analysis – the chemical modification of the proteins by S-carboxy-methylation under strongly alkaline conditions[23,24]. Unfortunately, the covalent introduction of the highly polar carboxymethyl group drastically modifies the electrophoretic mobilities, in particular the isoelectric points of the proteins[5,6,24,25]. Moreover the carboxymethyl group possesses strong immunogenic properties[26], thus making a meaningful comparison with the unmodified cytokeratins in many respects rather difficult. It is then a stroke of luck that both of the studies mentioned above[3,4] on human hair proteins worked on the native, chemically unmodified alpha-keratins and thus allowed for the first time a direct comparison with cytokeratins.

ISOLATION OF NATIVE HARD ALPHA-KERATINS FROM HUMAN HAIR AND HAIR FORMING CELLS

The strategy used by Heid *et al.*[3] to obtain native hair alpha-keratins consisted in the isolation of hair-forming cells from the follicular base of plucked human anagen hairs. The reasoning behind this strategy – backed by numerous histochemical investigations[27–29], was that in those 'trichocyte preparations'[3], the alpha-keratins should still exist in a non-oxidized and non-crosslinked form. Moreover, a short incubation of the excised lower part of the hair follicles (transsected about 2 mm above the follicular base) in a high salt buffer (10 mmol/l Tris–HCl, 140 mmol/l NaCl, 1.5 mol/l KCl, 5 mmol/l EDTA, 0.5% w/v Triton X-100, pH 7.6) – commonly used to extract soluble proteins from tissues – enabled the authors to manually remove both the outer and the inner root sheath, thus leaving the lowermost central core of trichocytes available for keratin extraction[3]. It should be mentioned that, recently, Jones and Pope[30] used a similar approach for the enrichment of hair-forming cells. Subsequently, however, these authors used S-carboxymethylation for protein analysis.

Alternatively, Heid *et al.*[3] also used human hair tips as a source for keratin extraction. To this purpose the hairs were reduced to a fine powder in a steel ball mill, cooled with liquid nitrogen. Depending on whether one- or two-dimensional gel electrophoretic analysis of the proteins was intended, both potential keratin sources were directly dissolved in the corresponding sample buffers [1DE: 5% SDS, 10 mmol/l β-mercaptoethanol, 10 mmol/l Na_2HPO_4 x $2H_2O$, 10% glycerol, pH 6.8[31]; 2DE: 9.5 mol/l urea, 0.5% SDS, 0.5% β-mercaptoethanol, 5% Nonidet P-40, 2% of a special mixture of ampholites with a high resolution power of pH 5–8 (modified according to reference 32); for the solubilization of powdered hairs, 5% β-mercaptoethanol was used].

After boiling (only in the case of 1DE) and homogenization, the samples were centrifuged and the keratin-containing supernatants were deep frozen until use. In the investigation by Lynch *et al.*[4] only human hair clippings were used as starting material for keratin extraction. The composition of the urea/β-mercaptoethanol extraction buffer was essentially comparable to that of the 2DE sample buffer described by Heid *et al.*[3], except that the pH was raised to 9.6. This high pH previously also used by other authors[30], produces a swelling of the hairs and was expected to favor an efficient reduction of S–S bonds by unfolding the compact keratin structures.

It should be mentioned that, in both studies, hair alpha-keratins from different animal species, i.e. cow and sheep[3]; rabbit, mouse and sheep[4] as well as hard alpha-keratin preparations from human nails[4], were used for comparison with human hair alpha-keratins.

ANALYSIS OF ONE- AND TWO-DIMENSIONAL ELECTROPHORETIC PATTERN OF NATIVE HAIR ALPHA-KERATINS

One-dimensional analysis of SDS/β-mercaptoethanol extracted alpha-keratins from human trichocyte preparations led to the detection of two groups of proteins, migrating in a molecular weight range of either 56–60 kDa or 42–44 kDa. Thus the observed MW range is largely consistent with that observed for soft keratins (40–70 kDa,[33]). The high MW group of proteins consisted of three distinct bands, whereas the smaller group of proteins was resolved into two bands[3]. Two-dimensional analysis using an ampholite system which optimally spreads proteins in a pH range of 5–8 resulted in a much clearer picture (Figure 1a). The high MW protein family (56–60 kDa) was clearly resolved into four distinct keratin subunits of relatively high isoelectric point values (6.0–7.2). According to their localization in the gel they were designated Hb1, Hb2, Hb3 and Hb4 (H for hair and b for basic). Similarly the 42–44 kDa protein family was also resolved into four easily visible proteins

15

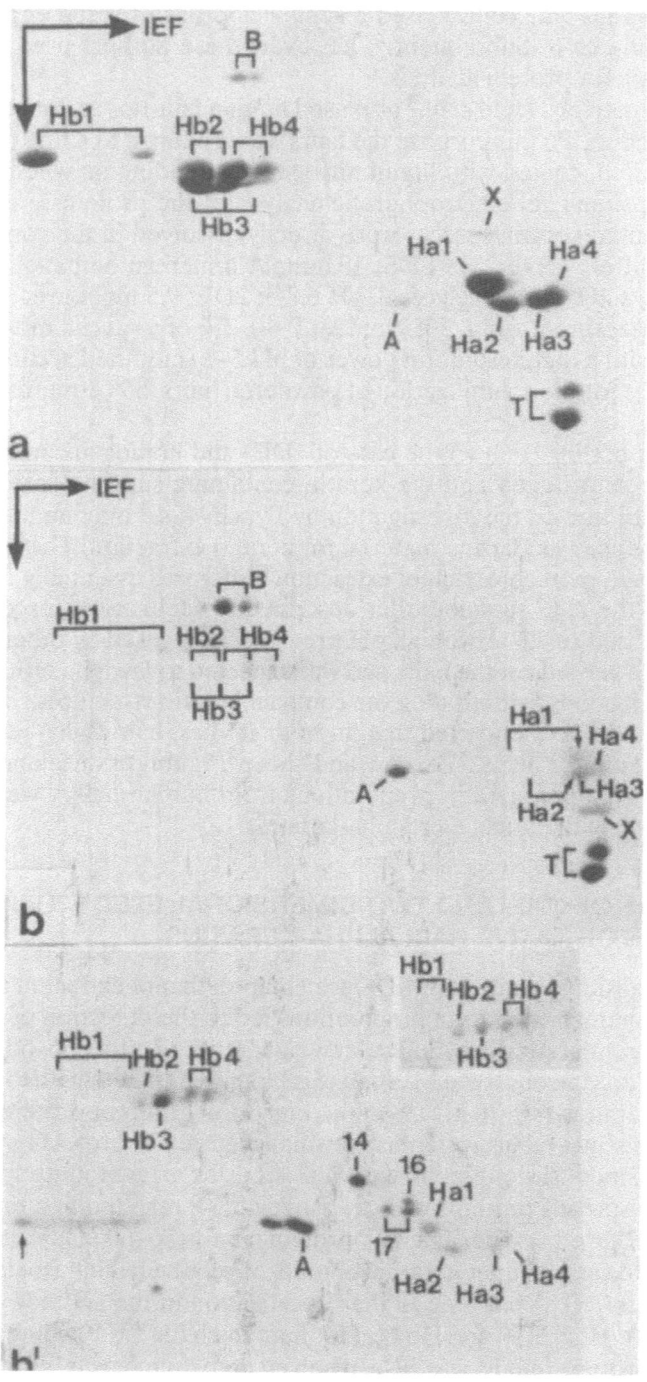

which, however, appeared in a more acidic pH range (4.8–5.2). They were therefore designated Ha1, Ha2, Ha3 and Ha4 (a for acidic). Consistently, especially the members of the basic subfamily exhibited two or more fairly easily visible satellite spots of isoelectric variants, a feature which is also characteristic for cytokeratins under appropriate focusing conditions[33]. In this context it is worth mentioning that essentially comparable two-dimensional keratin patterns were obtained from bovine and ovine trichocyte preparations, except some more or less pronounced species-dependent variations in the positions of keratins Hb2 and especially Ha1 and Ha2[3].

Therefore in terms of detectable keratin subunits, these characteristic patterns of native hair alpha-keratins with the observed division into a basic and acidic subfamily are in principle in complete agreement with the results obtained with S-carboxymethylated wool alpha-keratins (see Chapter 2[5,6]). However, even a superficial inspection of the corresponding gels reveals how drastically the introduction of carboxymethyl groups interferes with the charge properties and hence with the mobility of the individual proteins of both subfamilies. Therefore, a direct correlation between S-carboxymethylated wool alpha-keratin subunits 7a, 7b, 7c and 5 (type I) and 8a, 8b, 8c1 and 8c2 (type II) and the human native hair alpha-keratin subunits Ha1, Ha2, Ha3 and Ha4 and Hb1, Hb2, Hb3 and Hb4 cannot be made.

Most interestingly, virtually all subunits of the basic and the acidic keratin subfamilies of the human trichocyte preparations could also be detected in two-dimensionally resolved extracts of mature hair (Figure 1b). However, in contrast to the keratins present in hair-forming cells, the keratins from mature hair clearly displayed mainly the more acidic isoelectric variants of each individual keratin subunit. Since exactly these satellite spots were found to be strongly labeled after incubation of human trichocyte preparations in a medium containing ^{32}P-orthophosphate, the authors concluded that, *in vivo*, the hair alpha-keratins are subject to an increased phosphorylation as the trichocytes move away from the follicular base[3].

At this point it is interesting to compare these results with those obtained by Lynch *et al.*[4]. As mentioned before, these authors used only mature hair for the isolation of keratins. After one-dimensional resolution of the proteins solubilized at high pH, they also describe a high and a low MW family, however, their subsequent two dimensional resolution led only to three relative-

Figure 1 Two dimensional electrophoresis of human alpha-keratins isolated from hair forming cells (trichocytes) (a), mature hair (b), or synthesized in an *in vitro* translation system from human hair follicle mRNA (c). The samples were analyzed by isoelectric focusing in the first dimension (IEF) and by SDS-polyacrylamide gel electrophoresis in the second dimension (downward arrow). The following marker proteins were used: B, bovine serum albumin; A, alpha-actin (in a and b); beta- and gamma-actin (in c); T, tropomyosin; X (in a and c) represents unidentified material. For the designation of the hair alpha-keratins, see text. Note that in c also root sheath epithelia cytokeratins numbers 14, 16 and 17 are detectable amongst the translation products (see also text). The insert in c shows that the different keratin subunits vary in intensity in different experiments. (Reproduced with permission from ref. 3)

17

ly basic proteins (MW 60, 59, 56 kDa) and two acidic proteins (MW 44 and 46 kDa). In accordance with results obtained by Heid et al.[3], an essentially comparable protein pattern was observed with keratin extracts from sheep wool and in addition from human nails. A closer inspection of the gels suggests that, in the study by Lynch et al.[4], the basic subunits Hb2 and Hb4 do not seem to be resolved from each other, and apparently also the acidic subunits Ha1 and Ha4 migrate together. Most probably the discrepancy in the number of detectable subunits between the two laboratories is due to the increased phosphorylation of the keratin subunits observed by Heid et al. in mature hairs[3]. Figure 1b clearly shows that the accumulation of the more acidic isoelectric variants of the individual keratin subunits may simulate the presence of only three and two distinct proteins in the basic and acidic subfamilies, respectively. This phenomenon is certainly even more accentuated if the ampholite system used is not optimally calibrated for the appropriate resolution of the proteins.

Collectively, however, both studies have shown that native hard alpha-keratins can be isolated in sufficient amounts both from hair-forming cells and the mature hair under conditions which also solubilize soft keratins. Apparently, the extraction procedures at neutral or slightly alkaline pH led to a selective solubilization of the hard alpha-keratins, i.e. the low sulfur keratin fraction, whereas some immunological data by Lynch et al.[4] suggest that a shift to strongly alkaline extraction conditions also solubilizes at least trace amounts of native high sulfur proteins. The hard alpha-keratins can be successfully analyzed by one- or two-dimensional gel electrophoresis without prior S-carboxymethylation. Moreover, the studies have confirmed previous findings with S-carboxymethylated wool alpha-keratins in that also native hair alpha-keratins of different species can be divided into a basic type II and an acidic type I subfamily, each consisting of four individual keratin subunits.

FURTHER CHARACTERIZATION OF NATIVE HUMAN HAIR ALPHA-KERATINS

A characteristic feature of SDS/β-mercaptoethanol or urea/β-mercaptoethanol solubilized cytokeratins of a distinct epithelium or epithelial cells is their ability to reform 8–10 nm filaments in vitro after dialysis against weakly reducing buffers of low ionic strength[34-36]. From numerous investigations with isolated keratin subunits it is now well established that the successful in vitro reformation of intact filaments requires the presence of at least one member of the type I and type II family[36,37]. In the study by Heid et al.[3], both total basic and acidic hard alpha-keratins were isolated by preparative gel electrophoresis, dissolved in urea/β-mercaptoethanol, mixed in approximately equal amounts and dialyzed against a buffer containing 50 mmol/l Tris–HCl, 200 mmol/l DTE, pH 7.6. Following this, electron microscopic inspection indeed revealed the characteristic formation of 8–10 nm filaments besides protofilament structures[3]. However, as emphasized by the authors, unlike the in vitro restoration of 8–10 nm filaments from cytokeratins[34–37], the *in vitro* assembly of hard alpha-keratins from hair required the presence of substantially higher amounts of the reducing agent. In view of the relatively high content of cysteine residues in hair alpha-keratins (1–3 mol%[5,6]), this measure is apparently necessary to prevent the precocious arrest of filament assembly due to the pronounced tendency to form S–S bonds. Considering the recently demonstrated 'promiscuity' of cytokeratins with regard to their ability to assemble *in vitro*[37], it would be interesting to know whether hair alpha-keratins of one type are also able to form filaments with cytokeratins of the opposite type. As yet those experiments have not been made.

In vitro translation studies with total mRNA of terminally differentiating epithelia such as the epidermis have shown that not every subunit present in the epidermal keratin pattern is encoded by mRNA of its own[38]. Detailed protein analysis of fractionated epidermis, in combination with comparative peptide mappings, have revealed that those subunits which are not translated *in vitro* are indeed secondarily derived stratum corneum equivalents of encoded keratin subunits[38,39]. There is strong evidence that the seemingly controlled post-translational modifications at the transition from the granular to the cornified layer proceeds via the proteolytic degradation of the strongly basic carboxyterminal tail of encoded keratins[40], thus giving rise to smaller derivatives which are progressively more acidic than their encoded precursors[38,39,41].

Although similar to the epidermis, the hair follicle also represents a terminally differentiating system, a comparable degradation mechanism of distinct keratin subunits is not likely to occur in this tissue since, in terms of both number and size, the keratin subunits present in the trichocytes at the follicular base are not different from those of the mature hair[3]. As already mentioned, the only maturation-associated post-translational modification of hair alpha-keratins seems to be an increased phosphorylation[3]. On the other hand this strongly suggests that all keratin subunits of the hair are genuine translation products. Indeed *in vitro* translation experiments with mRNA, isolated by Heid *et al.* from human hair follicle bases, confirmed that virtually all keratin members of both subfamilies can be identified among the *in vitro* translation products (Figure 1c)[3]. It should be mentioned in this context that previous *in vitro* translation experiments, conducted with mRNAs from mouse hair follicles and sheep wool follicles, had already provided evidence that hair alpha-keratins are not subject to post-translational cleavage of larger precursors, but are genuinely synthesized in their finished size[42,43].

Finally, co-electrophoresis studies carried out by Heid *et al.*[3] with hair alpha-keratins and a large number of cytokeratins of various epithelial tissues and cells demonstrated that apparently none of the hair alpha-keratins is identical to any of the human cytokeratins. This led the authors to complete their previously established catalog of 19 human cytokeratins[33] by the eight hair alpha-keratins, thus raising the total number of presently known genuine human keratins to 27 individual members. Interestingly, the hair alpha-keratins belong either to the least basic or the most acidic members of the respective type II and type I subfamilies (Figure 2).

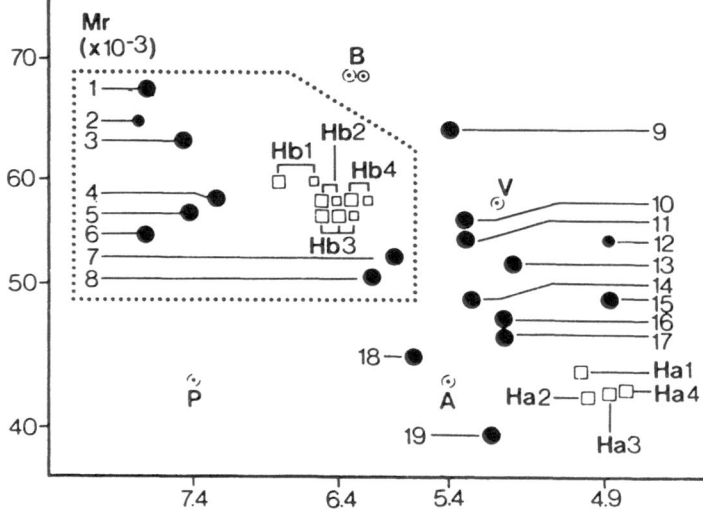

Figure 2 Schematic presentation of human alpha-keratins from hair forming cells (open squares) and human epithelial cytokeratins (filled circles). (Reproduced with permission from ref. 3)

IMMUNOLOCALIZATION OF HAIR ALPHA-KERATINS

In both the investigations by Heid et al.[3] and Lynch et al.[4], immunohistochemical studies were carried out with either polyclonal or monoclonal antibodies against native human hair alpha-keratins. However, prior to the discussion of these results it should again be recalled that potentially antibodies against cytokeratins may crossreact with hard alpha-keratins and vice-versa[17,44]. An impressive example for this phenomenon is the monoclonal antibody Kg 8.13, which recognizes an epitope common to type II basic cytokeratins and, surprisingly, also present in the type I cytokeratin 18[45]. As shown by Heid et al.[3], this antibody stains virtually all components of the hair follicle, i.e. the outer and inner root sheath, the hair cuticle and cortex, and most importantly also the matrix cells of the entire bulbar region in a comparable intensity. In contrast a polyclonal antibody against human callus keratin was found to react only with the outer and inner root sheath and the hair cuticle[4].

At this point it is necessary to include some elucidative remarks on what is presently known on the keratin expression in the outer and inner root sheath of the human hair follicle. Studies by Moll et al.[46,47] and Heid et al.[3], with microdissected outer and inner root sheath preparations have shown that these structures contain keratins 5 and 14 and 6 and 16. (In embryonic hair follicles (20 weeks of pregnancy), keratin 17 is expressed instead of keratin 16[47]). Considering that the outer root sheath is continuous with the epidermis, the presence of keratins 5 and 14 is *per se* not surprising, since this keratin pair is characteristic of the basal cell layer of stratified epithelia[33,48]. We were recently able to show by means of *in situ* hybridization with specific cDNA clones, corresponding to mouse keratins 5 and 14[49–51] that the mRNAs of these keratins are indeed expressed in both the basal epidermal cell layer[50,51] and in the entire outer root sheath (Figure 3). In contrast, the

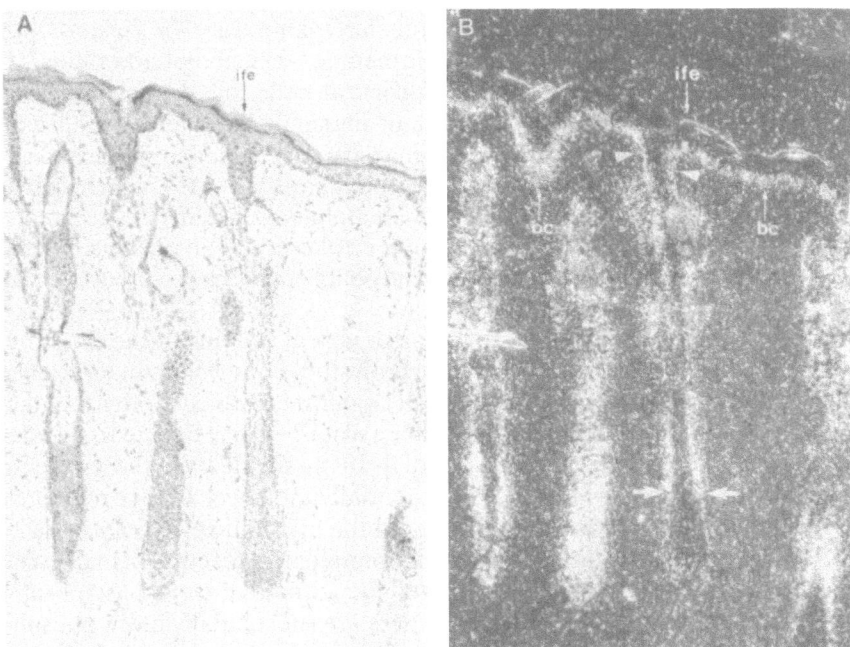

Figure 3 Transverse section of mouse back skin, *in situ* hybridized with a specific 3'-fragment of clone pkSCC60. This clone is complementary to the mRNA of the basal type II 60 kDa keratin of mouse epidermis, which corresponds to the human keratin no. 5 in the catalog of Moll *et al.*[33]. For *in situ* hybridization conditions, see references 50 and 51. A: Bright field illumination. Due to the low magnification, hybridization signals are barely visible. B: Dark field illumination reveals hybridization signals in the basal cell layer (bc) of the interfollicular epidermis (ife) and in the entire outer root sheath of the hair follicles. Arrowheads indicate the zone of the pilary canal. Arrows denote a zone where the outer root sheath undergoes an abrupt thickening at the height of the keratogenous zone of the hair cortex (see also ref. 4)

demonstration of the keratin pair 6 and 16 in outer and inner root sheath preparations is not readily explainable. This keratin pair is typical for cultured epidermal cells, and its synthesis *in vivo* is generally associated with a hyperproliferative state of a stratified epithelium[52]. At present it is not known whether the expression of keratins 6 and 16 is dependent on the hair cycle, in other words restricted to anagen hair follicles, nor is it known where this keratin pair is located within the outer and inner root sheath.

Indirect immunofluorescence studies by Heid *et al.* using a polyclonal antibody raised against the total acidic subfamily of human hair alpha-keratins revealed a strong reaction of the cuticular and cortical cells of the keratogenous zone of the hair shaft, whereas deep bulbar cells of the matrix were distinctly less stained. In addition, the antiserum also decorated the outer root sheath[3]. This staining pattern is somewhat different from that observed with a monoclonal antibody, AE13, from Sun's laboratory. In Western blots this antibody also reacted with the acidic members of hair alpha-keratins, and on tissue sections selectively stained cortical cells located several layers above the tip of the dermal papilla without any significant staining of the cells in between[4]. Essentially the same staining pattern of upper cuticular and cortical cells was observed with the monoclonal antibody AE3, which specifically reacts with the basic members of hair alpha-keratins in Western blots[4]. Since this antibody also recognizes type II cytokeratins[53], a positive reaction was also found in the outer root sheath, probably due to a crossreaction with keratin 5.

It has been suggested that the weak or absent staining of the lower bulbar cells of the hair follicle observed in both studies, as well as in a variety of investigations with monoclonal antibodies against S-carboxymethylated hard alpha-keratins from human hair and sheep wool[26,54] may be due to the electronmicroscopically observed paucity of 8–10 nm filaments in these cells[4,55]. However, as shown by Heid *et al.*[3], potentially the lower bulbar region can be stained as intensely as the remainder of the hair follicle with antibody Kg 8.13. One possible reason for the weak immunological reaction of matrix cells may be the fact that in all cases reported the antibodies were raised against alpha-keratins from mature hair, and these are substantially more phosphorylated than their low bulbar analogs[3]. Since there is evidence that serum antibodies against phosphoproteins are able to immunologically distinguish between the phosphorylated and the non-phosphorylated proteins[56], it cannot be excluded that the keratin antibodies used preferentially reacted in an advanced zone of the growing hair in which substantial phosphorylation of the keratins has already occurred.

Overall, the immunohistochemical studies with antibodies against native alpha-keratins, detecting either the basic or the acidic subunits, strongly indicate that the members of the two subfamilies are coordinately expressed during hair differentiation. However, the exact site of the induction of their expression still remains to be determined.

SUMMARY AND PERSPECTIVES

The first detailed description and analysis of the whole set of native hard alpha-keratins of the human hair has provided new evidence for the already widely accepted realization that these proteins represent a distinct subclass of epithelial cytokeratins which is highly conserved in mammals. As demonstrated by Lynch *et al.*, in a concomitant investigation of human nails, they seem to be generally involved in the formation of hardened cornified structures, and may therefore be regarded as molecular markers for hair/nail type differentiation.

Similar to cytokeratins, the hard alpha-keratins can be divided into two characteristic type I and type II subfamilies, each containing four individual members which are encoded by mRNAs of their own. The unambiguous identification of the whole set of proteins by gel electrophoretic methods requires sophisticated focusing conditions which have also shown that the different proteins undergo an increased phosphorylation during hair maturation. Reassociation studies in which collectively separated and solubilized type I and type II proteins were combined *in vitro*, revealed their capacity to assemble into 8–10 nm filaments provided, however, the reassociation conditions took into account the high cysteine content of the proteins. The presence of four protein subunits in each of the two subfamilies is indicative of the formation of an equal number of distinct keratin pairs, and preliminary immunohistochemical studies with antibodies recognizing either the basic or the acidic proteins in Western blots suggest that the oppositely charged proteins appear coordinately in the keratogenous zone of the forming hair shaft.

These new insights in the field of hard alpha-keratin composition, synthesis and localization raise a variety of new questions. It is evident that further studies will have to deal with the identification of the four possible pairs of hard alpha-keratins. It will then be necessary to elucidate whether the presumptive keratin pairs are expressed simultaneously or in a stepwise manner within the lower bulbar region and whether there is a subsequent segregation of distinct pairs into cuticular, cortical and – if present – medullary structures. However, the understanding of hair differentiation will be incomplete without a similarly detailed analysis of keratin expression in the outer and inner root sheath and, most importantly, in the lowermost germinative region of the hair bulb.

It can be predicted that the strategy for the resolution of these questions is largely committed. It will certainly involve recombinant DNA techniques to elucidate both the nucleotide and amino acid sequences of the different hard alpha-keratins and their respective mRNAs or genes. These will provide an arsenal for the generation of highly specific gene probes and antibodies, which in turn will be a prerequisite to gaining further knowledge of the complex differentiation pathways of the hair from the hair follicle germinative cells.

ACKNOWLEDGEMENTS

I am grateful to W. Heid and H.J. Stark for helpful discussion, and W.W. Franke for permission to reproduce Figures 1 and 2.

REFERENCES

1. Montagna W, Parakkal PF. *The Structure and Function of Skin*, pp. 172–258. New York and London: Academic Press, 1974
2. Chapman RE. Hair, Wool, quill, nail, claw, hoof and horn. In *Biology of the Integument*, vol. 2: *Vertebrates* (Bereiter-Hahn J, Matoltsy AG, Richards S eds), pp. 293–317. Berlin, Heidelberg, New York, Tokyo: Springer, 1986
3. Heid HW, Werner E, Franke WW. The complement of native alpha-keratin polypeptides of hair-forming cells: a subset of eight polypeptides that differ from epithelial cytokeratins. *Differentiation*, **32**, 101–119, 1986
4. Lynch MH, O'Guin WM, Hardy C, Mak L, Sun T-T. Acidic and basic hair/nail ('hard') keratins: their colocalization in upper cortical and cuticle cells of the human hair follicle and their relationship to 'soft' keratins. *J Cell Biol* **103**, 2593–2606, 1986
5. Rogers GE. Genes for hair and avian keratins. *Ann NY Acad Sci*, **19**, 403–425, 1985
6. Powell BC, Rogers GE. Hair keratin: composition, structure and biogenesis. In *Biology of the Integument*, vol. 2: *Vertebrates*. (Bereiter-Hahn J, Matoltsy AG, Richards S, eds), pp. 695–721. Berlin, Heidelberg, New York, Tokyo: Springer 1986
7. Rogers GE. Keratin genes. In *Eukaryotic Genes: Their Structure, Activity and Regulation*, (Maclean N, Gregory JP, Flavell RA, eds), 415–430. London: Butterworth, 1983
8. Fraser RBD, Mac Rae TP. Molecular structure and mechanical properties of keratins. In *The Mechanical Properties of Biological Material*, Vincent JFV, Currey JD eds), pp. 211–246. London: Society for Experimental Biology, 1980
9. Gough KH, Inglis AS, Crewther WG. Amino acid sequences of alpha-helical segments from S-carboxymethylkerateine-A. Complete sequence of a type I segment. *Biochem J*, **173**, 373–385, 1978
10. Hogg DMC, Dowling LM, Crewther WG. Amino acid sequences of alpha-helical segments from S-carboxymethylkerateine A. *Biochem J*, **173**, 353–363, 1978
11. Sparrow LG, Inglis AS. Characterization of the cyanogen bromide peptides of component 7c, a major microfibrillar protein from wool. *Proc 6th Int Wool Text Res Conf, Pretoria, 1980*, vol. 2, pp. 237–246
12. Crewther WG, Dowling LM, Gough KM, Inglis AS, Parry DAD. Primary structure of a microfibrillar protein from wool. *Abstr Proc 12th Int Congr Biochem. Perth*, P0S: 004–205
13. Crewther WG, Dowling LM, Inglis AS. Amino acid sequence data from a microfibrillar protein of alpha-keratin. *Proc 6th Int Wool Text Res Conf, Pretoria*, vol. 2, 1980, pp. 79–91
14. Crewther WG, Dowling LM, Gough KH, Marshall RC, Sparrow LG. The microfibrillar proteins of alpha-keratin. In *Fibrous Proteins: Scientific, Industrial and Medical Aspects*, vol. 2 (Parry DAD, Creamer LK, eds), pp. 151–159. London: Academic Press, 1980
15. Fraser RBD, MacRae TP, Rogers GE. *Keratins – Their Composition, Structure and Synthesis*, pp. 56–82. Illinois: Charles Thomas, 1972
16. Baden HP, Goldsmith LA, Fleming B. A comparative study of the physicochemical properties of human keratinized tissues. *Biochem Biophys Acta*, **322**, 269–278, 1973
17. Weber K, Osborn M, Franke WW. Antibodies to merokeratin from sheep wool decorate cytokeratin filaments in nonkeratinizing epithelial cells. *Eur J Cell Biol*, **23**, 110–114, 1980

18. Weber K, Geisler N. The structural relation between intermediate filament proteins in living cells and the alpha-keratins of sheep wool. *EMBO J*, **1**, 1155–1160, 1982
19. Weber K, Geisler N. Intermediate filaments-from wool alpha-keratins to neurofilaments: a structural overview. In *Cancer Cells*, vol. 1: *The Transformed Phenotype* (Levine A, Topp W, Vande Woude G, Watson JD, eds), pp. 153–159. New York: Cold Spring Harbor Laboratory, 1984
20. Crewther WG, Dowling LM, Steinert PM, Parry AD. Structure of intermediate filaments. *Int Biol Macromol*, **5**, 267–274, 1983
21. Ward KA, Edwards KJ, Sleigh MJ. The structure of the wool keratin microfibrillar genes. *Proc Aust Biochem Soc*, **15**, 70, 1983
22. O'Donnel IJ, Thompson EOP. Studies on reduced wool: the isolation of a major component. *Aust J Biol Sci*, **17**, 973–989, 1964
23. Crewther WG. Primary structure and chemical properties of wool. *Proc 5th Int Wool Text Res Conf. Aachen*, **1**, 1–101, 1976
24. Gillespie JM. The structural proteins of hair: isolation, characterization, and regulation of biosynthesis. In *Biochemistry and Physiology of Skin* (Goldsmith LA, ed.), pp. 475–510. New York: Oxford University Press, 1984
25. Marshall RC. Characterization of the proteins of human hair and nail by electrophoresis. *J Invest Dermatol*, **80**, 519–524, 1983
26. French PW, Hewish DR. Localization of low-sulfur keratin proteins in the wool follicle using monoclonal antibodies. *J Cell Biol*, **102**, 1412–1418, 1986
27. Barnett RJ, Seligman AM. Histochemical demonstration of protein-bound sulfhydryl groups. *J Natl Cancer Inst*, **13**, 905–925, 1953
28. Hardy MH. The histochemistry of hair follicles in the mouse. *Am J Anat*, **90**, 285-335, 1952
29. Montagna W, Eisen AZ, Rademacker AH, Chase HB. Histology and cytochemistry of human skin VI. The distribution of sulfhydryl and disulfide groups. *J Invest Dermatol*, **23**, 23–32, 1954
30. Jones LN, Pope FM. Isolation of intermediate filament assemblies from human hair follicles. *J Cell Biol*, **101**, 1569–1577, 1985
31. Laemmli UK. Cleavage of sructural proteins during the assembly of the head of bacteriophage T4. *Nature*, **227**, 680–685, 1970
32. O'Farrell PZ, Goodman HM, O'Farrell PH. High resolution two-dimensional electrophoresis of basic as well as acidic proteins. *Cell*, **12**, 1133–1142, 1977
33. Moll R, Franke WW, Schiller DL, Geiger B, Krepler R. The catalog of human cytokeratins: Patterns of expression in normal epithelia, tumors and cultured cells. *Cell*, **31**, 11–24, 1982
34. Steinert PM, Idler WW, Zimmerman SB. Self assembly of bovine epidermal keratin *in vitro. J Mol Biol*, **108**, 547–567, 1976
35. Franke WW, Schiller DL, Grund C. Protofilamentous and annular structures as intermediates during reconstitution of cytokeratin filaments *in vitro. Biol Cell*, **46**, 257–268, 1982
36. Eichner R, Sun T-T, Aebi U. The role of keratin subfamilies and keratin pairs in the formation of human epidermal intermediate filaments. *J Cell Biol*, **102**, 1767–1777, 1986
37. Hatzfeld M, Franke WW. Pair formation and promiscuity of cytokeratins: Formation *in vitro* of heterotopic complexes and intermediate-sized filaments by homologous and heterologous recombinations of purified polypeptides. *J Cell Biol*, **101**, 1826–1841, 1985
38. Schweizer J, Kinjo M, Fürstenberger G, Winter H. Sequential expression of mRNA-encoded keratin sets in neonatal mouse epidermis: basal cells with properties of terminally differentiating cells. *Cell*, **37**, 159–170, 1984

39. Bowden PE, Quinlan RA, Breitkreutz D, Fusenig NE. Proteolytic modification of acidic and basic keratins during terminal differentiation of mouse and human epidermis. *Europ J Biochem*, **142**, 29–36, 1984

40. Roop DR, Cheng CK, Titterington L, Meyers CA, Stanley JR, Steinert PM, Yuspa SH. Synthetic peptides corresponding to keratin subunits elicit highly specific antibodies. *J Biol Chem*, **259**, 8037–8040, 1984

41. Schweizer J, Winter H. Keratin polypeptide analysis of fetal and terminally differentiating newborn mouse epidermis. *Differentiation*, **22**, 19–24, 1982

42. Ward KA, Kasmavik SE. The isolation of wool keratin messenger RNA from sheep. *J Invest Dermatol*, **75**, 244–248, 1980

43. Bertolino AP, Gibbs PEM, Freedberg IM. *In vitro* biosynthesis of mouse hair keratins under the direction of follicular RNA. *J Invest Dermatol*, **79**, 173–177, 1982

44. Baden HP, Kubilus JK. A comparative study of the immunologic properties of hoof and nail fibrous proteins. *J Invest Dermatol*, **83**, 327–331, 1984

45. Gigi O, Geiger B, Eshhar Z, Moll R, Schmid E, Winter S, Schiller DL, Franke WW. Detection of a cytokeratin determinant common to diverse epithelial cells by a broadly cross-reacting monoclonal antibody. *EMBO J*, **1**, 1429–1437, 1982

46. Moll R, Fanke WW, Volc-Platzer D, Krepler R. Different keratin polypeptides in epidermis and other epithelia of human skin: a specific cytokeratin of molecular weight 46,000 in epithelia of the pilosebaceous tract and basal cell epitheliomas. *J Cell Biol*, **95**, 285–295, 1982

47. Moll R, Moll J, Wiest W. Changes in the pattern of cytokeratin polypeptides in epidermis and hair follicles during skin development in human fetuses. *Differentiation*, **23**, 170–178, 1982

48. Sun T-T, Eichner R, Schermer A, Cooper D, Nelson WG, Weiss RA. Classification, expression and possible mechanisms of evolution of mammalian epihelial keratins: a unifying model. In *Cancer Cells*, vol. 1 *The Transformed Phenotype*, pp. 169–176. New York: Cold Spring Harbor Laboratory, 1984

49. Knapp B, Rentrop M, Schweizer J, Winter H. Nonepidermal members of the keratin multigene family: cDNA sequences and in situ localization of the mRNAs. *Nucleic Acids Res*, **14**, 751–763, 1986

50. Rentrop M, Knapp B, Winter H, Schweizer J. Differential localization of distinct keratin mRNA-species in mouse tongue epithelium by in situ hybridization with specific cDNA probes. *J Cell Biol*, **103**, 2583–2591, 1986

51. Knapp B, Rentrop M, Schweizer J, Winter H. Three cDNA sequences of mouse type I keratins: cellular localization of the mRNA in normal and hyperproliferative tissues. *J Biol Chem*, **262**, 938–945, 1987

52. Weiss RA, Eichner R, Sun T-T. Monoclonal antibody analysis of keratin expression in epidermal diseases: a 48 and 56 kD keratin as molecular marker for hyperproliferative keratinocytes. *J Cell Biol*, **98**, 1397–1406, 1984

53. Woodcock-Mitchell J, Eichner R, Nelson WG, Sun T-T. Immunolocalization of keratins polypeptides in human epidermis using monoclonal antibodies. *J Cell Biol*, **95**, 580–588, 1982

54. Ito M, Tazawa T, Shimizu N, Ito K, Katsuumi K, Sato Y, Hashimoto K. Cell differentiation in human anagen hair and hair follicles studied with anti-hair keratin monoclonal antibodies. *J Invest Dermatol*, **86**, 563–569, 1986

55. Hashimoto K, Shibazaki S. Ultrastructural study on differentiation and function of hair. In *Hair* (Kobori T, Montagna W eds), pp. 23–57. Tokyo: University of Tokyo Press, 1976

56. Nairn AC, Detre JA, Casnellie JE, Greengard P. Serum antibodies that distinguish between the phospho- and dephospho-forms of a phosphoprotein. *Nature (Lond)*, **299**, 734–736, 1982

57. Steinert PM, Parry DAD, Racoosin EL, Idler WW, Steven AC, Trus BL, Roop DR. The complete DNA and deduced amino acid sequence of a type II mouse epidermal

keratin of 60,000 Da: analysis of sequence differences between type I and type II keratins. *PNAS*, **81**, 5709–5713, 1984

3

The mammalian tongue filiform papillae: a theoretical model for primitive hairs

D Dhouailly* and T-T Sun**

*UA CNRS 682, Université Joseph Fourier, Grenoble France
**Department of Dermatology, New York University School of
Medicine, USA

ABSTRACT

The dorsal surface of the mammalian tongue is covered with numerous projections called filiform papillae. Immunohistochemical staining and immunoblotting data indicate that the interpapillary epithelium expresses esophageal-type keratins while the papillary epithelium expresses skin- and hair-type keratins. The hard keratins of mouse tongue are indistinguishable from the keratins of the pelage, while the hard keratin of human tongue corresponds to a minor hair-related keratin. Thus, the filiform papillae are constructed by combining two populations of keratinocytes that undergo skin and hair types of differentiation. They can therefore be interpreted as primary cutaneous appendages. Variations in the detailed lingual papillary structure among the different mammalian species, from a simple anterior/posterior type of compartmentalization (rodents) to a complicated concentric construction (primates) lead to propose a theoretical model to understand how mammalian hairs may have evolved from reptilian scales.

INTRODUCTION

Many integumental structures of lower vertebrates have been suggested as ancestral to the hairs[1,2]. One hypothesis is that mammalian hairs may have been derived from complex epidermal modifications of the mechanoreceptor sense organs, based on the fact of the sensory function of some hairs in modern mammals. One other hypothesis, which does not exclude the former, is that hairs may have evolved from the hinge region of therapsidian scales. The caudal integument of mice and rats could be a remnant of that condition, as it possesses scales with hairs erupting at the posterior half of each scale.

Although a relationship between mammalian hairs and reptilian scales is generally assumed, the absence of relevant paleontological data has precluded any detailed consideration of this problem. Furthermore the morphogenetic events in hair development are difficult to relate to any possible evolutionary sequence. But heterospecific dermal–epidermal recombinants involving embryonic tissues from mouse and lizards have shown that the first steps of dermal–epidermal interactions during the embryonic development of mammalian hairs and actual reptilian scales have remained close enough to be understable between epithelial and mesenchymal cells belonging to these two classes of vertebrates[3]. Thus, we can presume that the early events during hair development are the remnants of those which may have occurred during the morphogenesis of paleontological reptilian scales.

However, the chief difficulty in thinking about the evolution of the first hairs resides in accounting for the genesis of the hair's complicated structure with its six concentric sheaths of epithelial cells, through a continuous series of hypothetical morphological steps, from a simple scaled structure. Indeed, a scale is only a fold of the epidermis, comprising an anterior and a posterior part. Another point to be taken into account is the distribution of keratins in the integument. In lower vertebrates there exists only one class of keratin polypeptides, the alpha ('soft') type. In reptilians, there are two types of keratins, alpha and beta, which are distributed in an alternate horizontal or vertical fashion, according to the various species. In mammals, all the keratin polypeptides are of the alpha-type but it has been confirmed recently[4,5] that the hair ('hard') keratins are significantly distinct from the epidermal ('soft') keratins. The hair-type keratins seem to be involved only in the formation of hardened cornified structures, and may therefore be regarded as molecular markers for 'hair/nail' type differentiation or 'hard' keratinization. Thus, as several antibodies have been raised in different laboratories[4,5] (see also Serre et al., this volume) against the various hair keratins, they can be used to detect those markers of differentiation in various tissues.

By studying the actual mammals for transient structures between scales and hairs, we became interested in the lingual filiform papillae for two reasons. First, several authors have suggested, based on ultrastructural data the presence of hard type keratins in the tongue epithelium[6,7]. Moreover, in rodents those papillae are of a simple scale-like structure (Figure 1), while in primates the filiform papillae are morphologically complex. Each primary human filiform papilla is composed of several secondary papillae, with each forming long, cornified threads curved towards the pharynx (Figure 7). This structure is even magnified in the case of the human disease called 'black hairy tongue', where hair-like projections occur on the dorsal tongue surface. By using the AE13 antibody, which is specific for the 44–46 kDa acidic hair keratins[4], we have been able to show that the posterior half of the mouse lingual filiform papillae was AE13-positive (Figure 2), suggesting the presence of hair-type keratins in the dorsal tongue[8]. This antibody staining has been found also in rabbit (Figure 4), cat, human (Figure 7) and monkey tongue filiform papillae. Anti-hair antibody staining has again been detected in human, and in cow, lingual dorsal epithelium by other authors (Moll et al., poster and abstract presented at this meeting).

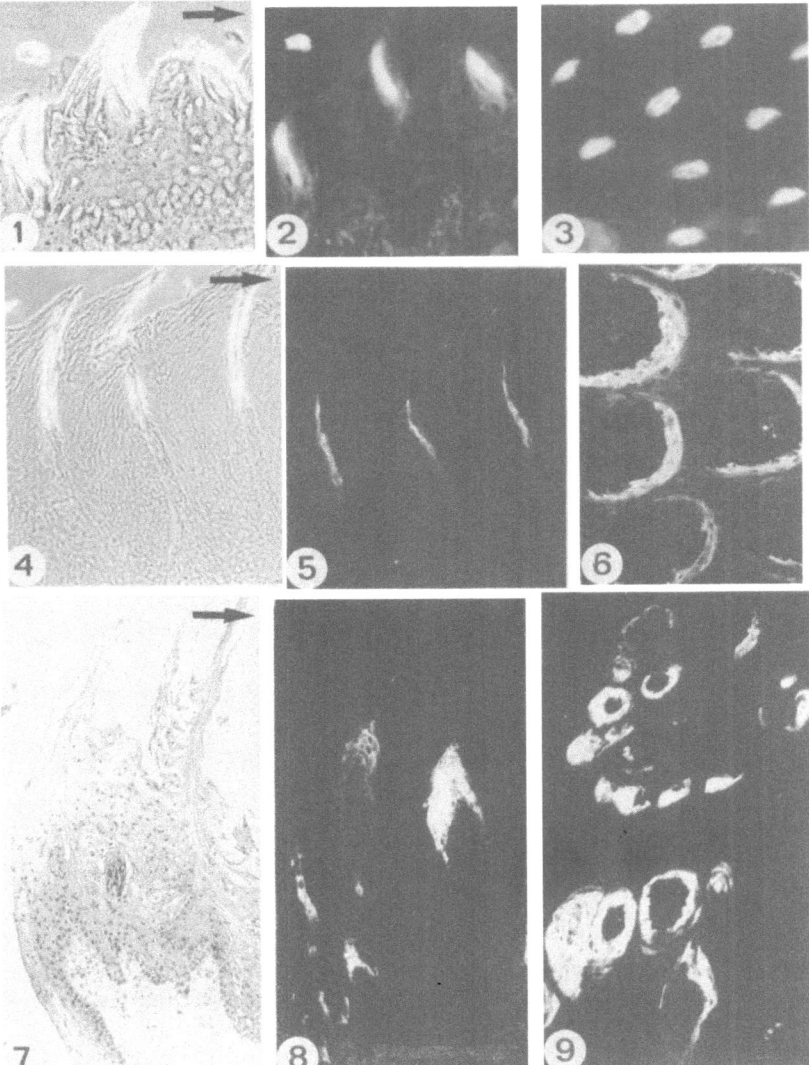

Figures 1–9   Detection of hair-type keratins in lingual dorsal epithelium by indirect immunofluorescent staining with the AE13 antibody. Longitudinal (Figures 1, 2, 4, 5, 7 and 8) and
horizontal (Figures 3, 6, 9) sections. The arrows point towards the pharynx.

In mouse tongue, the AE13 antibody decorates the half posterior part of the papilla (Figure
2). In horizontal section this posterior part appears as a simple straight structure (Figure 3).
In rabbit tongue, the AE13 antibody decorates a semi-cylindrical structure (Figures 5 and 6)
in the posterior part of the filiform papilla.

In human tongue, the AE13 antibody stains the central part of each secondary papilla (Figure
8). In a horizontal section of two primary filiform papillae (Figure 9), each secondary papilla sectioned near to its base shows a ring of AE13-positive cells around a dermal core, while
more distal sections show a full cord of AE13-positive cells.

31

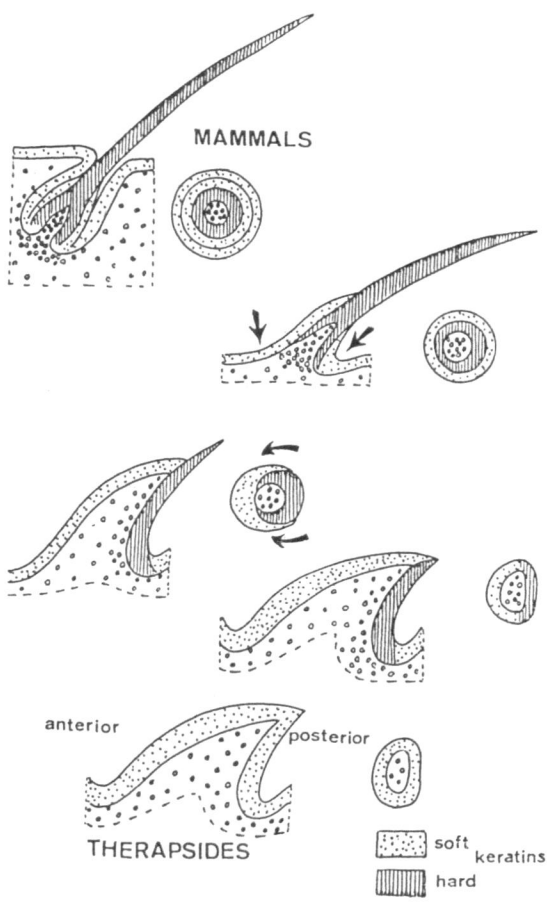

Figure 10 A theoretical model showing how hairs may have evolved from the posterior part of scales from paleontological reptiles (Therapsides). E: epidermis D: dermis

In order to define the biochemical basis of this immunohistochemical staining reaction, the tongue keratins have been analyzed by one and two dimensional immunoblotting[9]. The results show that the hard keratins of mouse lingual dorsal epithelium co-migrate with authentic mouse hair keratins, but that the AE 13-reactive keratin of human tongue does not correspond to any previously described human hair keratin. By using S-carboxymethylation, this new human keratin, with a 51 kDa molecular weight, has been identified as being a minor polypeptide involved in normal hair keratin pattern[9].

This study has been completed using the AE2 antibody, specific for skin-type keratins K10, K1 and 2 and the KA5 antibody specific for K10, as well as by using the AE8 antibody, which is specific for the esophageal-type keratin number 13. The results show that the interpapillary epithelium expresses mainly esophageal-type keratin, while the papillary epithelium expresses mainly skin- and hair-type keratins. To precisely determine the relative location of cells expressing skin- and hair-related keratins within the lingual papillae, we stained horizontal sections (cut parallel to the tongue surface). The results indicate that in the case of mouse tongue, the anterior, half is decorated with the AE2 antibody, while the posterior half is stained by the AE13 antibody. This posterior half has a simple, straight structure (Figure 3). In the case of rabbit tongue, the posterior AE13-positive cells form a semi-cylindrical structure (Figure 6), while in human tongue, the AE2 and AE13 (Figure 9) antibodies, respectively, decorate outer and inner 'rings' of cells, surrounding a mesenchymal core, at the base of each secondary papilla. Furthermore, a horizontal section from the mid-height of a secondary papilla shows only a full cord of AE13-positive cells. Such a concentric structure has some resemblance to a hair follicle.

Thus, the lingual filiform papilla may be considered as a primitive type of cutaneous appendage. Its structure varies according to different species, while the structure of the hair follicles is similar in all species of mammals. During evolution, however, the selective pressure on tongue papillae may have been different from the selective pressure on pelage hairs. The actual variations in lingual filiform papillae may be related to functional differences, such as lapping water or grooming the fur. However, variations in the distribution of hair-type keratins in lingual dorsal epithelium among different mammalian species, ranging from a simple scale-like to a more complex concentric hair-like structure had led us to propose a model for hair origins (Figure 10).

In our opinion, the formation of hairs may not have evolved from à simple elongation of scale tips, or from a rod of cells which may have grown out of the scale hinge region, but from a gradual transformation of the posterior half scale epidermis, through a semi-cylindrical to a progressively more complete cylindrical structure. The last step could have been the invagination of the hair base into the dermis, to form the hair follicle proper.

REFERENCES

1. Elias H, Boctner S. On the phylogeny of hair. *Am Mus Novit* **1820**: 1–15, 1957
2. Maderson PFA. When? Why? and How? Some speculations on the evolution of the vertebrate integument. *Am Zool* **12**; 159–171, 1972
3. Dhouailly D. Dermo-epidermal interactions during morphogenesis of cutaneous appendages in amniotes. *Front Matr Biol* **4**; 86–121, 1977
4. Lynch MH, O'Guin WM, Hardy C, Mak L, Sun TT. Acidic and basic hair/nail 'hard' keratins: their colocalization in upper cortical and cuticle cells of the human hair follicle and their relationship to 'soft' keratins; *J Cell Biol* **103**; 2593–2606, 1986
5. Heid HW, Werner E, Franke WW. The complement of native alpha-keratin polypeptides of hair-forming cells: a subset of eight polypeptides that differ from epithelial cytokeratins. *Differentiation* **32**; 101–119, 1986

6. Farbman AT. The dual pattern of keratinization in filiform papillae of rat tongue. *J Anat* **106**; 1233–242, 1970
7. Hume WJ, Potten CS. The ordered columnar structure of mouse filiform papillae. *J Cell Sci* **22**; 149–160, 1976
8. Dhouailly D, Sun TT. Mammalian tongue epithelium expresses three keratin pairs characterizing 'hair', 'skin' and 'esophageal' types of keratinocyte differentiation. *J Cell Biol* **103**; 203a, 1986
9. Dhouailly D, Xu C, Manabe M, Sun TT. Three distinct populations of dorsal tongue keratinocytes express keratin markers for hair- skin- and esophageal-types of differentiation. *J Biol Biochem* (submitted)

4

Comparative electrophoretic analysis of sulfur containing proteins of hair bulb, keratogenous zone and hair shaft

C Nappe, M Kermici and P Boré

L'Oréal
Laboratoires de Recherche Fondamentale
1 Avenue Eugène Schueller
93600 Aulnay-sous-bois
France

ABSTRACT

The S-alkylated hair proteins show characteristic electrophoretic patterns. This study described the evolution of these proteins at different states of maturation corresponding to: bulb (b), keratogenous zone (kz) and fiber (f).

The proteins are solubilized and S-carboxymethylated by $2[^{14}C]$iodoacetic acid and analyzed by SDS-PAGE and two-dimensional electrophoresis. This study reveals the presence of fibrilar proteins (low sulfur proteins) with MW ranging from 67 to 45 kDa in b, kz, and f. Matricial proteins (high sulfur proteins) with MW from 30 to 14 kDa are detectable in kz and f. The comparison between b and kz electrophoretic patterns reveals two specific groups;A for b with MW higher than 45 kDa and B for kz with MW smaller than 45 kDa. A and B display different mobility at pH 8.9. At the three stages of differentiation studied, low sulfur proteins are present. High sulfur proteins, however, undergo modifications. They would result from an enrichment in sulfur of group B, which could be formed from A by hydrolysis during an earlier stage.

ABBREVIATIONS

SCM:	S-carboxymethylation
LSP:	Low sulfur proteins
HSP:	High sulfur proteins
MW:	Molecular weight
2-D:	Two-dimensional
SDS-PAGE:	Sodium dodecyl sulfate polyacrylamide gel electrophoresis

INTRODUCTION

A large number of physical and mechanical properties of hair (elasticity, tensile strength, etc.) seem to be related to its structure[1], and particularly to the arrangement of its constitutive proteins. Structural and chemical studies have shown that fibers are composed of keratinized cells, each of them containing microfibrils[2] arranged into an amorphous matrix. The microfibrils are composed of low sulfur proteins (LSP) and the matrix is characterized by its high sulfur content. Marshall and Gillespie[4] developed a technique to separate and analyze these proteins. After S-carboxymethylation (SCM) and analysis in SDS-polyacrylamide or two-dimensional gel electrophoresis, the proteins display a typical pattern[3,4] which can be modified for example after low sulfur diet[5] or in pathological cases such as trichothiodystrophy[6]. The maturation of hair corresponds to an increase in the number of intra- and inter-chain bonds like disulfur bridges and glutamyl–lysine crosslinks which stabilize the keratin structures and render them more insoluble[7]. But few data are available concerning the evolution of, and the relationship between, low sulfur proteins (LSP) and high sulfur proteins (HSP) during the maturation process of hair. The purpose of our study is to present the first results obtained from the analysis of SCM proteins extracted from bulb, keratogenous zone and hair fiber.

MATERIALS AND METHODS

Samples

Human anagen follicles were obtained by microdissection of human hair transplants. Outer and inner root sheaths were removed, and then the keratogenous zone was separated from the lower part of the bulb corresponding to germinative cells, as illustrated in Figure 1. Hair fibers were directly cut on the scalp.

Protein extraction and S-carboxymethylation

All samples were washed successively with petroleum ether, ethanol and water and then air-dried; 3 mg of hair sample was cut into small pieces. Twenty bulbs and 20 keratogenous zones were used for the study. Proteins were extracted by incubation at 37 °C for 18 h in a 50 mmol/l Tris-HCl buffer pH 9.3 containing 8 mol/l urea and 50 mmol/l dithiothreitol. Extracted proteins were S-carboxymethylated (SCM) by 6.5 μCi of 2[^{14}C]iodoacetic acid (specific activity 120 μCi/mmol, Amersham, France) according to Marshall and Gillespie[4].

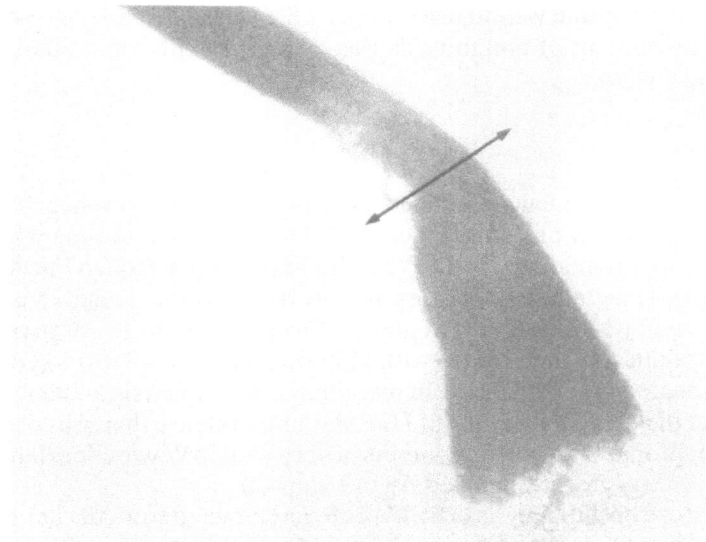

Figure 1 Anagen follicle following microdissection to remove inner and outer root sheaths. Bulb and keratogenous zone were separated as indicated in the figure.

Estimation of extracted proteins

Estimation of proteins was performed according to the colorimetric method of Bradford[8] using a 'Bio Rad Protein Assay' kit. Bovine serum albumin was used as a standard.

Electrophoretic analysis

Monodimensional electrophoresis was performed on polyacrylamide gel slab in SDS medium according to the Laemmli procedure[9] but using a stepwise separating gel (10–15% of acrylamide) as described by Marshall and Gillespie[4]. Three micrograms of each sample was used for this analysis. Two-dimensional electrophoresis was performed; in the first dimension in gel tube containing 8 mol/l urea at pH 8.9[10]. After 18 h migration at 50 V gels were equilibrated in Tris–HCl buffer containing 2.3% of SDS and then placed on the top of a gel slab. The second dimension is performed in SDS-PAGE (10–15% of acrylamide). Six micrograms was analysed. Gels were revealed by the fluorographic method of Laskey and Mills[11].

Amino-acid analysis

Hair bulbs, keratogenous zones (about 60 of each) and hair shafts were hydrolyzed *in vacuo* with constant boiling HCl at 108 °C for 22 h and freeze-

37

dried. The hydrolysate was adjusted to pH 7.8 and shaken with air to oxidize cystine. The content of amino acids was estimated with a modified 120 C amino acid analyzer.

RESULTS

The electrophoretic analysis of SCM proteins extracted from hair fiber revealed two groups of proteins (Figure 2c). The first group in the upper part of the gel corresponded to the LSP(2) with MW ranging from 67 to 45 kDa. This group was segregated into six spots in two-dimensional analysis and was characterized by a low mobility at pH 8.9. The group in the lower part of the gel corresponded to the HSP(2) with MW ranging from 45 to 14 kDa. HSP were segregated into eight spots in two-dimensional analysis and had a high mobility at pH 8.9. The labeling of HSP was more intense than was observed in the LSP group. Unresolved proteins of very high MW were located at the top of the gel (aggregates labeled Ag in Figure 2).

Electrophoretic analysis of SCM proteins extracted from the keratogenous zone presented, as in fiber analysis, LSP and HSP groups (Figure 2b). The two-dimensional analysis revealed that their polypeptide composition

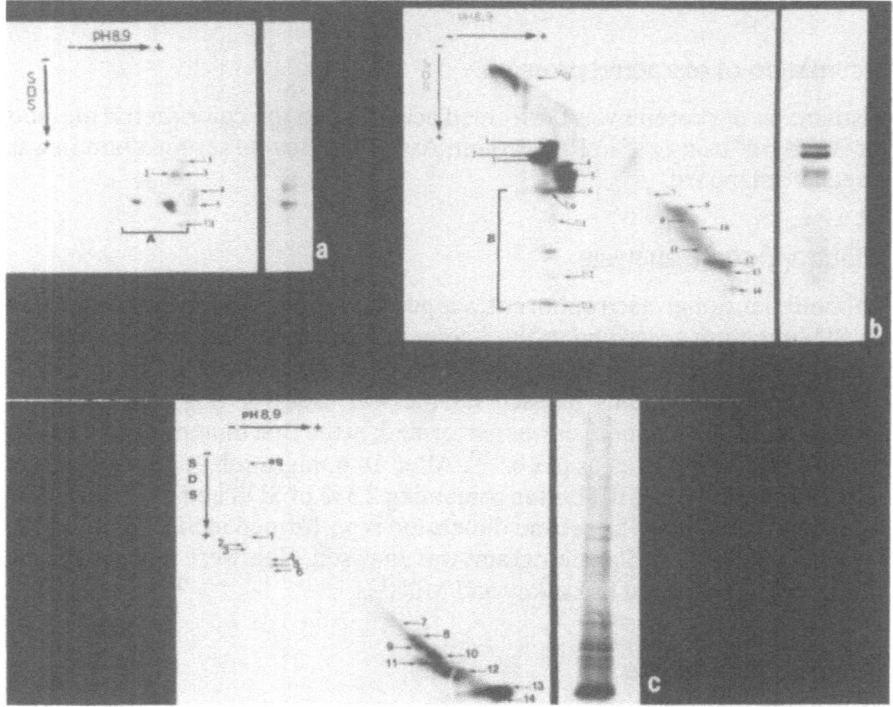

Figure 2 Autoradiographies of mono and bidimensional electrophoresis of SCM proteins extracted from: a: bulb, b: keratogenous zone, c: hair fiber

was the same as in hair fiber but with a modified intensity. Indeed, as opposed to hair fiber, the LSP displayed a very high intensity. Aggregates were present at the top of the gel. Nevertheless, the keratogenous zone was specifically characterized by a group of polypeptides (labelled B) with low MW (similar to HSP MW) but with low mobility at pH 8.9.

The electrophoretic analysis of bulb SCM proteins only revealed the LSP group (Figure 2a), with a range of MW and mobility similar to LSP extracted from hair fiber and the keratogenous zone. But two subunits corresponding to the highest MW, 67 and 65 kDa, were present but hardly detectable. The bulb was characterized by the presence of a group of polypeptides with MW about 45 kDa, and with low mobility at pH 8.9 (group A). No aggregates were revealed.

Amino acid composition reported in Table 1 shows that the cystine content is remarkably low (traces) in the bulbar zone compared to the keratogenous zone and hair shaft. Apart from cystine other amino acids also reveal modifications (especially aspartic acid and tyrosine).

Table 1 Amino-acid composition (as residues %) of hair bulb, keratogenous zone and hair shaft

	Bulb	Keratogenous zone	Hair shaft
Cysteic acid	1.4	1.5	0.9
Aspartic acid	9.4	6.9	5.3
Threonine	4.7	6.1	6.7
Serine	7.0	9.5	9.8
Glutamic acid	14.1	15.9	13.7
Proline	4.2	5.5	7.2
Glycine	5.2	4.1	4.1
Alanine	5.8	4.0	3.6
Valine	5.3	5.4	5.4
Cystine	traces	12.5	14.6
Methionine	traces	traces	0.2
Isoleucine	3.7	2.9	3.0
Leucine	8.8	7.3	6.5
Tyrosine	6.3	2.9	3.7
Phenylalanine	5.7	2.6	3.1
Lysine	7.3	4.3	3.3
Histidine	2.7	1.7	1.4
Arginine	8.4	6.9	7.5

DISCUSSION

Figure 3 is a schematic representation of the three different states of differentiation studied. The follicle undergoes differentiation with a regular sequence of events to form the fiber. Microscopic studies showed that structural modification takes place at different lengths of follicle[12]. We considered in our study the bulb, which contains the germinative cells and the elongation area corresponding to an early state of keratin aggregation, and the keratogenous zone characterised by cortex protein synthesis, and a marked change in shape of macrofibrils[12]. From our electrophoretic analysis, one might note four important points. The first one is that LSP are synthesized in the bulb, and did not seem to be modified in the keratogenous zone and in the fiber. This result is in agreement with Jones *et al.*[13] who found that cultured 'presumptive hair shaft' showed a continuing synthesis of LSP. The modification of the electrophoretic mobility due to the SCM, which provided different MW, the analysis of bulb SCM proteins in SDS-PAGE and the results given by Heid *et al.*[14] were similar.

The second point is that aggregates, corresponding to unresolved proteins with very high MW, were not detectable in the bulb but appeared in the keratogenous zone and in hair fiber (Figure 3). Their presence seemed to be related to a more advanced state of maturation.

The third point is that group A, found in the bulb, was not detectable in the other samples (Figure 3). The low mobility at pH 8.9 of this group of SCM proteins seemed to indicate that group A belonged to LSP. In the keratogenous zone, a group B appeared, with MW lower than group A but with the same mobility at pH 8.9. This fact suggested that group B could be formed from group A by hydrolysis. This interpretation is in agreement with the hypothesis of Rogers[15] and Gillespie[16].

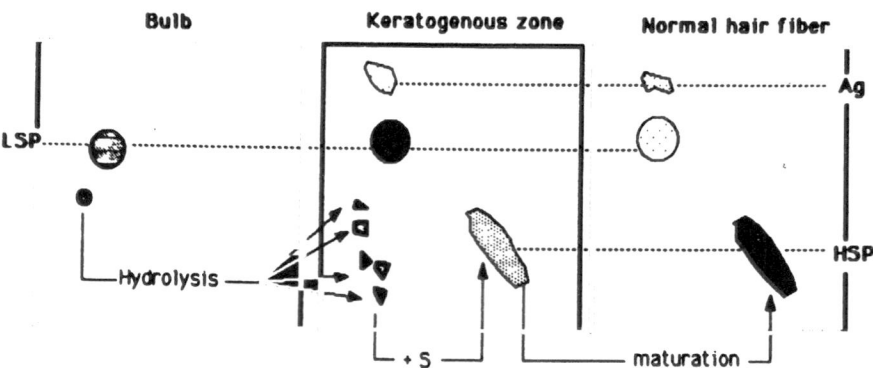

Figure 3   Schematic representation of maturation process hypothesis

The next point was that, in our experiment, the HSP appeared to be detectable in the keratogenous zone but with a low intensity compared to LSP. The HSP group in the fiber became more intense and group B disappeared. These observations, and the fact that group B had the same range of MW as the HSP group, could suggest that HSP come from group B. This hypothesis would suppose that the precursors (B) would be enriched in sulfur in the keratogenous zone. The amino acid composition seems to confirm this hypothesis; indeed the differences observed between the bulb and the keratogenous zone mainly consist of an enrichment in cystine in the keratogenous zone. According to Rogers[15] and Gillespie[16] one of the post-translational modifications might consist of the addition of cysteinyl residues to precursor forms represented in our study by group B. This hypothesis is also supported by the fact that Van Neste and Boré[17] suggested that *in vivo* there would be an active transport mechanism of cystine into the keratogenous zone through the inner root sheath.

Jones *et al.*[13] showed that cultured cells of the lower part of the human anagen hair shaft (corresponding to the bulb in our study) synthesized LSP but, in conflict with our results, also HSP. Nevertheless the synthesis of HSP was weak and decreased drastically after 3 days, whereas these authors found HSP in a presumptive hair shaft corresponding to bulb and keratogenous zone in agreement with our results. These observations suggest that LSP and HSP should follow a different synthesis pathway.

REFERENCES

1. Feughelman M. The relation between structure and mechanical properties of keratin fibers. *Appl Polymer Symp*, **18**, 757, 1971
2. Baden HP. Characterization of hair keratins. In *Hair Research: Status and Future Aspects* (Orfanos CE, Montagna W, Stuttgen G, eds), pp. 73–75, 1981
3. Marshall RC. Analysis of the proteins from single wool fibers by two dimensional polyacrylamide gel electrophoresis. *Text Research J*, 106–108, 1981
4. Marshall RC, Gillespie JM. Comparison of human hair by two dimensional electrophoresis. *J Forensic Sci Soc*, **22**, 377–388, 1982
5. Gillespie JM. The dietary regulated biosynthesis of high sulfur wool proteins. *Biochem J*, **98**, 669–677, 1966
6. Gillespie JM, Marshall RC. Comparison of the proteins of normal and trichothiodystrophic human hair. *J Invest Dermatol*, **80**, 195–202, 1983
7. Harding HWJ, Rogers GE. The occurrence of ε-(γ-glutamyl)lysine crosslinks in the medulla of hair and quills. *Biochem Biophys Acta*, **257**, 37–39, 1972
8. Bradford MM. A rapid and sensitive method for the quantification of microgram quantities of protein utilizing the principle of protein-dye binding. *Anal Biochem*, **72**, 248–254, 1976
9. Laemmli UK. Cleavage of structural proteins during the assembly of the head of bacteriophage T4. *Nature*, **227**, 680–685, 1970
10. Davis BJ. Disc electrophoresis. II: Method and application to human serum proteins. *Ann NY Acad Sci*, **121**, 404–427, 1964
11. Laskey RA, Mills AD. Quantitative film detection of ^{3}H and ^{14}C in polyacrylamide gels by fluorography. *Eur J Biochem*, **56**, 335–341, 1975
12. Orwin DF. Acid phosphatase distribution in the wool follicle. *J Ultrastruct Res*, **55**, 312–342, 1976
13. Jones LN, Fowler KJ, Marshall RC, Ackland ML. Studies of developing human hair shaft cells in vitro. *J Invest Dermatol*, **90**, 58–64, 1988
14. Heid HW, Werner E, Franke WW. The complement of native α-keratin polypeptides of hair forming cells: a subset of eight polypeptides that differ from epithelial cytokeratins. *Differentiation*, **32**, 101–119, 1986
15. Rogers GE. Enzymes and proteins of hair follicles. *Ann NY Acad Sci*, **83**, 408–428, 1959

16. Gillespie JM. In *The Biology of Skin and Hair Growth* (Lyne AG, Short BF, eds.), pp. 337–398, Sydney: Angus and Robertson, 1965
17. Van Neste D, Boré P. Trichothiodystrophie: une étude morphologique et bio-chimique. *Ann Dermatol Venereol*, **110**, 409–417, 1983

5

Four murine monoclonal antibodies specific for the inner root sheath in the human hair follicle

G Serre*, V Mils*, C Vincent*, A Conter*, S Michel,
J Kadouche*** and J-P Soleilhavoup**
*Laboratoire de Biologie Cellulaire, CHU Purpan, Toulouse, France
**Centre International de Recherches Dermatologiques (CIRD)
Sophia-Antipolis, Valbonne, France
***Société Clonatec, Paris, France

ABSTRACT

Hybridoma technology, which allows new differentiation antigens (AG) and thus tissular sub-populations to be defined, constitutes a major tool to study tissue differentiation. Towards this end, we produced murine monoclonal antibodies (MAB) to human epidermis, appendages and squamous epithelia. We present four MAB recognizing AG of the inner root sheath (IRS) of the human hair follicle (HF). The AG defined by three of these MAB are also expressed in the stratum granulosum (SG) of the epidermis.

The MAB were produced after immunization with human plantar stratum corneum (SC). Histological characterization was carried out by indirect immunofluorescence on smears and frozen or fixed tissues – skin and mucosae with stratified squamous epithelia from various anatomical sites – and on crosslinked envelopes (CLE) prepared from plantar SC. Immunochemical characterization was performed by ELISA using epidermal keratins as immunosorbent and by immunoblotting on SDS–PAGE-separated keratin polypeptides and on proteins extracted with Tris–SDS–2-mercaptoethanol from epidermis, plantar SC, gingival epithelium and from DETROIT-562, A431 and HT29 cell lines.

1.   The *G36-19* MAB labeled the SG within the epidermis, gingiva and hard palate, on frozen and fixed tissues. The labeling, cytoplasmic in the lower part of the SG, became pericellular in the upper part and disappeared in the SC. In the anagen HF, only the three layers of the IRS were labeled. In the same way, cytoplasmic in the first IRS cells, the labeling became closely membranous all along the IRS. On smears from hard palate and foot sole, a membrane-like microgranular and diffuse labeling was found. This pattern was found to be largely preserved on CLE

from plantar SC. The *G36-19*-defined AG was found to be absent in the non-cornified squamous epithelia. When assayed by ELISA or immunoblotting, *G36-19* showed no reactivity to any keratin, but recognized several non-keratin polypeptides ranging from 33.5 to 52 kDa.

2. The *F28-27* MAB showed the same histological and immunochemical characteristics as *G36-19*.

3. The *B17-21* MAB labeled SG, IRS and CLE in the same way but not the exfoliated corneocytes. Moreover, it was unreactive by immunoblotting on all the tested substrates.

4. The *G20-21* MAB recognized an AG exclusively expressed in the IRS cells.

Three of the MAB recognized original AG expressed in the CLE of the epidermal keratinocytes and also in an analogous structure of the IRS cells. Only the *G20-21* AG, carried by the same IRS cell structure, is specific of this differentiation pathway.

These four MAB are new differentiation markers, which allows an additional analogy between epidermal and IRS differentiation to be objectivated.

ABBREVIATIONS

2ME	2-mercaptoethanol
AG	antigen(s)
CLE	crosslinked envelope(s)
ELISA	enzyme-linked immunosorbent assay
HF	hair follicle
IRS	inner root sheath
MAB	monoclonal antibody(ies)
PAGE	polyacrylamide gel electrophoresis
PBS	phosphate buffered saline
PMSF	phenylmethylsulfonyl-fluoride
SC	stratum corneum
SDS	sodium dodecyl sulfate
SG	stratum granulosum
Tw	Tween 20

In order to define new differentiation antigens (AG) in human skin, we produced murine monoclonal antibodies (MAB) by immunization with human plantar stratum corneum (SC). We obtained a series of MAB directed against a large variety of epidermis and appendage components. Among them, three MAB specifically recognized the stratum granulosum (SG) in epidermis and the inner root sheath (IRS) in the hair follicle (HF) and one MAB recognized exclusively the IRS. We present the histological and immunochemical characterization of these MAB.

MATERIAL AND METHODS

Tissues, cells and cell lines

Normal human skin from various sites was obtained from patients undergoing amputation or plastic surgery (e.g. foot, leg, thigh, scalp, breast, arm). Normal human mucosae with stratified squamous epithelium came from patients undergoing surgery or from necropsies (e.g cornea, gingiva, esophagus, vagina, uterine, cervix). The tissue samples were either frozen-embedded at −80 °C or paraffin-embedded after fixation with ethanol, Bouin or Carnoy solutions. Human plantar SC was obtained by foot sole scraping from normal donors and pedicure patients. Corneocytes from the hard palate and plantar SC were collected by scraping. A431 cell-line was kindly provided by Dr Etievant (Laboratoire Pierre Fabre, Castres-F); HT29 by Dr Murat (Institut de Physiologie, Toulouse-F); MAJ Detroit 562 by Dr Ouhayoun (Laboratoire d'Odontologie, Paris-F).

Indirect immunofluorescence

Sections 4 μm thick were cut at −30 °C, air-dried and stored overnight at 4 °C. Smears from hard palate were used immediately after air-drying. Sections and smears were hydrated for 15 min in phosphate buffered saline, pH 7.4 (PBS), then incubated with MAB diluted in PBS (ascitic fluid or purified immunoglobulins) for 30 min at 37 °C in a moist chamber. After washing twice in PBS containing 0.05% Tween 20 (Tw), FITC-labeled antimouse IgG(H + L) antibodies diluted 1:50 in PBS were incubated on slides for 15 min at 37 °C. After two successive washings in PBS-Tw and PBS, the slides were mounted and observed on an Olympus BH2 microscope with UV epiillumination.

Enzyme-linked immunosorbent assay (ELISA)

A previously described indirect ELISA[1] using as immunosorbent human plantar SC keratin polypeptides solubilized in 8 mol/l urea, 1% w/w, 2-mercaptoethanol (2ME), 100 mmol/l Tris pH 7.4, was used to test the MAB.

Monoclonal antibody production

MAB were produced according to Köhler and Milstein[2] by fusing with polyethylene glycol 4000, the mouse myeloma SP2–0–AG 14 to splenocytes obtained from BALB/c mouse immunized with human plantar SC finely crushed in PBS buffer. Hybridoma supernatants were screened by indirect immunofluorescence on cryostat sections of normal human skin and by ELISA as described above for anti-keratin antibody activity. The supernatants reactive in one of the two tests were assayed with ELISA against actin, myosin, tubulin, tropomyosin, DNA, TNP and the hybridomas unreactive with these molecules were cloned twice. Then the MAB were produced in murine ascites. MAB isotypes were determined on cloned hybridoma supernatants by specific ELISA, and verified with radial immunodiffusion.

Protein extraction and crosslinked envelope preparation

Protein extracts from scalp epidemis, plantar SC and hard palate corneocytes were prepared as follows. Skin fragments were incubated for 5 min in PBS with 5 mmol/l EDTA, 0.4 mmol/l phenylmethylsulfonyl-fluoride (PMSF) at 60 °C, then for 5 min in 0.4 mmol/l PMSF, PBS at 4 °C[3]. Epidermis was cleaved from dermis and crushed in a Potter homogenizer directly in Laemmli sample medium[4]. Plantar SC was first crushed in a mortar, then in a homogenizer in the sample medium. In both cases, samples were incubated for 3 h at 25 °C, then hydrolyzed for 3 min at 100 °C.

Keratin polypeptides were extracted from isolated epidermis, gingival epithelium and from A431, Detroit 562 and HT29 cell-lines as described by Franke et al.[5] and from SC as described by Sun and Green[6]. Crosslinked envelopes (CLE) were prepared from plantar corneocytes, using SDS and 2ME, according to Sun and Green[7], and their purity verified by sodium dodecyl sulfate polyacrylamide gel electrophoresis (SDS–PAGE).

SDS–PAGE and immunoblotting

SDS–PAGE was carried out on 4–10% gels, according to Laemmli[4]. Proteins were transferred onto 0.22 μm nitrocellulose sheets in 20% methanol, 192 mmol/l glycine, 25 mmol/l Tris–HCl pH 8.3 buffer, with constant voltage for 2 h, according to Towbin et al.[8]. The blots were preincubated in PBS–Tw, then with MAB diluted in PBS–Tw for 1 h at 25 °C then overnight at 4 °C. The blots were rinsed twice for 10 min in 0.1% v/v Triton PBS–Tw, then for 10 min in 0.65 mol/l NaCl, 0.05% Tw, 10 mmol/l phosphate buffer and lastly for 20 min in PBS–Tw. They were then incubated with peroxidase-labeled sheep Fab fragments to mouse G immunoglobulins diluted 1:200 in PBS–Tw, for 90 min at 25 °C. After a rinsing sequence as above, staining was performed with 4-chloro-1-naphthol.

EE 21-06[9], a MAB to keratin polypeptides no. 1, 2, 9, 10 and 11 of the Moll catalog[10] was used as positive control in all experiments.

RESULTS

Histological characterization

G36-19 (IgG1 κ) and F28-27 (IgG1 κ)

In all respects, G36-19 and F28-27 displayed the same histological characteristics. Within the anagen HF they exclusively labeled the IRS. In the bulb of
the HF, the labeling was found to appear asynchronously in the three IRS
components: at first in the Henle layer, then in the cuticle of the IRS, lastly
in the Huxley layer. Light cytoplasmic and microgranular at the birth of the
IRS layers, mainly Henle's, the labeling rapidly became intense linear pericellular and closely membranous, producing a net-like pattern on tangential
sections. It persisted all along the IRS. Within gingiva, hard palate and all the
examined epidermal sites, G36-19 and F28-27 labeled the SG. This labeling,
as in the IRS, was found to be microgranular and cytoplasmic in the lower
part of the SG, to become pericellular in the upper part, and to disappear in
the SC. By contrast, in plantar epidermis the labeling weakly persisted all
along the SC and was found to be increased in the most superficial layers. On
smears of corneocytes from hard palate and from foot sole, the labeling was
found to be membranous-like microgranular regular and diffuse. In all the
examined non-cornified squamous epithelia, neither G36-19 nor F28-27 produced any labeling. On paraffin-embedded tissues their reactivity was found
to be preserved but sometimes decreased.

B17-21 (IgG1 κ)

Within the HF, B17-21 decorated the IRS exactly as G36-19 and F28-27 did.
Within the epidermis, it labeled the SG according to the same pattern as G36-
19 and F28-27. However, in plantar epidermis, B17-21 showed no increasing
intensity of labeling in the upper SC and, on plantar and hard palate smears,
it very weakly labeled only a few corneocytes. B17-21 was unreactive with all
the tested non-cornified squamous epithelia. On paraffin-embedded tissues
its reactivity was usually found to be preserved but, in some cases, decreased.

G20-21 (IgG1 κ)

G20-21 was always found to be unreactive towards epidermis, while it specifically recognized the IRS of the HF. In contrast with G36-19, F28-27 and
B17-21, it did not label the cuticle of the IRS, but only the Henle and Huxley layers with a pericellular linear and regular pattern. Moreover, the labeling intensity increased progressively from the lower to the upper part of the
IRS, and was found to be maximal on the desquamated IRS cells. G20-21
also produced apical microgranular cytoplasmic staining of secretory and
ductal cells of sweat glands. On plantar and hard palate smears it did not stain
corneocytes.

47

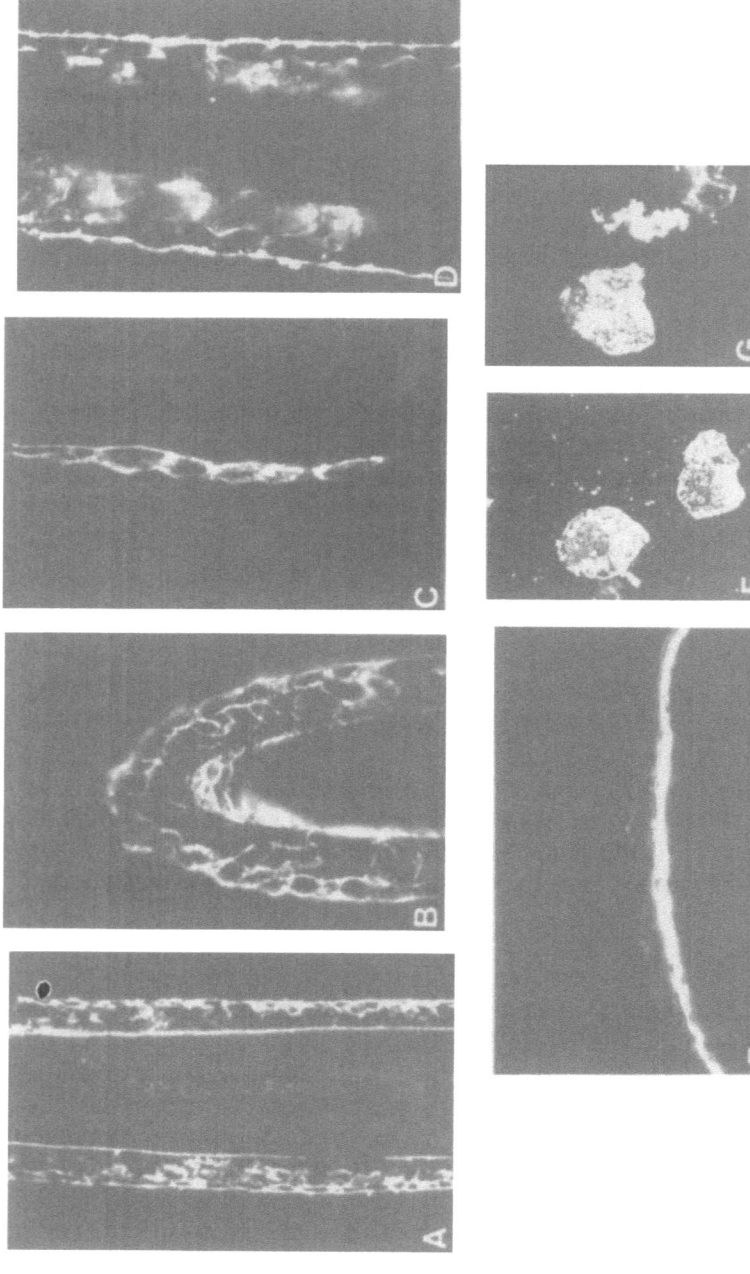

Figure 1 Immunohistological characteristics of G36-19 and G20-21 monoclonal antibodies towards human tissues and cells. **A–D**: cryostat sections of scalp; **E**: section of paraffin-embedded skin; **F**: smear from hard palate; **G**: cytocentrifugation of crosslinked envelopes purified from plantar SC. *G36-19* labels the three components of the mature IRS of the HF (**A, B**) and only the Henle layer at the birth of the IRS (**C**). *G20-21* labels the Henle and Huxley layers but not the cuticle of the IRS (**D**). *G36-19* exclusively labels the SG within the epidermis (**E**). On corneocytes (**F**), as on CLE (**G**), *G36-19* shows a regular microgranular membranous-like pattern

Immunofluorescence on crosslinked envelopes from plantar SC

When assayed on purified plantar CLE, G36-19, F28-27 and B17-21 decorated the quasi-totality of the cornified envelopes according to the same pattern as intact corneocytes. By contrast, G20-21 labeled no CLE.

ELISA

The four MAB were found to be unreactive with plantar SC keratin polypeptides, even at high concentrations and after a prolonged incubation (2 h at 37 °C plus overnight at 4 °C).

Immunoblotting

G36-19 and F28-27 (Figure 2)

The specificities of G36-19 and F28-27 were found to be quite similar. When assayed on plantar SC extract, both the MAB recognized a 33.5 kDa protein,

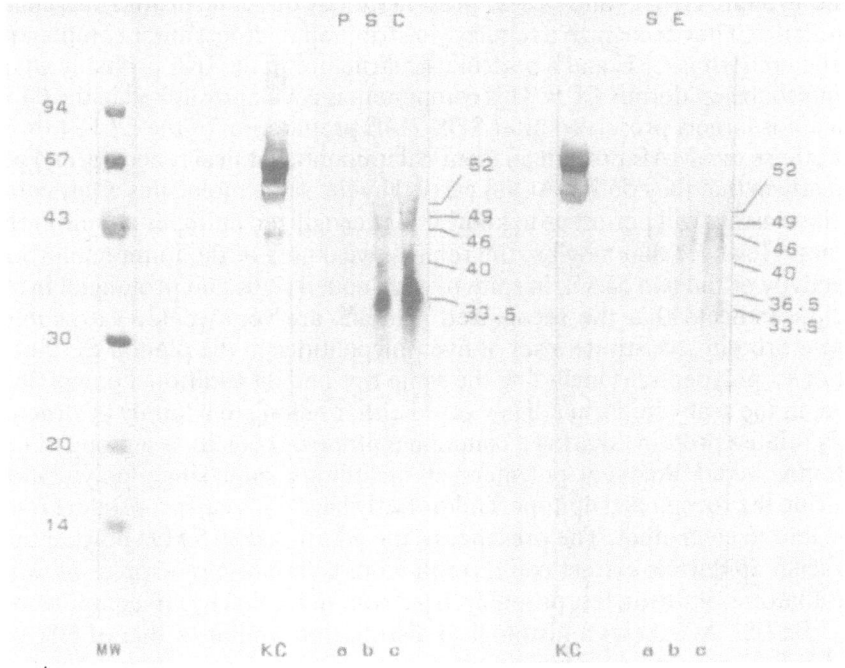

Figure 2   Immunoblotting reactivity of F28-27 monoclonal antibody on human epidermis extracts. Proteins extracted by Tris-SDS-2ME from human plantar stratum corneum (*PSC*) and from heat-cleaved scalp epidermis (*SE*) were run in a 10% polyacrylamide gel with increasing concentrations in three successive lanes (*a, b, c*), transferred onto nitrocellulose sheet and reacted with *F28-27* ascitic fluid diluted 1:100. Positive control with the monoclonal antibody EE21-06, specific for keratin polypeptides no. 1, 2, 9, 10, 11 of the Moll catalog was included (*KC*). Control proteins for molecular weight estimation (*MW*).

and more faintly four others of 40, 46, 49 and 52 kDa. On heat-cleaved scalp epidermis extract they recognised 52, 49 and 46 kDa proteins and more weakly 40, 36.5 and 33,5 kDa proteins. When assayed on keratins extracted from various epithelia and cell lines, these MAB never showed any reactivity.

B17-21

In the same experimental conditions, B17-21 never reacted on any substrate.

G20-21

This MAB has not yet been explored by immunoblotting.

DISCUSSION

G36-19, F28-27, B17-21 and G20-21 are specific markers of the IRS in the HF. The first three are also specific markers of the SG in the epidermis. Among them, G36-19 and F28-27 present exactly the same histological characteristics. They recognize a regularly distributed microgranular component of the epidermis CLE and a pericellular structure in the IRS probably analogous to the epidermis CLE. This component is covalently linked in the CLE since it is largely preserved after SDS-2ME preparation of the CLE. Moreover these two MAB present an identical immunochemical reactivity and we can affirm that they define AG(s) carried by the same molecules. Only competitive assays will permit us to know if the recognized epitopes are different or not. However that may be, the relative weakness of the immunoblotting reactivity of the two MAB, in spite of overloaded slabs and prolonged incubation, indicate that the recognized proteins are very weakly extractible. These proteins constitute a set of five polypeptides in the plantar SC and a set of six polypeptides including the same five and an additional one of 36.5 kDa, in the scalp epidermis. They could either belong to a family of structurally related proteins sharing a common epitope or constitute a group of covalently linked dimers or polymers, all including a same single polypeptide bearing the recognized epitope, and/or lastly have a precursor–product relationship to each other. The presence of the additional 36.5 kDa polypeptide on scalp epidermis extract could result from a variation of expression with the anatomical site or, less probably, from contamination by HF components.

B17-21 AG shows a histological distribution similar to that of G36-19 and F28-27 but differs in two points. Firstly, it labels very weakly a few corneocytes on smears from hard palate or foot sole, while all the CLE are very intensely labeled. Secondly it remains entirely non-reactive when assayed by immunoblotting. So, B17-21 defines a new AG of the CLE, masked on intact corneocytes, and possibly either conformational, or entirely linked to the CLE and absolutely non-extractible.

G20-21 is specifically expressed in the Henle and the Huxley layers of the IRS and not in the cuticle of the IRS. It defines a new AG specific for these two differentiation pathways. With regard to its labeling pattern, this AG is possibly associated with a CLE-like structure in these cells. Its immunochemical characterization remains to be performed.

In conclusion, G36-19, F28-27 and B17-21 differ from all the previously reported MAB against CLE antigens either by their histological and/or by their immunochemical characteristics[11-14]. They define new AG of the CLE of the epidermal keratinocytes which are also expressed in a CLE-like structure of the IRS cells. The AG are carried by epidermis protein components, which differ from the numerous components already described in normal and transformed keratinocytes[11-21]. These three MAB constitute an additional argument for the analogy which exists between the differentiation pathways of the epidermis and IRS of the HF. In contrast, G20-21 appears as a specific marker of the Henle and Huxley layer differentiation pathways.

ACKNOWLEDGEMENTS

We thank MF Isaia, MP Rue, S Bettinger, C Benat and N Rousseau for their valuable technical assistance, and Drs Etievant, Murat and Ouhayoun for giving cell lines. The work was supported in part by grants from the Association pour la Recherche contre le Cancer, the Ligue contre le Cancer and the Conseil Régional de Midi-Pyrénées.

Correspondence should be addressed to Dr Guy Serre, Laboratoire de Biologie Cellulaire, CHU PURPAN, Place du Dr Baylac, 31059 Toulouse Cedex, France.

REFERENCES

1. Serre G, Vincent C, Viraben R, Soleilhavoup JP. Naturally occurring autoantibodies to keratins in normal human sera. I: ELISA titration, immunofluorescence study. *J Invest Dermatol*, **88**, 21–27, 1987

2. Köhler GT, Milstein C. Continuous cultures of fused cells secreting antibody of predefined specificity, *Nature* **256**, 459–497, 1975

3. Dale BA, Perry TB, Holbrook KA, Hamilton EF, Senikas V. Biochemical examination of fetal skin biopsy specimens obtained by fetoscopy: Use of the method for analysis of keratins and filaggrin, *Pre Diag*, **6**, 37–44, 1986

4. Laemmli UK. Cleavage of structural proteins during the assembly of the head of bacteriophage T4. *Nature*, **227**, 680–685, 1970

5. Franke WW, Denk H, Kalt R, Schmidt E. Biochemical and immunological identification of cytokeratin proteins present in hepatocytes of mammalian liver tissue. *Exp Cell Res*, **131**, 299-318, 1981

6. Sun TT, Green H. Keratin filaments of cultured human epidermal cells. Formation of disulfide bonds during terminal differentiation. *J Biol Chem*, **253**, 2053–2060, 1978

7. Sun TT, Green H. Differentiation of the epidermal keratinocyte in cell culture: formation of the cornified envelope. *Cell*, **9**, 511–521, 1976

8. Towbin H, Staehelin T, Gordon J. Electrophoretic transfer of proteins from polyacrylamide gels to nitrocellulose sheets: procedure and some applications. *Proc Natl Acad Sci USA*, **76**, 4350–4354, 1979

9. Conter A, Ouhayoun JP, Mils V, Bettinger S, Vincent C, Kadouche J, Soleilhavoup JP, Serre G. EE21-06: un anticorps monoclonal contre les polypeptides kératine spécifiques des épithéliums malpighiens kératinisés. Congrès Annuel de Recherche Dermatologique, Bordeaux, 1987 (*Ann Dermatol Vénéréol*, in press)

10. Moll R, Franke WW, Schiller DL, Geiger B, Krepler R. The catalog of human cytokeratins: patterns of expression in normal epithelia, tumors and cultured cells. *Cell*, **31**, 11–24, 1982.

11. Ma ASP, Sun TT. Differentiation-dependent changes in the solubility of 195-kDa protein in human epidermal keratinocytes. *J Cell Biol*, **103**, 41–48, 1986.

12. Kubilus J, Kvedar J, Baden HP. Identification of new components of the cornified envelope of human and bovine epidermis. *J Invest Dermatol*, **89**, 44–50, 1987.

13. Baden HP, Kubilus J, Phillips SB. Characterization of monoclonal antibodies generated to the cornified envelope of human cultured keratinocytes. *J Invest Dermatol*, **89**, 454–459, 1987

14. Baden HP, Kubilus J, Phillips SB, Kvedar JC, Tahan SR. A new class of soluble basic protein precursors of cornified envelope of mammalian epidermis. *Biochim Biophys Acta*, **925**, 63–73, 1987.

15. Matoltsy AG, Balsamo CA. Study of the components of cornified epithelium of human skin. *J Biophys Biochem Cytol*, **1**, 339-360, 1955.

16. Kubilus J, Baden HP. Isolation of two immunologically related transglutaminase substrates from cultured human keratinocytes. *In Vitro*, **18**, 447–455, 1982

17. Kubilus J, Baden HP. Isopeptide bond formation in epidermis. *Mol Cell Biochem*, **58**, 129–137, 1984

18. Simon M, Green H. Participation of membrane-associated proteins in the formation of the cross-linked evelope of the keratinocyte. *Cell*, **36**, 827–834, 1984

19. Zettergren JG, Peterson LL, Wuepper DK. Keratolinin: the soluble substrate of epidermal transglutaminase from human and bovine tissue. *Proc Natl Acad Sci USA*, **81**, 238–242, 1984.

20. Nagae S, Lichti U, De Lucas LM, Yuspa SH. Effect of retinoic acid on cornified envelope formation: difference between spontaneous envelope formation in vivo or in vitro and expression of envelope competence. *J Invest Dermatol*, **89**, 51–58, 1987

21. Michel S, Schmidt R, Robinson SM, Shroot B, Reichert U. Identification and subcellular distribution of cornified envelope precursor proteins in the transformed human keratinocyte line SV-K14. *J Invest Dermatol*, **88**, 301–305, 1987

6

The dermo-epithelial interaction and the hair follicle

Ch M Lapiere
Department of Dermatology
CHU Liège
Tour de Pathologie
Sart Tilman, 4000 Liège, Belgium

ABSTRACT

Hair formation results of a complex cascade of cell–cell and cell–matrix interaction regulated by soluble mediators and various macromolecules. Variations in the composition and structure of the basement membrane zone and of the subepithelial connective tissues occur during the formation of the adnexae. The macromolecules composing these supporting structures have biological properties that might be involved in organogenesis.

The interaction between cells of the ectoderm and those of mesodermal origin is obvious during embryogenesis, in the formation of adnexae and later in postembryonic life in the persistence of the hair cycle. The epithelial–mesenchymal interaction will result in the formation of the basement membrane zone (BMZ), in the differentiation of the epidermis and its functional maturation and in the function of the connective tissue.

The BMZ extends from the basal pole of the keratinoblasts to the superficial layer of the dermis. The chemical nature, the physical organization and the biological significance of several of its constituents have been extensively investigated[1]. They can be interpreted as follows in terms of physical association to form the junction between the epithelial cells and their connective tissue support. The basal pole of the keratinocytes contains the membrane-bound and hemidesmosomes-associated bullous pemphigoid (BP) antigen[2] that interact with laminin in the lamina lucida of the BM. Laminin binds to itself and to type IV collagen of the lamina densa[3]. It also binds proteoheparan sulfate at the same location. The sublamina densa region is composed of proteoglycans, thin bundles of fibrils of collagen type III and I, fibronectin, acidic glycoproteins of the oxytalan fibers and the specific type VII collagen forming the anchoring fibrils probably similar to the EBA antigen[4]. The latter interacts with type IV collagen to ensure the adhesion of the BM to the dermis[5].

Beside their involvement in establishing the mechanical properties of the BM as a support most of the connective tissue and BM macromolecules display specific biological activities. For example the migration of keratinocytes is greatly enhanced on connective tissue macromolecules (type I or III collagen, fibronectin[6], etc.) as compared to BM macromolecules. Conversely, fibroblasts are more tightly bound to connective tissue than to basement membrane macromolecules. These cell–matrix interactions involving specific integrins[7] probably play a role in wound healing and perhaps also in the development and cycle of the hair follicle.

Keratinocytes in culture do not form a typical stratum corneum made of the differentiated types of keratins and cornified envelope proteins. Cultured on plastic, keratinocytes produce type IV collagen and laminin but do not organize them into a defined BM. Organotypical culture on a collagen gel increases the production of BM macromolecules except the BP antigen, but does not result in the formation of a visible BM. Explantation of the keratinocytes culture on the nude mouse results in both better differentiation of the stratum corneum[8] and the formation of a structured BM[9]. Such a BM could be formed *in vitro* by culture of keratinocytes in presence of a dermis[10]. An insoluble matrix of BM macromolecules also forms in culture when epithelial cells are in contact with fibroblasts, or with the extracellular matrix that they deposit *in vitro*[11]. These studies confirm and extend the findings of Briggaman *et al.*[12] of a production of BM components by epidermal cells and of the influence of the mesenchyme on epidermal differentiation including the formation of the BM.

A second type of specific dermo-epidermal interaction is involved in the differentiation and development of the appendages. Heterochronic, heterotopic and heterospecific dermo-epidermal recombination has allowed determination of the chronology of the interaction as summarized by Dhouailly in 1977[13]. The dermis causes the differentiation of the ectoderm into epidermis and sustains its proliferative activity. The epidermis modulates mesenchymal cells to induce them in appendage morphogenesis. This induced mesenchyme initiates the formation of the epidermal placodes and causes their transformation into rudiments of a specific quality determined by the epidermis. As far as hair is concerned the dermo-epithelial interaction is also required later for its continuous cycling. A significant information is located in dermal papillae that can induce the formation of a hair in contact with differentiated epidermis[14,15].

In the human embryo[16] the indifferent ectoderm is clearly defined as early as 7–8 days gestational age up to 1 month. At 4 weeks the periderm starts forming. At the end of the first trimester (8–10 weeks) a malpighian layer differentiates and anlage of epidermal appendages starts differentiating. At 9 weeks clusters of basal cells form the pregerms that develop in a cephalocaudal progression. During the first 2 months of the second trimester the pilosebaceous unit differentiates into hair pegs, solid cords of cells with a concave hair bulb and an enclosed dermal papilla. The sebaceous gland and apocrine glands develop from the hair peg. At 5 months the hair cone starts forming, the hair canal being already completed between 15 and 17 weeks. The first surface hair is visible at 16 weeks on the brows. Well after the epidermal appendages have formed keratinization begins in the interfollicular epidermis. As investigated mainly in rodents, several modifications occur in the connective tissue during the process of differentiation of the adnexae. Before the appearance of hair rudiments collagen I and III and fibronectin are uniformly distributed. They disappear during hair bud formation and surround at some distance the terminal hair bulb, except fibronectin that increases during hair bud formation[17]. All the BM macromolecules are present around the differentiating epidermis except the BP antigen that is constantly missing including in the functional dermal papilla[18] although basement membrane components are synthesized by dermal papillae cells[19]. These interactions between the mesenchyme and the differentiating epidermis suggest a developmental role for some of the connective tissue macromolecules.

The exchange of information between the epithelium and the mesenchyme also uses diffusible messages. Some of them have been isolated as the epithelial scatter factor secreted by fibroblasts[20] and a fibroblast anticontractile factor produced by the keratinocytes (Eisinger, 1987, personal communication). Epithelial cells also produce fibroblast activating factors, TGF beta, FGF-like polypeptides, etc. Interestingly some growth factors display a different type of activity when the cells are in contact with connective tissue or basement membrane macromolecules as EGF on fibroblasts[21]. The response of epithelial mammary cells to estrogens is modulated by with fibroblasts[22]. Such regulation processes might depend on a modification of the density or activity of membrane receptors of the receptive cells, as observed in the basal keratinocytes overlying the dermal condensates marking the first stage of hair follicle development[23].

It is most probable that a tightly regulated cascade of cell–cell and cell–matrix interaction operates to induce the differentiation of the cells resulting in the initial hair and its post-embyronic cycle.

REFERENCES

1. Martin GR, Timpl R. Laminin and other basement membrane components. *Ann Rev Cell Biol*, **3**, 57–85, 1987
2. Regnier M, Vaigot P, Michel S, Prunieras M. Localization of bullous pemphigoid antigen in isolated human keratinocytes. *J Invest Dermatol*, **85**, 187–190, 1985
3. Woodley DT, Rao CN, Hassell JR, Liotta LA, Martin GR, Kleinman HK. Interactions of basement membrane components. *Biochim Biophys Acta*, **761**, 278, 1983
4. Bruckner-Tuderman L, Schnyder UW, Winterhalter KH, Bruckner P. Tissue form of type VII collagen form human skin and dermal fibroblasts in culture. *Eur J Biochem*, **165**, 607–611, 1987
5. Keene DR, Sakai LY, Lunstrum GP, Morris NP, Burgeson RE. Type VII collagen forms an extended network of anchoring fibrils. *J Cell Biol*, **104**, 611–621, 1987
6. O'Keefe EJ, Payne RE, Russell N, Woodley DT. Spreading and enhanced motility of human keratinocytes on fibronectin. *J Invest Dermatol*, **85**, 125–130, 1985

7.   Ruoslahti E, Pierschbacher MD. New perspectives in cell adhesion: RGD and integrins. *Science*, **238**, 491–497, 1987
8.   Banks-Schlegel S, Green H. Formation of epidermis by serially cultivated human epidermal cells transplanted as an epithelium to athymic mice. *Transplantation*, **29**, 308–313, 1980
9.   Bohnert A, Hornung J, Mackenzie IC, Fusenig NE. Epithelial-mesenchymal interactions control basement membrane production and differentiation in cultured and transplanted mouse keratinocytes. *Cell Tissue Res*, **244**, 413–429, 1986
10.   Woodley DT, Regnier M, Prunieras M. In vitro basal lamina formation may require non-epidermal cell living substrate. *Br J Dermatol*, **103**, 397–404, 1980
11.   Delvoye P, Pierard D, Noel A, Nusgens B, Foidart JM, Lapière ChM. Fibroblasts induce the assembly of the macromolecules of the basement membrane. *J Invest Dermatol* (in press)
12.   Briggaman RA, Dalldorf FG, Wheeler CE. Formation and origin of basal laminina and anchoring fibrils in adult human skin. *J Cell Biol*, **51**, 384–395, 1971
13.   Dhouailly D. Dermo-epidermal interactions during morphogenesis of cutaneous appendages in amniotes. *Front Matrix Biol*, **4**, 86–121, 1977
14.   Cohen J. Transplantation of hair papillae. *Symp Zool Soc Lond*
15.   Oliver RF. The induction of hair follicle formation in the adult hooded rat by vibrissa dermal papillae. *J Embryol Exp Morphol*, **23**, 219–236, 1970
16.   Holbrook KA. Human epidermal embryogenesis. *Int J Dermatol*, **18**, 329–356, 1979
17.   Mauger A, Emonard H. Hartmann DJ, Foidart JM, Sengel P. Immunofluorescent localization of collagen types I, III and IV, fibronectin, laminin and basement membrane proteoglycan in developing mouse skin. *Arch Dev Bioe*, **196**, 295–302, 1987
18.   Westgate GE, Shaw DA, Harrap GJ, Couchman JR. Immuno-histochemical localization of basement membrane components during hair follicle morphogenesis. *J Invest Dermatol*, **82**, 259–264, 1984
19.   Couchman JR. Rat hair follicle dermal papillae have an extracellular matrix containing basement membrane components. *J Invest Dermatol*, **87**, 762–767, 1986
20.   Stoker M, Gherardi E, Perryman M, Gray J. Scatter factor is a fibroblast-derived modulator of epithelial cell mobility. *Nature*, **327**, 239, 1987
21.   Colige A, Nusgens B, Lapière Ch M. The effects of EGF on human skin fibroblasts is modulated by the extracellular matrix. *Arch Dermatol Res* (in press)
22.   Haslam SZ. Mammary fibroblast influence on normal mouse mammary epithelial cell responses to estrogen in vitro. *Cancer Res*, **46**, 310–316, 1986
23.   Green MR, Couchman JR. Distribution of epidermal growth factor receptors in rat tissues during embryonic skin development, hair formation, and the adult hair growth cycle. *J Invest Dermatol*, **83**, 118–123, 1984

7

Isolation, culture and in vitro behavior of cells isolated from papillae of human hair follicles

AG Messenger

Department of Dermatology
Royal Hallamshire Hospital
University of Sheffield
Sheffield, S10 2JF, UK

ABSTRACT

The dermal papilla is a connective tissue structure situated at the base of the hair follicle. Together with the fibrous sheath surrounding the follicle, the papilla is derived from an aggregation of mesenchymal cells which appears at an early stage of embryological development. Differentiation of hair follicle epithelium is dependent on inductive signals from the dermal papilla, both during embryogenesis and in the adult follicle. To study dermal papilla function in more detail methods have been developed for culturing cells from isolated papillae of various mammalian species, including man. Human papilla cells tend to display distinctive *in vitro* morphology and behavior. Like rat vibrissa papilla cells, they readily form multilayered aggregates, particularly when plated onto collagen gels. Papilla cells derived from human beard follicles grow more rapidly than scalp follicle cells (doubling times 40 h and 70–80 h respectively).

This appears to be an inherent property which is unaffected by exogenous testosterone. Both *in vivo* and *in vitro*, human dermal papilla cells synthesize an extracellular matrix containing interstitial collagens and basement membrane proteins. Cultured cells also release IGF-1 (Somatomedin C) into serum-free supernatants, although the relevance of this finding to *in vivo* function has not been established. Attempts to show that human papilla cells retain the ability to induce hair growth, using *in vitro* models, have so far been unsuccessful. However, it has been shown that rat vibrissa cells will induce hair growth when implanted into the intact animal, and further studies with human cells are in progress. The use of cell culture models in hair biology is at an early stage of development, but it is hoped that they will considerably expand the scope of future research.

INTRODUCTION

In recent years there has been an upsurge of interest in the hair follicle, largely fueled by the advent of pharmacological agents which modulate hair growth. However, our understanding of how these drugs work has been severely hampered by the lack of knowledge of the regulatory processes governing normal hair growth, and also of the pathogenesis of the various disorders we are trying to treat. A particular problem in hair research has been the absence of suitable laboratory models. Animal models have, of course, been used for many years, but these can be cumbersome, they provide only limited information and are not necessarily applicable to human hair growth. An alternative approach which is being explored in a number of centers is to use tissue culture. While it cannot yet be claimed that we have a true *in vitro* model of the hair follicle it is now possible to culture hair follicle cells of both epithelial and dermal derivation. My own particular interest, and the subject of this presentation, is the culture of cells from the human dermal papilla. Although the dermal papilla is a tiny structure we believe it plays a crucial role in regulating growth and differentiation in the hair follicle. The ability to culture papilla-derived cells, therefore, is a prerequisite of a more complete *in vitro* model of the hair follicle and also provides the opportunity to study the molecular basis of dermal papilla function in much greater depth than have previously been possible.

ANATOMY

The dermal papilla is a connective tissue structure situated at the base of the hair follicle. In anagen follicles the papilla invaginates the epithelial hair bulb matrix, remaining in contact with the fibrous sheath surrounding the follicle via a narrow stalk at its base. The papilla itself is composed of specialized fibroblast-like cells and, in larger terminal follicles, a central capillary loop. During anagen, papilla cells lie in an extracellular matrix rich in mucopolysaccharides[1] and basement membrane proteins[2,3] and display ultrastructural features indicative of synthetic activity[4]. The extracellular matrix gradually diminishes during catagen and disappears almost completely as the follicle enters telogen. However, the cellular population of the dermal papilla is believed to remain constant throughout the hair cycle and apposition with the base of the hair follicle epithelium is maintained. Synthesis of extracellular matrix is resumed as the epithelial matrix grows down to invest the papilla with the onset of the next anagen phase.

Function of the dermal papilla

To appreciate the function of the dermal papilla, we have to go back to the embryological development of the hair follicle. The epithelial component of the follicle first appears as a crowding of cells in the basal layer of the fetal

58

epidermis. At about the same time, mesenchymal cells begin to aggregate immediately beneath the epidermis at this point. As the hair peg develops these aggregated mesenchymal cells organize into the presumptive dermal papilla and fibrous sheath[5]. There is a wealth of evidence that, though certain characteristics of the fully developed follicle may be determined by factors intrinsic to the epithelium, the signals responsible for initiating follicle development and for instructing the epithelium to form a hair follicle are derived from the mesenchymal component (reviewed in refs 6 and 7). Indeed, a follicle will not form if the aggregation of mesenchymal cells is prevented[8].

One of the intriguing features of hair biology is that anagen development in the adult follicle closely resembles the embryological events. This raises the possibility that the papilla possesses functions similar to its mesenchymal precursor. Evidence that this is indeed the case has mainly come from the work of Oliver on the rat vibrissa follicle[9–11]. The beauty of this model, first developed by Cohen[12], is that, by reflecting the cheek pad of the animal, various manipulations can be performed on the lower part of individual vibrissa follicles *in situ*.

After the cheek pad has been replaced the constant spatial organization of vibrissa follicles allows the result of the procedure to be easily observed. Oliver showed that removal of the dermal papilla from a vibrissa follicle resulted in temporary cessation of hair growth. However, a new dermal papilla then developed from the fibrous sheath and hair growth resumed. The next step was to excise the complete hair bulb. If less than one-third of the lower follicle was removed a papilla was again formed from the fibrous sheath and a new matrix developed from the outer root sheath. If more than one-third of the lower follicle was amputated the fibrous sheath failed to produce a new papilla and no matrix development occurred. However, matrix development could be induced by implanting an isolated dermal papilla into the lower end of such a follicle and then a new hair would grow. In further experiments Oliver was able to demonstrate that follicular structures were also formed when isolated dermal papillae were associated with a follicular epidermis which was then implanted into the skin. These studies have clearly demonstrated that the dermal papilla is responsible for inducing and maintaining matrix differentiation in adult follicles, at least in the rat vibrissa follicle, and also suggest that the lower part of the fibrous sheath may share some of these properties.

Whether the dermal papilla determines other aspects of hair growth such as the duration of anagen is uncertain although there is some evidence to suggest that hair diameter is dependent on the size of the papilla[13]. This may be relevant when we come to consider androgen responses. The nature of the inductive signals from the papilla to the matrix epithelium is unknown. We know that there are heterotypic contacts between mesenchymal and epithelial cells during embryonic development[14] and the rat whisker experiments have also indicated that direct apposition is necessary for interaction to occur between adult papilla implants and the follicular epithelium. However, other factors such as the composition of the extracellular matrix and perhaps paracrine growth factors may also be important.

Dermal papilla cell culture

My own interest in the dermal papilla arose out of work I had been doing on the pathogenesis of alopecia areata. I had reached the stage where, in order to pursue this work, I needed some form of model for the human hair follicle. At about this time Jahoda and Oliver published a method for culturing cells from isolated rat whisker dermal papillae[15]. This encouraged me to develop the following method for isolating dermal papillae from human hair follicles and for establishing cell cultures from the papilla explants[16].

ISOLATION AND CULTURE OF HUMAN DERMAL PAPILLAE

1.   Anagen hair follicles are dissected out of biopsied tissue. Plucked follicles are not satisfactory as they rarely yield a dermal papilla. I usually use scalp tissue which can be obtained when various minor lesions such as nevi are being surgically excised (follicles can, of course, be obtained from other sites; male beard skin is particularly useful as the follicles are large and easily manipulated). The hair bulbs are then excised and placed in culture medium in a second Petri dish.

2.   The hair bulb epithelium is then separated from the dermal papilla and the fibrous sheath by gentle pressure with a 21G needle. Separation occurs easily and proteolytic enzymes are not necessary.

3.   The fibrous sheath is then opened using the sharp bevelled edge of the needle tip and by further gentle manipulation the dermal papilla can usually be persuaded to protrude through the opening. The papilla is then transected across its stalk and transferred to a third Petri dish.

These steps are performed using a stereomicroscope equipped with transmitted illumination and zoom magnification. The papilla explants can then be cultured in the Petri dish but I prefer to transfer them to a culture flask using a Pasteur pipette. It is important that the flask is then left undisturbed in the incubator for about 7 days by which time most of the papilla explants have attached to the bottom of the flask and cells will have started to migrate onto the substrate. The cells spread slowly and it may take up to 6 weeks before they can be subcultured as a single cell suspension. Subsequent passages are generally performed at 2-week intervals.

In order to characterize the cells grown from human dermal papillae we have studied a number of their *in vitro* properties. Where possible we have tried to relate these properties to the *in vivo* situation and in some experiments we have also compared papilla cells with dermal fibroblasts cultured from the same biopsy tissue.

MORPHOLOGY AND BEHAVIOR

Although there is some variation between different cell lines, cultured human dermal papilla cells display fairly consistent morphological and behavioral features. The cells tend to be flattened and spread-out in shape rather than having the spindle-cell shape of dermal fibroblasts. This is most prominent at the edges of expanding colonies. After subculture papilla cells typically form aggregates and clumps which become multilayered before reaching confluence, whereas dermal fibroblasts grow as monolayers forming into parallel arrays. The degree to which papilla cells aggregate in vitro is variable and appears to be more prominent in slowly growing cell lines. However, if papilla cells are seeded as a single-cell suspension onto collagen gels, aggregation occurs very rapidly and consistently to produce large clumps of cells scattered over the gel surface[17]. Fibroblasts, on the other hand, usually remain evenly distributed when seeded onto collagen gel. Papilla cells cultured from rat whisker follicles[18] and from sheep wool follicles display similar aggregative behavior, suggesting that this property is of fundamental functional significance. The resemblance to mesenchymal aggregation during follicular morphogenesis is striking, and is in accord with the view that these adult cells retain certain embryological characteristics.

CELL GROWTH

In their initial studies, Jahoda and Oliver reported that rat whisker papilla cells grew more slowly in culture than dermal fibroblasts[15]. They felt that this may reflect the low proliferative activity of dermal papilla cells in vivo. We have found that human cells derived from scalp follicles also grow slowly in vitro compared with parallel lines of dermal fibroblasts. Their longevity is also less than that of fibroblasts; senescence of cultured papilla cells usually occurs after 5 to 10 passages whereas most fibroblast lines will survive at least 12 passages and often more. However, we have noted differences in the growth potential of papilla cell lines depending on their site of origin[19]. Cells derived from male beard follicles (doubling time c. 40 h) grow more rapidly than scalp follicle cells (doubling time 70–80 h). This appears to be an intrinsic property; the in vitro growth of papilla cell lines from androgen-dependent and androgen-independent follicles (e.g. occipital scalp) is unaffected by the addition of testosterone in physiological concentrations to the culture medium. The possibility that androgen-dependent responses in the hair follicle are mediated via the dermal papilla is currently being studied as human papilla cells have been shown to possess androgen receptors and 5-alpha reductase activity[20].

SYNTHETIC ACTIVITY

We can get some idea of the type of compounds synthesized in the dermal papilla by using various methods such as histochemistry, immunohistochemistry and electron microscopy. These techniques have certain limitations, however, and we hope that cell culture will provide much more information on the molecular biology of dermal papilla function. To use cultured cells for this purpose it will be important to establish whether they retain their *in vivo* phenotype and, where possible, we have tried to compare the synthetic activity of the cultured cells with the parent tissue. The work carried out so far has concentrated mainly on extracellular matrix; we also have some preliminary data on the synthesis of growth factors.

EXTRACELLULAR MATRIX

Collagen fibres can be seen within the dermal papilla at electron microscopy although they are not as prominent as in the dermis. Types I and III collagen can also be demonstrated in the human dermal papilla and the fibrous sheath by immunofluorescence using the appropriate antibodies. Staining of human papilla cell cultures with the same antibodies reveals positive staining of cytoplasm and of extracellular fibrillar material from a very early stage of the primary culture (7 days) through to late subcultures. These findings are the same as for dermal fibroblasts, and can be confirmed by standard biochemical techniques when sufficient cells are available. I have stressed that this is the case for the human dermal papilla because the rat whisker papilla appears to be different. Little or no interstitial collagen can be seen in the rat papilla by immunofluorescence and rat cells only begin to synthesize collagens I and III after about 3 weeks in culture[3]. However, Couchman found that rat papilla cells synthesize collagen IV in early primary culture as well as other basement membrane proteins. This compares with the parent tissue where the extracellular matrix of the dermal papilla stains strongly for collagen IV and for laminin in both rat and man. The precise localization of this material has not been studied using immunoelectron microscopy, but it has long been known that interrupted basement membrane-like structures occur around cells in the dermal papilla[21]. We have found that cultured human papilla cells also stain with antibodies to collagen IV at immunofluorescence. Fluorescence is seen in the cytoplasm and on fibrillar extracellular material, particularly in the vicinity of cell aggregates. Positivity for collagen IV varies considerably between different cell lines; in some lines over 90% of cells have been positive, whereas in other lines positive cells are scanty. Immunofluorescent staining for laminin is less consistent, but we have obtained positive results in two of the six lines studied. None of the papilla cell lines studied has stained for Factor VIII-related antigen, indicating that they are not of endothelial derivation.

DO PAPILLA CELLS MAKE BASEMENT MEMBRANE STRUCTURES IN VITRO?

At electron microscopy we have seen electron-dense extracellular material deposited beneath the cells in a linear fashion strongly resembling basement membrane. Cells make contact with this material via well-defined attachment plaques and the undersurface of the cells is also rich in pinocytotic activity and coated pits.

Proteoglycans and glycosaminoglycans form the other major component of the dermal papilla extracellular matrix. Their biological role in relation to hair growth is unknown, although it is worth noting that hypertrichosis may be a feature of various disorders, such as pretibial myxoedema and certain of the mucopolysaccharidoses, in which these compounds are deposited in the skin in increased amounts. Using standard biochemical methods we have found that cultured papilla cells incorporate radiolabeled precursor into hyaluronic acid and sulphated glycosaminoglycans. We are currently trying to identify the synthesis of specific proteoglycans in the dermal papilla *in vivo* and *in vitro* in more detail, but these studies are not far enough advanced for me to present the results at this stage.

GROWTH FACTORS

The evidence that growth factors are involved in controlling hair growth is limited. There are receptors for epidermal growth factor in the hair follicle[22] but the administration of epidermal growth factor to mammalian species inhibits hair growth, notably in the sheep, where large doses cause shedding of the fleece[23]. However, the possibility that papilla-derived growth factors influence epithelial behavior in the hair follicle is attractive, and we are currently looking at the synthesis of a number of growth factors by cultured cells. At the present time I can only present data on one such growth factor: Insulin-like growth factor 1 (IGF-1). IGF-1 is widely distributed in the body and has a number of biological actions. These are not restricted to growth promotion and include the enhancement of differentiation in certain tissues. For example, IGF-1 stimulates glycosaminoglycan synthesis in cartilage, and is also believed to mediate the action of growth hormone (reviewed in ref. 24). To date we have studied IGF-1 synthesis using a sensitive radioimmunoassay in five papilla cell lines. All released IGF-1 into serum-free culture supernatant in biologically significant amounts. Interestingly, the most active cell line in terms of IGF-1 synthesis was derived from male chest follicles. Whether IGF-1 has a role in hair growth remains to be seen although it has been shown to stimulate epidermal cell growth *in vitro*[25].

INDUCTION OF HAIR GROWTH

The ultimate test that cultured dermal papilla cells retain their *in vivo* function would be to demonstrate that they have the ability to induce hair matrix differentiation. This has clearly been shown to be the case for rat papilla cells; using the vibrissa model, Jahoda and his colleagues implanted cultured cells into the lower ends of follicles from which the lower halves had been amputated. The implantation of papilla cells resulted in the formation of a hair bulb matrix and the restoration of hair growth. In contrast, fibroblasts failed to induce hair growth[26]. Recently, the same group has claimed that cultured vibrissa papilla cells will induce follicular neogenesis from overlying epidermis when implanted directly into rat ear skin. Moreover, these follicles produced a vibrissa-like hair, suggesting that the site-dependent properties of hair follicles are determined by the connective tissue. This is at variance with previous views on epidermal specificities and we await publication of their methods with interest. Attempts to show that human dermal papilla cells can induce hair growth have so far been restricted to *in vitro* models and, to the best of my knowledge, have been unsuccessful. We have tested three model systems:

1. A feeder layer system in which epidermal keratinocytes were co-cultured with mitomycin C-treated dermal papilla cells or dermal fibroblasts. Epidermal prekeratins were analyzed after 1 or 2 weeks but no differences were observed with either feeder layer type.

2. A skin equivalent model. Epidermal keratinocytes were cultured on collagen gels incorporating dermal papilla cells or dermal fibroblasts. After 2 weeks the gels were examined histologically. Some downward budding from the reconstructed epidermis was seen into gels incorporating papilla cells, but these did not convincingly resemble hair follicles.

3. An organ culture model. Segments of the lower part of human follicles (minus the hair bulb) were embedded in collagen gels either alone or in close association with isolated dermal papillae. In further experiments the hair follicle segments were associated with cultured papilla cells or dermal fibroblasts. Budding of epithelium from the outer root sheath, usually at the lower 'hair bulb' end of the explant, occurred after about 5 days. These buds took the form of columns of cells and sometimes formed cyst-like structures. Histologically, none showed evidence of hair matrix differentiation.

Induction of hair growth using rat papilla cells has so far only been achieved when the cells are reintroduced into the intact animal and the failure of these *in vitro* experiments is perhaps not too surprising. There are technical difficulties in extending the animal experiments to man, although they are not insurmountable. However, there are potential hazards to be considered, particularly if we are thinking about re-introducing cultured cells into man, and some other model system, e.g. performing recombinant experiments on tissue transplanted onto athymic nude mice, may be preferable.

CONCLUSIONS

The procedure for culturing human dermal papilla cells is now well established and is being performed in a number of centers. These cells possess distinctive properties which resemble those of the parent tissue. However, much remains to be done; in particular we need to know whether these cells retain the ability to induce hair matrix differentiation and for how long the phenotype is maintained in culture. The ability of cultured rat papilla cells to induce vibrissa growth declines after about three passages, and this imposes limits on the usefulness of any single cell line. Once these problems are overcome the potential applications of cell culture techniques for studying hair biology and hair disease are considerable. Interactions between mesenchymal and epithelial cells are also of general biological interest in many tissues. Finally, we may be able to use cultured cells for studying the action of drugs which modify hair growth, and in the development of new forms of treatment.

ACKNOWLEDGEMENTS

This work would not have been possible without the help of others; in particular I would like to acknowledge the contributions of Kathy Elliott, Jennifer Senior, Lisa Cadwood, Alistair Strain, Anne Temple, Diane Holland and Valerie Randall.

REFERENCES

1. Montagna W, Chase HB, Malone JD, Melaragno HP. Cyclic changes in polysaccharides of the papilla of the hair follicle. *QJ Microscop Sci*, **93**, 241–245, 1952
2. Couchman JR, Gibson WT. Expression of basement membrane components through morphological changes in the hair growth cycle. *Dev Biol*, **108**, 290–298, 1985
3. Couchman JR. Rat hair follicle dermal papillae have an extracellular matrix containing basement membrane components. *J Invest Dermatol*, **87**, 762–767, 1986
4. Young RD. Morphological and ultrastructural aspects of the dermal papilla during the growth cycle of the vibrissal follicle in the rat. *J Anat* **131**, 355–365, 1980
5. Pinkus H. Embryology of hair. In The Biology of Hair Growth (Montagna W, Ellis RA, eds), pp. 1–32. New York: Academic Press, 1958
6. Billingham RE, Silvers WK. Studies on the conservation of epidermal specificities of skin and certain mucosas in adult mammals. *J Exp Med*, **125**, 429–446, 1967
7. Sengel P. *Morphogenesis of Skin*. Cambridge: Cambridge University Press, 1976
8. Jacobson CM. A comparative study of the mechanisms by which X-irradiation and genetic mutation cause loss of vibrissae in embryo mice. *J Embryol Exp Morphol*, **16**, 369–379, 1966
9. Oliver RF. Whisker growth after removal of the dermal papilla and lengths of the follicle in the hooded rat. *J Embryol Exp Morphol* **15**, 331–347, 1966
10. Oliver RF. The experimental induction of whisker growth in the hooded rat by implantation of dermal papillae. *J Embryol Exp Morphol* **18**, 43–51, 1967

11. Oliver RF. The induction of hair follicle formation in the adult hooded rat by vibrissa dermal papillae. *J Embryol Exp Morphol*, **23**, 219–236, 1970

12. Cohen J. The transplantation of individual rat and guinea pig whisker papillae. *J Embryol Exp Morphol*, **9**, 117–127, 1961

13. Ibrahim L, Wright EA. A quantitative study of hair growth using mouse and rat vibrissal follicles. I Dermal papilla volume determines hair volume. *J Embryol Exp Morphol*, **72**, 209–224, 1982

14. Hardy MH, Van Exan RJ, Sonstegard KS, Sweeny PR. Basal lamina changes during tissue interactions in hair follicles, an *in vitro* study of normal dermal papillae and vitamin A-induced glandular morphogenesis. *J Invest Dermatol*, **80**, 27–34, 1983

15. Jahoda C, Oliver RF. The growth of vibrissa dermal papilla cells *in vitro*. *Br J Dermatol*, **105**, 623–627, 1981

16. Messenger AG. The culture of dermal papilla cells from human hair follicles. *Br J Dermatol*, **110**, 685–689, 1984

17. Messenger AG, Senior HJ, Bleehen SS. The *in vitro* properties of dermal papilla cell lines established from human hair follicles. *Br J Dermatol*, **114**, 425–430, 1986

18. Jahoda CAB, Oliver RF. Vibrissa dermal papilla cell aggregative behaviour *in vivo* and *in vitro*. *J Embryol Exp Morphol*, **79**, 211–224, 1984

19. Randall VA, Messenger AG. *In vitro* properties of dermal papilla cells cultured from beard and scalp hair follicles. *J Endocrinol*, **108**, 120, 1986

20. Murad S, Hodgins MB, Simpson NB, Oliver RF, Jahoda C. Androgen receptors and metabolism in cultured dermal papilla cells from human hair follicles. *Br J Dermatol*, **113**, 768, 1985

21. Hashimoto K, Shibazaki S. Ultrastructural study on differentiation and function of hair. In *Biology and Disease of Hair* (Kobori T, Montagna W, eds) pp. 23–57. Baltimore: University Park Press, 1976

22. Green MR, Couchman JR. Distribution of growth factor receptors in rat tissues during embryonic skin development, hair formation and the adult hair growth cycle. *J Invest Dermatol*, **83**, 118–123, 1984

23. Moore GPM, Panaretto BA, Robertson D. Inhibition of wool growth in merino sheep following administration of mouse epidermal growth factor and a derivative. *Aust J Biol Sci*, **35**, 163–172, 1982

24. Underwood LE, D'Ercole AJ, Clemmons DR, Van Wyk JJ. Paracrine functions of Somatomedins. *Clin Endocrinol*, **15**, 59–77, 1986

25. Pittelkow MR. Somatomedin C is a growth factor for human prokeratinocytes *in vitro*. *Br J Dermatol*, **113**, 769–770, 1985

26. Jahoda CAB, Horne KA, Oliver RF. Induction of hair growth by implantation of cultured dermal papilla cells. *Nature*, **311**, 560–562, 1984

8

A new in vitro culture system to produce a fully differentiated epidermis from human hair follicle outer root sheath cells

M-C Lenoir, BA Bernard, G Pautrat, M Darmon and B Shroot

Centre International de Recherches Dermatologiques (CIRD)
Sophia Antipolis
F-06565 Valbonne Cedex, France

ABSTRACT

During wound healing, interfollicular epidermis can be regenerated from the outer root sheath of hair follicles, showing that the cells of this structure can shift toward an interfollicular epidermal phenotype. Similarly, it has been shown that a multilayered epithelium originating from outer sheath cells can be obtained *in vitro* by culturing hair follicles. However, in the culture systems developed so far, the phenotypical shift was incomplete since the cells retained some of their original characteristics and did not acquire several key markers of terminally differentiated epidermis. In this paper we describe a new tissue culture method for obtaining a multilayered epithelium from outer sheath cells. This is performed by implanting human hair follicles vertically into dermal equivalents and then raising the culture to the air–liquid interface. The morphological, immunological and biochemical features of the *in vitro* reconstructed tissue are very similar to those observed in normal interfollicular epidermis, including those specific for terminally differentiated keratinocytes. In particular, the basic 67 kDa keratin (normally absent in conventional cultures and in freshly isolated hair follicles) is present and detectable from the first suprabasal layers, as in normal skin. Thus, under appropriate *in vitro* conditions, outer root sheath cell differentiation can be modulated so as to express an interfollicular epidermal phenotype as occurs *in vivo* during wound healing.

In other respects the possibility of producing large quantities of living skin equivalents by implanting a number of hair follicles in large lattices provides the pharmacologist with an easy and quantitative system for studying the effects and metabolization of drugs. This system is easy to set up and very flexible. Preliminary data show that biopsies of this *in vitro* reconstructed epidermis can be serially passed in freshly cast dermal equivalents. This epidermis can also be cryopreserved without loss of viability. This system could thus also represent a promising and suitable alternative source for autologous keratinocytes for the treatment of burns and other surgical use.

In excised wounds and after split-skin surgical removal of epidermis, epidermal repair occurs from the specialized appendages of human skin such as sweat glands, sebaceous glands and hair follicles. These appendages provide sources of keratinocytes, contributing to the epithelial renewal by migrating and undergoing mitosis. It is thus appropriate to use the outer root sheath of human hair follicle as a source of proliferating keratinocytes. This goal has been achieved and such cultures have been used for studies on differentiation, transformation and carcinogenesis[1,2]. Several methods have been developed for establishing primary cultures of human hair follicles[3-6]. However, yield and reproducibility were poor[3,4]. Additionally, biochemical analyses revealed that cultured hair follicle cells synthesized the same set of keratin polypeptides as freshly isolated hair follicles, although they stratified and apparently differentiated[5,8]. This suggests that the phenotypic transition towards an epidermal-like phenotype was limited to a multistratified morphology, since biochemical markers specific for interfollicular epidermis did not appear. This is in contrast with what happens *in vivo* during epidermal regeneration after wounding.

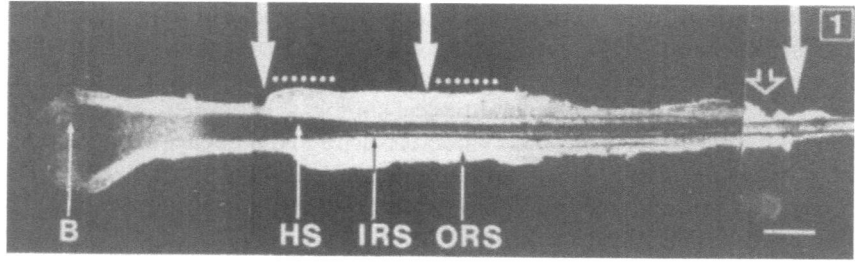

Figure 1 Plucked anagen hair follicle, with the bulb (B), hair shaft (HS), inner root sheath (IRS), and outer root sheath (ORS). Arrows indicate where hair follicle is sectioned for implantation. Open arrow-head locates the opening of the sebaceous gland duct. Dotted lines represent the portions which are actually inserted into the collagen lattice. Bar represents 250 μm

The aim of the present study was to design a culture system which would improve the growth of outer root sheath cells and thus make possible a full phenotypic transition towards interfollicular epidermis. In order to achieve this goal, hair follicles (Figure 1) were implanted vertically into freshly cast dermal equivalents[9,10] which were brought to the air–liquid interface onto a grid, after 5 days of culture under immersion. At that time a narrow fringe of tissue had appeared around the hair follicles. The area of this newly grown epithelium increased with time and completely covered the dermal equivalents by days 13 to 15 (Figure 5). A good outgrowth was observed at day 13 in 83.3% of the cultures performed from the hair follicles of the 30 volunteers tested. Although it is almost impossible to have direct evidence of the origin of this outgrowth, this regenerative tissue probably originated from the outer root sheath cells[3,7], which, in the absence of the sebaceous gland (Figure 1) and beside the inner root sheath cells of the hair follicle section, represent the vast majority of the cells in direct contact with the dermal equivalent.

Stained paraffin sections of the regenerated epithelium (Figure 2) obtained after 28–30 days of culture suggested that, in spite of a slight hyperplasia, not only stratification, but also terminal epidermal differentiation had occurred. A granular layer with numerous keratohyalin granules and a horny layer were present. Moreover, a dense material evoking a basement membrane was deposited at the 'dermal–epidermal' junction and basal cells had a cuboidal shape, as normally found *in vivo*, but very rarely in culture. These features were very similar to those observed in normal skin, and contrasted strikingly with the morphology of the outer root sheath from which the culture originated.

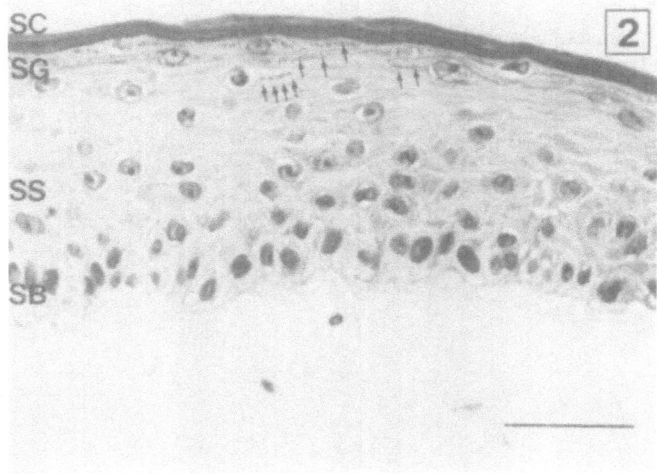

Figure 2 Morphology of reconstructed epidermis obtained after 28 days of culture. Cultures were fixed in 10% formalin and processed for embedding in paraffin. Vertical sections were stained with haemalum-phloxine-saffron. (SB: stratum basale; SS: stratum spinosum; SG: stratum granulosum; SC: stratum corneum.) Note the perpendicular orientation of the basal cells and the numerous keratohyalin granules (arrows). Bar represents 50 µm

Sections were stained with antibodies specific for basement membrane components and with antibodies specific for the various stages of epidermal differentiation (Lenoir *et al.*, submitted). Results showed that (i) a basement membrane was present at the dermal–epidermal junction, and (ii) interfollicular keratinocyte terminal differentiation took place in this system, in a

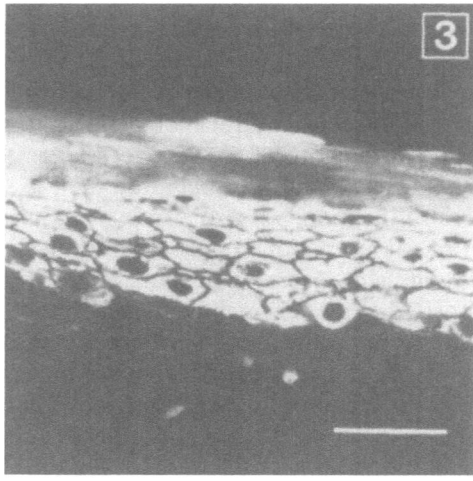

Figure 3 Immunofluorescence localization of the 67 kDa keratin in a vertical frozen section (5 μm) of the reconstructed epidermis

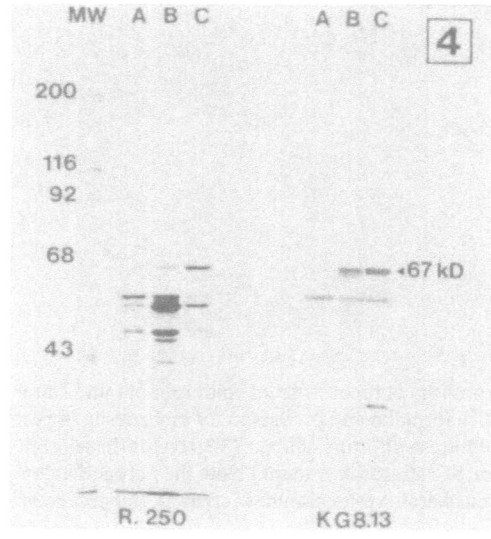

Figure 4 Identification of the 67 kDa keratin (67 kDa), in cellular extracts of hair follicle (A), reconstructed epidermis (B), and normal human epidermis (C). Proteins were separated by polyacrylamide gel electrophoresis, stained by Coomassie blue staining (R250), and identified by immunoblotting with KG8.13 monoclonal antibody. Note the similarity of the results obtained with the *in vitro* reconstructed epidermis and normal human epidermis protein extracts. MW: molecular weight markers

way very similar to that observed in normal skin. This was confirmed by electron microscopy.

Specifically, the 67 kDa keratin was quantitatively expressed in the reconstructed epidermis and had a characteristic suprabasal location as in normal skin (Figure 3). To ascertain that the keratin detected by immunofluorescence was indeed the 67 kDa keratin, and not a cross-reacting keratin, total cellular proteins of freshly plucked hair follicle, human epidermis and *in vitro*-reconstructed epidermis were prepared by urea extraction, analyzed and compared by polyacrylamide gel electrophoresis and immunoblotting. On gels, the basic 67 kDa keratin was indeed detected in the *in vitro* reconstructed epidermis (Figure 4b), as in normal epidermis (Figure 4c), *but not* in freshly isolated hair follicles (Figure 4a). This keratin polypeptide was further identified by immunoblotting with KG8.13 monoclonal antibody.

The advantages of using human hair follicles as a source of keratinocytes have been recently reviewed elsewhere[11]. Drawbacks, however, were low yield and low reproducibility. Since our main goal was to study whether outer root sheath cells were able to acquire *in vitro* an interfollicular epidermal phenotype, as happens during split-skin wound healing, a prerequisite was to improve the culture system. By implanting hair follicle explants, in an upright position, into a freshly cast dermal equivalent, we tried to mimic the natural

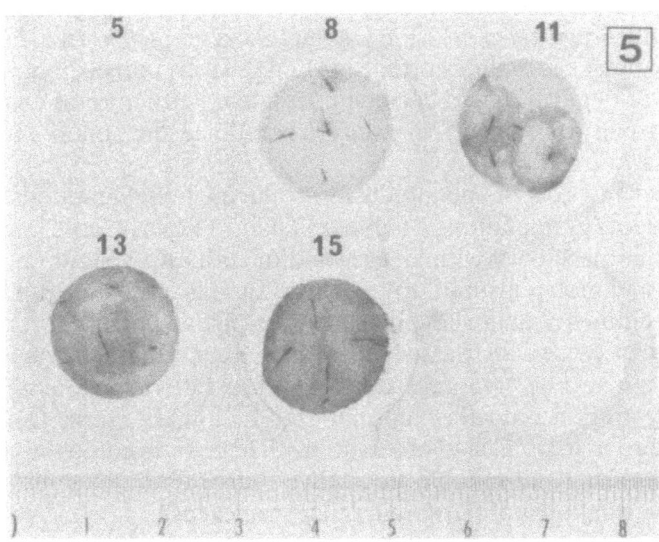

Figure 5 Kinetics of outgrowth of epidermal sheet after hair follicles were implanted into a dermal equivalent. Hair follicles were cultured for indicated periods (in days), then, cultures were fixed in 10% formalin and stained with Nile Blue sulfate (Sigma) at a final concentration of 1/10,000 in PBS. After 30 min incubation at 37 °C, the cultures were rinsed for 2 x 15 min in PBS before being photographed

topography and environment of the hair follicle. Moreover, the beneficial effect on keratinocyte differentiation of air-exposure of the dermal equivalent system had been recently documented[12–14]. The results of our study show that abundant cultures can be readily obtained with this new tissue culture system. Indeed, 1 cm^2 can be covered by epithelial outgrowth from only one hair follicle within 10–12 days, whichever the donor was (Figure 5).

During this epithelialization process, cultured outer root sheath cells clearly undergo a phenotypical shift towards an interfollicular keratinocyte phenotype.

In this respect, it has recently been shown by light and electron microscopy[15], by immunofluorescence with specific monoclonal antibodies[16], and by one- and two-dimensional gel electrophoresis[6] that the outer root sheath cells of anagen hair follicle display a specific keratin set different from that of epidermis. Particularly, the 67 kDa is not represented in this set. Actually, these cells follow a specific differentiation pathway, resulting in the keratinization of innermost cells and trichilemmal keratinization[16]. On the contrary, in our tissue culture system, morphological criteria and differentiation markers such as the 67 kDa keratin, involucrin, membrane-bound transglutaminase and filaggrin (Lenoir et al., submitted) demonstrated that the cells have acquired an interfollicular epidermal phenotype rather than a hair follicle one. Since the outer root sheath cells do not follow in situ the same differentiation pathway as interfollicular keratinocytes, we have to assume that the epidermal phenotypical expression is somehow repressed in vivo, maybe because of the presence of the keratinized Henle's layer. Indeed, it is only when Henle's layer degenerates to become a less dense structure in anagen hair follicle that outer root sheath cells start to keratinize and undergo trichilemmal keratinization[16].

In other respects the possibility of producing large quantities of living skin equivalents by implanting a number of hair follicles in large lattices provides the pharmacologist with an easy and quantitative system for studying the effects and metabolism of drugs. This system is easy to set up and very flexible. Preliminary data show that biopsies of this in vitro reconstructed epidermis can be serially passed in freshly cast dermal equivalents. This epidermis can also be cryopreserved without loss of viability and has been successfully grafted onto the nude mouse (Lenoir, Bernard, Démarchez, Darmon, Shroot, unpublished observation). This system could thus also represent a promising and suitable alternative source for autologous keratinocytes for the treatment of burns and other surgical use.

REFERENCES

1.	Vermorken, AJM, Verhagen H, Vermeesch-Markslag AMG, Wirtz P, Bernard BA, Asselineau D, Lenoir MC, Kimenai PM, Shroot B. Differentiation of keratinocytes in vitro; a new culture vessel mimicking the in vivo situation. Mol Biol Rep, 10, 205–213, 1985

2. Vermorken AJM, Goos CMAA, Hukkelhoven MWAC, de Bruyn CHMM. Human hair follicles in metabolic studies. In *Models in Dermatology* (Maibach H, Lowe N eds), vol 2, pp. 198–208, Basel: Karger, 1985

3. Weterings PJJM, Vermorken AJM, Bloemendal H. A method for culturing human hair follicle cells. *Br J Dermatol*, **104**, 1–5, 1981

4. Wells, J. A simple technique for establishing cultures of epithelial cells. *Br J Dermatol*, **107**, 481–482, 1982

5. Limat A, Noser FK. Serial cultivation of single keratinocytes from the outer root sheath of human scalp hair follicles. *J Invest Dermatol*, **87**, 485–488, 1986

6. Stark H, Limat A, Breitkreutz D, Fusenig NE. Keratin patterns expressed by human hair follicle cells *in vivo* persist *in vitro*. *J Invest Dermatol*, **87**, 169a, 1986

7. Weterings PJJM, Vermorken AJM, Bloemendal H. Protein biosynthesis in cultured human hair follicle cells. *Mol Biol Rep*, **6**, 153–158, 1980

8. Weterings PJJM, Verhagen H, Wirtz P, Vermorken AJM. Differentiation of human scalp hair follicle keratinocytes in culture. *Virch Arch (Cell Pathol)*, **45**, 255–266, 1984

9. Bell E, Ivarsson B, Merrill C. Production of a tissue-like structure by contraction of collagen lattices by human fibroblasts of different proliferative potential *in vitro*. *Proc Natl Acad Sci USA*, **76**, 1274–1278, 1979

10. Bell E, Ehrlich HP, Buttle DJ, Nakatsuji T. Living tissue formed *in vitro* and accepted as skin-equivalent tissue of full thickness. *Science*, **211**, 1052–1054, 1981

11. Vermorken AJM. Culture techniques and potential research-applications of human hair follicle cells *in vitro*. *Alt Laborat Anim*, **13**, 8–37, 1985

12. Asselineau D, Bernard BA, Bailly C, Darmon M. Epidermal morphogenesis and induction of the 67 kDa keratin polypeptide by culture of human keratinocytes at the liquid–air interface. *Exp Cell Res*, **159**, 536-539, 1985

13. Asselineau D, Bernard BA, Bailly C, Darmon M, Pruniéras M. Human epidermis reconstructed by culture: is it normal? *J Invest Dermatol*, **86**, 181–185, 1986

14. Coulomb B, Saiag P, Bell E, Breitburd F, Lebreton C, Heslon M, Dubertret L. A new method for studying epidermalization in vitro. *Br J Dermatol*, **114**, 91–101, 1986

15. Ito M. The innermost cell layer of the outer root sheath in anagen hair follicle: light and electron microscopy study. *Arch Dermatol Res*, **279**, 112–119, 1986

16 Ito M, Tazawa T, Shimizu N, Ito K, Katsummi K, Sato Y, Hashimoto K. Cell differentiation in human anagen hair and hair follicles studies with anti-hair keratin monoclonal antibodies. *J Invest Dermatol*, **86**, 563–569, 1986

9

Non-keratinocyte cells in hair follicles (with special emphasis to human hair follicles)

J-P Ortonne

Department of Dermatology, Hôpital Pasteur, BP No. 9
06002 Nice Cedex, France

ABSTRACT

The three dendritic cell populations present in epidermis, i.e. Langerhans cell, Merkel cell and melanocytes, also occur in hair follicles. Langerhans cells have been demonstrated by both indirect immunofluorescence and electron microscopy in the upper part of the outer root sheath of hair follicles. Their presence in the hair matrix is still a matter of discussion. Very little is known on the biology of follicular Langerhans cells. Merkel cells may be associated with various types of hair including vellus hair, sinus hair, vibrissae or whiskers. They form organized intraepithelial associations with axon terminals. This is also the case of the tactile hair disk, which is usually, but not constantly, in relation to the hair follicles.

Hair follicle melanocytes synthesize the melanin pigments responsible for the hair color. This follicular compartment of melanocytes is anatomically, and at least to some extent, physiologically distinct from the epidermal one.

INTRODUCTION

The three dendritic cell populations present in epidermis, i.e. Langerhans cell (LC), Merkel cell (MC) and melanocytes (M) also occur in hair follicles. There is a striking contrast between our knowledge on follicular M and hair follicle-associated MC whereas, very few data are available on follicular LC. Although some works describe the distribution of LC in hair follicles, very little is known of their biological functions in this particular site, and it is impossible to draw a precise comparison between epidermal and follicular LC. More is known about follicular MC. Hairs in the skin of man and mammals function as organs of touch, although this does not represent their exclusive function. It is clear that MC play an important role in these biological processes and are involved in the sensory innervation of several types of hair follicles.

Follicular M produce melanin pigments which are responsible for hair color. These M are anatomically, and to some extent physiologically, different from epidermal M.

LANGERHANS CELLS

Several studies have been carried out on the distribution of Langerhans cells in the normal pilosebaceous system.

By light microscopy, gold chloride[1,2] or ATPase +[3-6] dendritic cells have been demonstrated in the pilary canal, the outer root sheath of the hair follicle between the infundibulum and the hair bulge, and the various parts of the sebaceous gland. The first ultrastructural proof of the presence of Langerhans cells with characteristic Birbeck granules in the outer root sheath of hair follicle was obtained by a study on guinea pig skin[7]. In an electron microscopic investigation of the normal human pilosebaceous system[8], LC were also observed in the outer root sheath of the hair follicle between the infundibulum and the hair bulge, but they could not be found in the other parts of the hair follicle. LC were also present in the excretory ducts of sebaceous glands[8]. The ultrastructural features of these cells were identical with those described in human epidermis. In these two ultrastructural studies[7,8], no LC were found below the bulge of the hair follicles either in man or in guinea pigs whereas another study reported the occurrence of a few LC in the hair matrix of healthy persons[9]. The reason for this discrepancy is unknown. These conflicting findings may be due to the fact that the number of LC in the hair bulbs of healthy persons is very low, or that these cells are not constantly present in this area[10].

More recent studies using the monoclonal antibody OKT 6[10.11], or NA 1/34[12] confirmed the results obtained by EM, and gave additional quantitative data. Schematically, OKT 6 positive cells were numerous in the infundibular part of the hair follicles, but their number decreased markedly at the level of the sebaceous gland, and no OKT 6 positive cells could be demonstrated below the point of attachment of the arrector pili muscle[10,11]. To summarize, there is a general agreement on the occurrence of LC in the upper part of the outer root sheath of hair follicles. Their presence in the hair matrix is still a matter of debate.

Very little is known on the biology of follicular LC. No functional study of this LC subpopulation has been specifically performed.

MERKEL CELLS

Merkel cells (MC) may be associated with various types of hair, including vellus hair, sinus hair, vibrissae or whiskers[13,14]. The structure of sinus hair follicle is complex, distinguished in particular by the presence of a large cavernous venous sinus and a conspicuous ring sinus and bulge. In the vibrissal or sinus hair or whisker of mammals, MC may be observed, nestled into the external root sheath. In addition, the tactile hair disk (THD), which contain many MC–neurites complexes is usually, but not constantly, in relation to the hair follicles.

MC AND VELLUS HAIR[14]

Vellus hairs are short, very fine, soft, silky, usually unpigmented and unmedullated. They are found on many seemingly hairless areas of the human body such as the forehead, eyelids, bald scalp and most areas erroneously referred to as glabrous[15].

In these types of hair, MC are located in the collar-like protrusions of the hair follicles below the opening of the sebaceous gland. In the vellus hair in man and monkeys, these MC are always associated with nerve endings.

In addition to these intraepithelial MC, there are other MC associated with palisade-like nerve endings below the sebaceous gland, in the connective tissue portion of the hair follicle. MC associated with nerve endings are also present in the nerve fascicle close to the vellus hair, or in the connective tissue portion of the vellus hair follicle.

MC AND SINUS HAIR, VIBRISSAE OR WHISKERS

The vibrissae or sensory hair of mammals possess intraepithelial MC–nerve complexes. They are produced from special follicles containing erectile tissue. There are no strictly comparable follicles in man. There are large groups of MC in the epithelial swelling of the hair follicle[16]. This is well demonstrated by electron microscopic investigations which reveal several hundred MC in sinus hair follicles[17–19]. These cells are located in the basal cell layer of the upper region of the external root sheath and are arranged in a close-meshed cuff[17–19]. In this region, in contrast to regions of epidermis, the MC appear flattened and elongated and are frequently observed to abut the basal lamina[20]. In this location, they have a lobulated pale nucleus, and contain typical MC granules. Intermediate filaments and mitochondria are found in their cytoplasm. MC are attached to adjacent outer root sheath cells by occasional desmosomes. Finger-like cytoplasmic projections of the MC in the hair sheath may be observed[21]. The MC–nerve complex in the upper portion of the sensory hair has been studied in detail. The nerve is intimately apposed to the MC and develops an ending with many mitochondria, neurofilaments, myelin figures and lipid[19,21]. The MC are totally surrounded by epithelial cells or neural processes.

MC are also present in the upper region between the blood sinus and the epidermis[16]. In this area the follicular epithelium forms ridges which run parallel to the axis of the hair. The basal layer of the epithelium ridges contain many MC which are structurally identical to epidermal MC.

Using the fluorescent dye quinacrine to label MC, it has been possible to visualize two separate clusters of quinacrine fluorescent cells around sinus hairs[20]. The first cluster consists of a collar of many MC which completely surrounds the sinus hair shaft as it traverses the epidermis. In the rat whisker pad these clusters consist of up to 200 or more MC[20]. There is a marked polarization of the MC, as might be expected of a directional sensor. Based on light microscopy observations, it may be suggested that MC outline the surface of an obliquely cut conical section[20]. In rat vibrissae the second cluster consists of a cylindrical cuff of MC in the upper region of the external root sheath. The MC are arranged periodically in slightly staggered array. The fluorescent band is bounded by about 25–36 MC along the longitudinal margins and about 10–18 MC along the upper transverse margin[20]. Similar observations have been performed on rabbit vibrissae using monoclonal antibodies to anticytokeratin 8 as MC marker (personal observation).

The pattern described above corresponds to the distribution of MC around sinus hairs as described by previous electron microscopic studies.

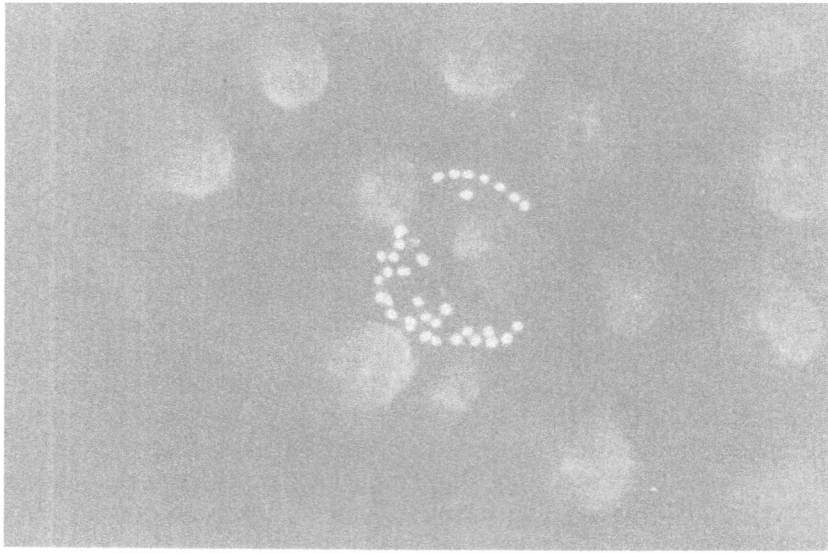

Figure 1 Rabbit split epidermis. Ring-cluster of Merkel cell surrounding an hair follicle in rabbit hairy skin. A monoclonal antibody reacting with cytokeratin 8 is used to detect Merkel cell

THE TACTILE HAIR DISK (THD)

THD is a specialized disk of epidermis found in the hairy skin of mammals[22]. Although in some species this structure is not always associated with a hair (e.g. the cat)[23], in others there is a direct association between these two structures. In many mammals, the tylotrich hair follicle (TDF) is caudal to the

78

hair[24] but in man its position is not constant[25]. This justifies the description of THD in this chapter.

THD is an epithelial thickening containing many MC–neurite complexes[26]. TDF are structurally similar in different species. In many mammals they are associated with tylotrichs or specialized hair. This association is fairly constant in the rat, mouse, and guinea pig, whereas in cat and man there is little or no relationship between TDF and hairs[27]. (Every fourth or fifth hair on the human trunk is associated with a THD[25]).

There are slight variations in the gross appearance and size of THD among species. In the cat, rat and some other species, THD can easily be seen with the naked eye, especially after depilation[27]. In the hairy skin of adult rats, THD are 100–300 μm in diameter and 3–5 mm apart[28] and are elevated approximately 40 μm above the surrounding skin[29]. In man, TDF vary widely in prominence from subject to subject[30] and are frequently difficult or impossible to identify with the dissecting microscope[27].

The external surface of TDF may have a slightly rounded eminence with interruption of the normal skin markings at this level. Under the dissecting microscope, THD has a different pigmentation from surrounding skin. There is a cluster of blood vessels within it, which can be easily recognized after clearing the stratum corneum with a drop of oil. The density of distribution of THD is of 1–2/sq cm in human skin[31], and they occur at intervals of about 1 to 2 mm in mice, 3 to 5 mm in rats and guinea pigs, 5 to 10 mm in rabbits and cats[27,28].

The microscopic anatomy of THD is quite similar in all species examined[23,26,27,29,31,32]. THD are characterized by an epidermal thickening. This is due to a pseudostratified columnar layer of cells filled with fibrils, all oriented perpendicularly to the skin surface. This additional layer is superficial to the epidermal basement membrane. There are many hemidesmosomes at the basement membrane zone, below columnar cells. Merkel cells are identified at the dermal–epidermal junction, often protruding into the upper dermis. These MC are interspersed at frequent intervals between the columnar epithelial cells and the basement membrane.

One disk may contain as many as 50 MC[23]. A nerve, losing its myelin sheath, enters into close contact with each MC. There is a synaptic specialization of the membranes between the neurite and MC, and occasionally MC granules have been seen to fuse with the specialized area of membranes[23].

The dermis below the disk is occupied by many large capillaries and myelinated nerve fibers. These nerve endings originate from a very large myelinated branching nerve fiber. By electron microscopy, MC of the THD are shown to be identical to MC in other sites.

Physiological studies have demonstrated that THD is a highly sensitive sensor to signal the central nervous system with a long stream of action potentials when pressure is applied in a certain direction to its associated hair[27]. The action potentials are sent as long as an animal remains in contact with an object. The exact role in signaling sensation in humans is undetermined[27].

79

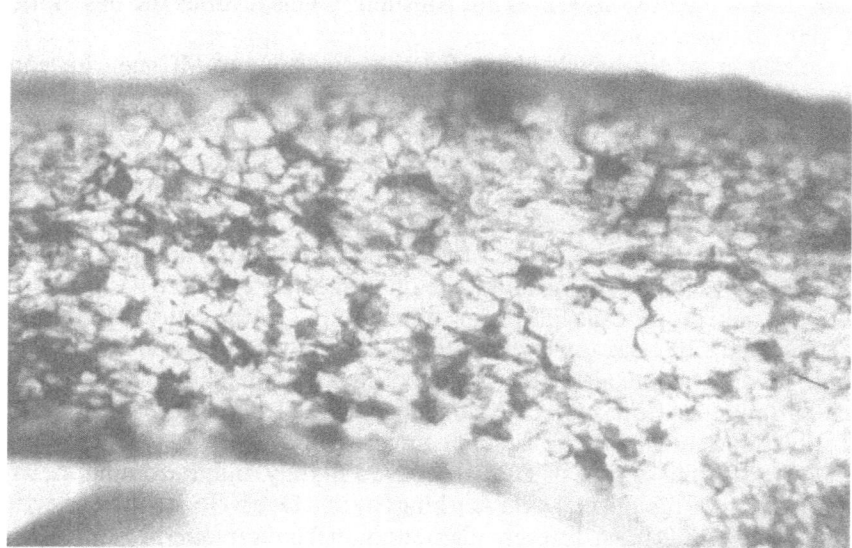

Figure 2 Dopa-positive melanocytes in the outer root sheath of a hair follicle during the healing of a pure epidermal wound induced by suction

The basic mechanism by which mechanical force is transduced into neural action potentials within THD is not yet clear. The specific function of the MC is still a matter of speculation. The recent immunohistochemical demonstration of neuropeptides and of neuron-specific enolase in MC may suggest a neuroendocrine function[33]. However, in the MC–axon complex there is no general agreement whether the MC or the axon ending represent the prime transducer element[33].

MELANOCYTES

In active hair follicles, melanocytes characteristically occur in the wall of the pilary canal (infundibulum) and in the pigmented part of the bulb, close to the upper part of the dermal papilla. Usually no active melanocytes are observed in other locations. However, dopa-positive melanocytes have been observed in outer root sheaths of hair follicles after irradiation with X-rays[34], after dermabrasion[35], after exposure to ultraviolet rays[36] and after oral photochemotherapy[37,38]. Amelanotic melanocytes (dopa-negative) have been observed along the outer root sheath of the middle and lower part of the follicle, between the basal portion of the tall epithelial cells which form the outer peripheral layer[35]. In connection with the distribution of these active and inactive melanocytes, Staricco[35] divided the hair follicle into four parts: portions A and D, i.e. melanotic portions, constitute, respectively, the upper part of the follicle (infundibulum) and the upper part of the bulb in contact with the upper papilla. Portion B comprises the middle and lower follicles and possesses amelanotic melanocytes. Portion C is the generally amelanotic outer root sheath of the bulb and the hair matrix below Montagna's critical level.

The melanocyte population of the skin can be considered as a bicompartmental system composed of an epidermal and a follicular compartment[39]. Several clinical situations may suggest that these two subpopulations of melanocytes have a relative independence. Indeed, senile white hair often occurs on a scalp epidermis with a normal melanin pigmentation. On the other hand, body hairs often keep their normal color in a fully depigmented lesion of vitiligo[40].

It is clear, however, that exchanges may occur between these two compartments, which are not closed systems. This has been demonstrated under certain circumstances in which one of the two melanocyte compartments is altered or destroyed. After dermabrasion (removal of the epidermis and the infundibulum follicle), amelanotic melanocytes divide in the middle portion of the hair follicle, become active (dopa-positive) and migrate upward from the outer root sheath to the infundibulum and later into the basal layer of the healing surrounding epidermis[34]. A similar process occurs during epidermal wound healing after pure epidermal destruction by suction (Ortonne et al., personal observations). Evidence for such exchanges have also been obtained from the study of repigmentation of vitiligo skin during oral photochemotherapy[37,38]. Elegant experiments performed in the white skin of trichrome guinea pigs suggest that melanocytes injected intradermally incorporate into the hair bulbs and migrate upwards into the outer root sheath[41]. It is not yet clear, however, if there are other melanocyte precursors distinct from the amelanotic melanocytes present in the outer root sheath of hair follicles. It has been suggested that a reservoir of melanocytes exists in hair follicles of C57 black mice, but its existence has not yet been demonstrated[42].

Less evidence exists to suggest migration of melanocytes from the epidermis into the hair follicles. In most cases, after destruction of hair melanocytes by various physical agents (X-ray, freezing, etc.), regenerated hair follicles remain depigmented, giving rise to white hair[43,44]. However, few experiments suggest that such exchanges exist.

In the guinea pig, an autograft of full-thickness black skin is left during 7 days in white skin. Then the graft is removed. This is followed by the appearance of pigmentation due to active melanocytes in the healing wound. Within a few months white hair grows as well as black hair[45]. This may be due either to the persistence in the wounds of pigmented hair bulbs from the graft, or to a migration of isolated melanocytes from the pigment grafts which colonize the regrowing white hair bulbs. In man, after induction of a pure dermal wound, removing the middle and lowest portion of hair follicles, regrowing hair is still pigmented. It is possible that the melanocytes present in this hair originate from the overlying epidermis[46]. Another experiment performed in trichrome guinea pigs suggests that epidermal and follicular melanocytes are interchangeable. After injection of epidermal cells from a pigmented zone of the skin into a superficial epidermal and follicular wound induced in a white patch of the same animal, a growth of pigmented hair occurs, suggesting that the grafted melanocytes have been incorporated into the healing hair follicles[47]. Similar results have been obtained in a more recent study[41]. Although elegant, these experiments do not give conclusive evidence for the occurrence of movement of melanocytes from the epidermis towards the hair bulb.

Hair bulb melanocytes differ from those in the epidermis only in some respects. They synthesize larger melanosomes than the epidermal melanocytes[48]. Follicular melanocytes are active only during a specific phase of hair production, namely anagen stages III through VI. Ultrastructural changes in melanocytes are related to the hair cycle, and in hair follicles of C57 black mice early anagen is associated with several modifications[42]: increase in volume of the cytoplasm, increase in dendritiness, development of the Golgi complex and rough endoplasmic reticulum, and finally increase in size and number of melanosomes.

During catagen and telogen, the melanocytes contain only a few small premelanosomes. They exhibit scanty cytoplasm with less well-developed Golgi complexes and rough endoplasmic reticulum and nuclei with prominent heterochromatin patterns. It has also been observed that the shape and internal structure of the melanosomes can change during the black hair cycle. The fate of bulb melanocytes after the hair growing phase has not yet been clarified. Radiation studies[49], and light microscopic histological studies[50] have shown that resting hair follicles have 'precursor melanocytes'. These cells have been suggested as the source of bulb melanocytes in the growing phase. Results of an ultrastructural study on mouse hair follicles in each stage of the hair cycle suggest that some bulb melanocytes may have survived to undergo dedifferentiation during catagen and telogen. Thereafter, they may undergo proliferation and differentiation, and repopulate the bulb during early anagen[42]. The pigmentation of hair follicles follows sequences of events identical to those seen in interfollicular epidermis.

Hair melanocytes transfer melanosomes to follicular epithelial cells. Medullary cells receive their melanin from melanocytes in the upper part of the hair bulb, in a manner similar to that described for the epidermis[51,52]. Melanosomes are also transferred to immature cortical cells[53].

Due to their larger size, melanosomes are usually distributed singly, whatever the ethnic background is. As the process of keratinization continues, melanin granules, along with other cytoplasmic remnants, become embedded in keratin. The cuticle cells contain few or no melanosomes. Usually, no melanin is seen in the cells of the inner root sheath. The distribution of melanosomes in the upper part of the outer root sheath resembles that in epidermis. In the lower part of the sheath the majority of cells contain only a small amount of melanin pigment.

The responses of epidermal and follicular melanocytes to exogenous or endogenous stimuli differ slightly. It has been demonstrated that the activity of follicular melanocytes is strongly modified by ovariectomy, estrogen administration or pregnancy. On the other hand, hormones have apparently little influence on the activity of epidermal melanocytes[52]. This is also the case for alpha-MSH. The reasons for these differences are unknown. Clinical examples also suggest that follicular melanocytes are more sensitive to nutritional influences[54].

Due to their anatomical localization, follicular melanocytes are less exposed to environmental factors than are epidermal melanocytes. This is the case for UV radiations. Although PUVA is known to affect hair growth and hair pigmentation, it is likely that, in normal conditions, UV rays have very little effect on the determinism of constitutive hair pigmentation.

The activity of melanocytes is under genetic control. Genes act within melanocyte or outside the pigment cells through their environment. Follicular melanocytes have a quite different environment from that of epidermal melanocytes, and thus are exposed to quite different regulating factors. Some genes apparently express their effect more strongly in follicular melanocytes. This is the case for allelic series affecting pheomelanogenesis. Their mode of action is not yet fully understood.

Hair pigmentation is determined by the quality and quantity of the melanosomes transferred from melanocytes to cells of the cortex of hair follicles. It is regulated by various factors including the number of melanocytes, the rate of synthesis of melanosomes, the degree and type of melanization within melanosomes as well as the mode of their transfer to, and their degradation within, keratinocytes[55].

According to the classic view, eumelanins which are insoluble in acid and alkali and contain nitrogen but no sulfur, give the dark brown to black colors, whereas pheomelanins, which are soluble in alkali and possess both nitrogen and sulfur, give yellow to reddish-brown colors. Recent advances in the biochemistry of melanins and the ultrastructure of melanosomes, together with the development of new techniques to characterize better the biochemical structure of melanins present in melanogenic tissues, including hair[56], suggest that the biological situation is more complex. Indeed, it is likely that most natural melanins are copolymers (mixed type melanins) of eumelanins and pheomelanins.

Elegant methods allow the measurement of tyrosinase activity, the key enzyme involved in melanin synthesis, in human hair bulbs. In addition, it is possible to analyze quantitatively the content and the class of melanin pigments in human hair without isolation of melanins from these tissues. This method is based on the determination by high-performance liquid chromatography of degradation products formed after permanganate oxidation of eumelanin and hydriodic acid hydrolysis of pheomelanin[56]. Several studies have tried to correlate hair color with the type of melanogenesis in follicular melanocytes evaluated by these biochemical techniques, and analyzed ultrastructurally to define the melanosome morphology[57,58]. They have led to rather surprising results.

It has been demonstrated that visual differentiation of hair color does not always reflect the melanogenesis type in human hair follicles, and does not correlate with the absolute contents of eumelanins and pheomelanins in tissues. Furthermore there is a lack of correlation between the dopa-oxidase and tyrosine hydroxylase activities of tyrosinase and hair color although high tyrosinase activity has been reported in red hair bulbs[59,60]. This suggests that other factors of the pigment pathway are also responsible for the control of hair color. However, chemical analysis of melanins, i.e. the ratio of eumelanins to pheomelanins, corresponds well to the fine structural differentiation of eumelanogenesis and pheomelanogenesis. Follicles specified as pheomelanic by chemical analysis (low ratio of eumelanin and pheomelanin) correspond to the following colors: fire red and light red. They contain spherical-granular melanosomes (pheomelanosomes). 'Eumelanin' follicles containing ellipsoidal-lamellar melanosomes (eumelanosomes) correspond to black and dark to light brown colors. However, follicles with 'mixed-type' melanogenesis contain both types of melanosomes and are associated with a wide variety of hair color including blonde, blonde-brown, medium light-brown, medium dark-brown, light red, dark-red and fire red.

Senile white hair shows a decreased number, or an absence, of functioning melanocytes. There is no detectable tyrosinase activity by chemical analysis. Furthermore, white hair bulbs do not contain immunoreactive tyrosinase antigen.

REFERENCES

1. Breathnach AS. The distribution of Langerhans' cells within the human hair follicles and some observations on its staining properties with gold chloride. *J Anat*, **97**, 73–80, 1963
2. Breathnach AS, Birbeck MS, Everall JD. Observations bearing on the relationship between Langerhans' cells and melanocytes. *Ann NY Acad Sci*, **100**, 223, 1963
3. Baker RW, McKee-Protopapas S, Habowsky JE. The Langerhans cell in hairless mouse epidermis. *Scan Electron Microsc*, **1**, 457–465, 1983
4. Khalil HM, Nitiuthai S, Allen JR. Alkaline phosphatase-positive Langerhans cells in the epidermis of Cattle. *J Invest Dermatol*, **79**, 47–51, 1982
5. Wolff K. Histologische Beobachtungen aus der normalen menschlichen Haut bei der Durchführung fermet-histochemischer Untersuchungen mit Adenosintriphosphat. *Arch Klin Exp Derm*, **216**, 1, 1963
6. Wolff K, Winkelmann RK. Non-pigmentary enzymes of the melanocyte-Langerhans' cell system, *Advances in Biology of Skin*. Vol. 8, pp. 135–167. Oxford: Pergamon Press, 1967
7. Breathnach AS, Goodwin EP. Electron microscopy of non-keratinocytes in the basal layer of white epidermis of the recessively spotted guinea-pig. *J Anat*, **99**, 377, 1965
8. Jimbow K, Sato S, Kukita A. Langerhans cells of the normal human pilosebaceous system. *J Invest Dermatol*, **52**, 177–180, 1969
9. Sato S, Kukita A, Jimbow K. Electron microscopic studies of dendritic cells in the human grey and white hair matrix during anagen. *Pigment Cell*, **1**, 20–26, 1973

10. Wiesner-Menzel L, Happle R. Intrabulbar and peribulbar accumulation of dendritic OKT-6 Positive cells in alopecia areata. *Arch Dermatol Res*, **276**, 333–334, 1984

11. Kohchiyama A, Hatamochi A, Ueki H. Increased number of OKT-6 -positive dendritic cells in the hair follicles of patients with alopecia areata. *Dermatologica*, **171**, 327–331, 1985

12. Thomas JA, Biggerstaff M, Sloane JP, Easton DF. Immunological and histochemical analysis of regional variations of epidermal Langerhans cells in normal human skin. *Histochem J*, **16**, 507–519, 1984

13. Breathnach AS. The mammalian and avian Merkel cell. In *The Skin of Vertebrates*. (Spearman RIC, Riley PA, eds), Linnean Society Symposium Series, **9**, 283–291, 1979

14. Iggo A. Electrophysiology of cutaneous sensory receptors. In *The Skin of Vertebrates*. (Spearman RIC, Riley PA, eds), Linnean Society Symposium series, **9**, 255–270, 1979

15. Montagna W. General review of the anatomy, growth and development of hair in man. In *Biology and Disease of the Hair*. (Kobori T, Montagna W, eds) Tokyo: University of Tokyo Press, 1975

16. Halata Z. Sensory innervation of various hair follicles. In *The Skin of Vertebrates*. (Spearman RIC, Riley PA, eds), Linnean Society Symposium series, **9**, 303–307, 1979

17. Halata Z, Munger BL. Sensory nerve endings in Rhesus monkey sinus hairs. *J Comp Neurol*, **192**, 645–663, 1980

18. Hartschuh W, Weihe E. Fine structure analysis of the synaptic junction of Merkel cell–axon complexes. *J Invest Dermatol*, **75**, 159–165, 1980

19. Patrizi G, Munger BL. The ultrastructure and innervation of rat vibrissae. *J Comp Neurol*, **126**, 423–436, 1966

20. Nurse CA, Mearow KM, Holmes M, Visheau B, Diamond J. Merkel cell distribution in the epidermis as determined by quinacrine fluorescence. *Cell Tissue Res*, **228**, 511–524, 1983

21. Andres KH. Zur Feinstruktur des rezeptoren am sinushaaren. *Z Zellforsch*, 75, 339–365, 1966.

22. Pinkus F. Uber einen bisher unbekannten Nepenapparat am Haarsystem des Menschen. *Haarscheiben Dermatol*, **9**, 465–469, 1902

23. Iggo A, Muir AR. The structure and function of a slowly adapting touch corpuscle in hairy skin. *J Physiol (London)*, **200**, 763–796, 1969

24. Mann ST, Straile WE. Tylotrich (hair) follicle: association with a slowly adapting tactile receptor in the cat. *Science*, **147**, 1043–1045, 1965

25. Kawamura T, Nichiyama S, Ikeda S, Tajima K. The human Haarscheibe, its structure and function. *J Invest Dermatol*, **42**, 87–90, 1964

26. Winkelmann RK, Breathnach AS. The Merkel cell. *J Invest Dermatol*, 60, 2–15, 1973

27. Smith KR Jr The Haarscheibe. *J Invest Dermatol*, **69**, 68–74, 1977

28. Straile WE. Sensory hair follicles in mammalian skin: the tylotrich follicle. *Am J Anat*, **106**, 133–147, 1960.

29. English KB. Morphogenesis of Haarscheiben in rats. *J Invest Dermatol*, **69**, 58–67, 1977

30. Tamponi M. Nuovo contributo alla conoscenze del "disco del pelo" (Haarscheibe de Pinkus) con particolare riguardo alla sua iconografia macroscopia. *Arch Ital Dermatol Venereol Sessuol*, **15**, 378–394, 1939

31. Smith KR. The structure and function of the Haarscheibe. *J Comp Neurol*, **69**, 41–46, 1967

32. Nillson BY. Structure and function of the tactile hair receptors on the cat's foreleg. *Acta Physiol Scand*, 77, 396–416, 1969

33. Hartschuh W, Jweihe E, Reinecke M. The Merkel cell. In *The Biology of the Integument* Vol. 2: *Vertebrates*. Springer-Verlag, Berlin, 605–620, 1986

34. Montagna W, Chase HB. Histology and cytochemistry of human skin. X-irradiation of the scalp. *Am J Anat*, **99**, 425–446, 1956

35. Staricco RG. Amelanotic melanocytes in the outer sheath of the human hair follicle and their role in the repigmentation of regenerated epidermis. *Ann NY Acad Sci*, **100**, 239–255, 1963

36. Staricco RG, Miller-Millinska T. Activation of the amelanotic melanocyte in the outer root sheath of the hair follicle following ultraviolet exposure. *J Invest Dermatol*, **32**, 163–164, 1962

37. Ortonne JP, MacDonald DM, Micoud A, Thivolet J. PUVA induced repigmentation of vitiligo: histoenzymological (split dopa) and ultrastructural study. *Br J Dermatol*, **101**, 1–13, 1979

38. Ortonne JP, Schmitt D, Thivolet J. PUVA induced repigmentation of vitiligo. Scanning electron microscopy of hair follicles. *J Invest Dermatol*, **74**, 40–42, 1980

39. Ortonne JP, Benedetto JP. Mélanocytes épidermiques et mélanocytes folliculaires. *Ann Genet Sel Anim*, **13**, 17–26, 1981

40. Mosher DB, Fitzpatrick TB, Ortonne JP. Abnormalities of pigmentation. In *Dermatology in General Medicine*. (Fitzpatrick TB, Eisen AZ, Wolff K, Freedberg IM, Austen KF, eds), pp. 568–629. New York: McGraw-Hill, 1979

41. Surleve-Bazeille JE, Gauthier Y. Fate of non-tumorous melanocytes injected within the dermis. Annual experimental study. Pigment Cell Research (in press)

42. Sugyiama S, Kukita A. melanocyte reservoir in the hair follicles during the hair growth cycle: an electron microscopic study. In *Biology and Diseases of the Hair*. (Kobori T, Montagna T, eds), pp. 181–200. Baltimore: University Park Press, 1976

43. Chase HB, Rauch H. Greying of hair. II. Response of individual hairs in mice to variations in X-irradiation. *J Morphol*, **87**, 381–392, 1950

44. Taylor AC. Survival of rat skin and changes in hair pigmentation following freezing. *J Exp Zool*, **110**, 77–112, 1949

45. Voulot C. Mise en évidence d'une mélanisation des bulbes pileux au cours du phénomène d'extension pigmentaire. *CR Acad Sci Paris*, **262**, 2646–2649, 1966

46. Inaba M, Anthony J, McKinstry C. Histologic study of the regeneration of axillary hair after removal with subcutaneous tissue shaver. *J Invest Dermatol*, **72**, 224–231, 1979

47. Pepper FJ. Pigmentation in a white haired region of the hooded rat as a result of cell transplantation. *J Morphol*, **98**, 367–387, 1956

48. Toda K, Pathak MA, Parrish JA, Fitzpatrick TB. Alteration of racial differences in melanosome distribution in human epidermis after exposure to ultraviolet light. *Nature*, **236**, 143–145, 1972

49. Potten CS. The X-irradiation of melanocyte precursor cell in resting hair follicles. In *Pigmentation, Its Genesis and Biologic Control*. (Riley V, ed), pp. 433–440. New York Appleton Century Crofts, 1972

50. Silver AF, Chase HB, Potten CS. melanocyte precursor cell in the hair follicle germ during the dormant stage (telogen). *Experientia*, **25**, 299–301, 1968

51. Jimbow K, Quevedo WC Jr, Fitzpatrick TB, Szabo G. Some aspects of melanin biology 1950–1975. *J Invest Dermatol*, **67**, 72–89, 1976

52. Snell RS. Hormonal control of hair color. In *Pigmentation: its Genesis and Biologic Control*. (Riley V, ed), pp. 193–205. New York: Appleton Century Crofts, 1972

53. Kinebuchi S, Kobori T, Hori Y. Behavior of melanosomes in melanocytes and keratinocytes of Japanese skin and Black hair. In *Biology of Normal and Abnormal Melanocytes*. (Kawamura T, Fitzpatrick TB, Seiji M, eds), pp. 191–208. Tokyo: University of Tokyo Press, 1971

54. Ortonne JP, Mosher DB, Fitzpatrick TB. *Vitiligo and Other Hypomelanoses of Hair and Skin*. (Monograph). New York: Plenum Press, 1983

55. Ortonne JP, Thivolet J. Hair melanin and hair color. In *Hair Research, Status and Future Aspects*. (Orfanos C, Montagna G, Stüttgen G, eds), pp. 146–162. Berlin: Springer, 1981

56. Ito S, Jimbow K. Quantitative analysis of eumelanin and pheomelanin in hair and melanomas. *J Invest Dermatol*, **80**, 268–272, 1983
57. Jimbow K, Ishida O, Takahashi H, Ito S. Hair color and type of melanogenesis in human hair: characterization based on chemical analysis of eumelanin and pheomelanin and ultrastructural analysis of melanosome structure. In *Structure and Function of Melanin*. (Jimbow K, ed.), **1**, 26–36, 1984
58. Jimbow K, Ishida O, Ito S, Hori Y, Witkop CJ, King RA. Combined chemical and electron microscopic studies of pheomelanosomes in human red hair. *J Invest Dermatol*, **81**, 506–511, 1983
59. Lloyd T, Garry FL, Manders EK, Marks JG. The effect of age and hair colour on human hair bulb tyrosinase activity. *Br J Dermatol*, **116**, 485–489, 1987
60. Townsend D, Olds DP, King RA. Dopa-oxidase activity in human hairbulbs measured by high-performance liquid chromatography. *J Invest Dermatol*, **86**, 570–572, 1986

10
The human hair follicle: a target for androgens

C Sultan, K Bakkar and AJM Vermorken
Unité de Recherche sur la Biochimie des Stéroides, INSERM U 58 (Pr
B. Descomps),
Laboratoire de Biochimie Endocrinienne du Développement et de la
Reproduction, CHU Montpellier, France

ABSTRACT

The human hair follicle changes that are brought about by androgens are well known and the pilosebaceous units are generally the targets of androgens. However, the way in which androgens may act to influence hair follicles differentiation and function remains unclear.

Cultured human hair follicle keratinocytes in the Epicult™ dishes permitted investigation of androgen metabolism. Cultured keratinocytes showed that testosterone was mainly converted into androstenedione, although a slight amount of 5α-reduced metabolites (especially androsterone) was formed. This testosterone metabolism was comparable with that of freshly isolated hair follicles. Testosterone is converted into either dihydrotestosterone, which is a more potent androgen than testosterone itself, or androstenedione, less active than testosterone: the action of androgens on hair follicles appears to be controlled by the relative strength of these two metabolic reactions.

In order to study the relative importance of dihydrotestosterone in hair growth, we developed the hamster flank organ test, since it contains androgen-dependent hair follicles: we found a linear relationship between the percentage of dihydrotestosterone formed by the hamster flank organ and the number of hairs in the histological preparation. Testosterone metabolism is also affected by the availability of cofactors such as NAD and NADPH. Our recent studies in idiopathic hirsutism show that, not only 5α-reductase, but also another NADPH-dependent enzymatic transformation (3α-hydroxysteroid dehydrogenase) is increased in hair follicles hyperreactive to androgens. Hence, the activity of G6PD enzyme (which provides NADPH) could be important in determining the response of hair follicles to androgenic stimulus. The low 5α-reductase activity of the fully differentiated cultured keratinocytes compared to that of actively proliferating keratinocytes confirms this hypothesis.

INTRODUCTION

Human skin and its appendages, especially the pilo-sebaceous structures, are target organs for hormones. The growth, texture and pigmentation of hair is affected by different endocrine factors acting on the hair follicle[1]. The present review deals mainly with androgens, but estrogens are also known to have a slight stimulatory effect on pubic and axillary hair growth. This is shown by the growth of pubic hair following induction of puberty in hypogonadal patients using small doses of estradiol alone. The estradiol effect may be mediated by androgen receptor induction or by increases in IGF_I, which, along with other growth factors, probably acts in synergy with androgens in stimulating hair growth, as in the case of growth hormone. It has recently been suggested that IGF_I is produced by the hair follicle itself.

Androgen-induced changes in hair follicles are well known, but the mechanisms by which they occur are mostly still unclear. In this review we examine data from hair follicle studies that appear to have a particular bearing on the influence of androgens on hair follicle differentiation and function[2]. The character and extent of this influence differ according to the location of the hair follicle:

1. hair follicles in the distal portion of the limbs are not androgen-dependent;

2. those in the scalp are not androgen-dependent, but are sometimes inhibited by androgens;

3. pubic and axillary hair follicles are affected by low levels of androgens;

4. body hair and beard are affected by high levels of androgens.

HAIR GROWTH

Several factors influence the extent of hair growth:

1. the length of the anagen, which varies according to the location (3 months for the moustache, 3 years for the scalp);

2. the percentage of hair in the anagen (90% of scalp hair, 60% of beard hair);

3. the linear growth rate, which varies according to body location, e.g. 0.21 mm per day for thigh hair, 0.45 mm per day for pubic and scalp hair;

4. hair diameter, sexual hair being thicker (80 μm) than scalp hair (60 μm);

5. terminal hair growth density; e.g. the greater apparent density of sexual hair in men than in women is due to differences in the density of completely terminal hair rather than to differences in the density of the pilosebaceous units.

HORMONE INFLUENCES

Ebling[3] has stated that hormonal influences on the follicular cycle, which in terms of evolution are related to the adaptive function of molting, must be clearly distinguished from the specific role of androgens in inducing sexual and other adult hair, whose adaptive function is to delay sexual signals until puberty.

It should be noted that, apart from puberty, the control of hair growth by the endocrine system is indirect, insofar as it does not initiate hair follicle activity, but rather accelerates or delays the onset of cyclic events, whatever the intrinsic mechanisms may be.

ANDROGENS

Sexual hair development appears to be related to plasma androgens (testosterone) in a dose-dependent manner. However, the relationship involves more than just the levels of androgens, there are other androgen parameters which contribute to the stimulation of sexual hair: the free fraction of testosterone is sometimes more closely related to hair growth than is the total.

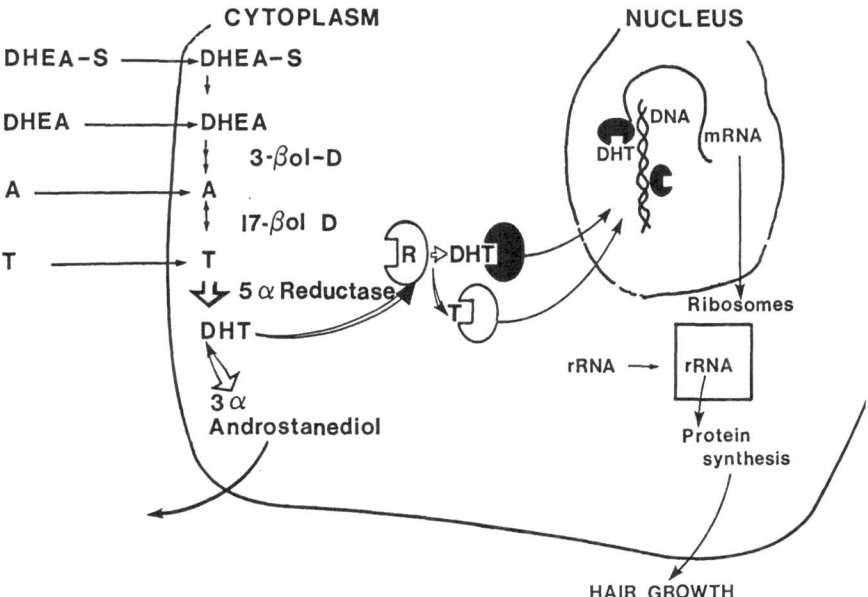

Figure 1 Metabolism and mechanism of action of androgens within hair follicles

Moreover, androgen metabolism is known to occur in hair follicles, whose capacity for this metabolism is greater than the level of available testosterone.

91

Testosterone (T) is reduced to dihydrotestosterone (DHT), via the enzyme 5α-reductase (Figure 1). Furthermore, androgen response by a given target organ requires the presence of a specific intracellular receptor, either residing in the nucleus, or transferred to it from the cytoplasm. If this receptor is lacking, the response of target cell is impaired[4].

Androgen metabolism and receptor binding of testosterone (T) or dihydrotestosterone (DHT) are thought to be the initial biochemical determinants of androgen action in hair follicles, but since most work has been done on plucked hair follicles[5–7] and cultured keratinocytes[8,9], it remains to be determined whether these cells are representative of the target cells upon which androgens act to cause hair growth.

Androgen metabolism in hair cells appears to be particularly directed toward inactivation of T to 17-ketosteroids rather than to DHT formation. However, the major determinant of androgen action in hair cells is DHT. *In vitro* data indicate that the relative intracellular potency of androgens in hair is 78% DHT, 21% T. As suggested by Hay[10], the regulation of intracellular DHT formation may be strongly affected by 17β-hydroxysteroid dehydrogenase, which converts T into Δ4-androstenedione. The T sensitivity of hair in different parts of the body could be regulated by differences in the relative amounts of 5α-reductase and 17β-hydroxysteroid dehydrogenase, which would determine the rate of intracellular DHT formation. These two pathways are thought to affect each other via changes in substrate availability and to regulate androgen activity correspondingly in hair follicles. Thus, the ratio 5α-reductase/17β-hydroxysteroid dehydrogenase appears to be a marker for epithelial differentiation into androgen target cells. Moreover, the availability of cofactors such as NAD and NADPH has an effect on T metabolism. We recently showed[11] that in idiopathic hirsutism, hair follicles that are hypersensitive to androgens show an increase not only in 5α-reductase but also in another NADPH-dependent enzyme, i.e 3β-hydroxysteroid dehydrogenase. Consequently, the androgen response of hair follicles could be affected by the activity of glucose-6-phosphate dehydrogenase, which provides NADPH. This hypothesis is supported by the low 5α-reductase activity in fully differentiated cultured keratinocytes compared to that in proliferating keratinocytes.

REGIONAL SPECIALIZATION OF HAIR FOLLICLE CELLS WITH RESPECT TO ANDROGEN METABOLISM

Facial and body hair

The most obvious examples of androgen-dependent hair are the male beard and moustache. Reduction of T by 5α-reductase appears to be necessary for the growth of facial hair. In the 5α-reductase deficiency syndrome, for instance, the beard is absent or sparse. Further support for the involvement of 5α-reductase is provided by the finding that in patients with celiac disease, characterized by high T levels and low DHT levels, the rate of beard growth is related to the plasma DHT concentration. Insofar as hair density appears to be correlated solely with T, the transformation of vellus follicles to produce beard hair may not be initiated by the same factors as those affecting subsequent growth.

Androgen receptor involvement is further supported by the fact that facial hair does not occur in the case of androgen insensitivity syndrome. i.e. testicular feminization, where no androgen receptors are found in target tissues. Moreover, the growth of thigh hair clearly involves androgen receptors, since the final length of the hair in hirsute women is significantly reduced by cyproterone acetate, which competes with DHT for the androgen receptor. The diameter, amount of pigmentation, and extent of medullation are also reduced.

Axillary and pubic hair

Axillary and pubic hair are clearly androgen-dependent. Pubic hair does not appear to require testicular androgens. In children with adrenal insufficiency, pubarche is effective. When the adrenal output is adequate, low androgen levels can stimulate the growth of pubic and axillary hair.

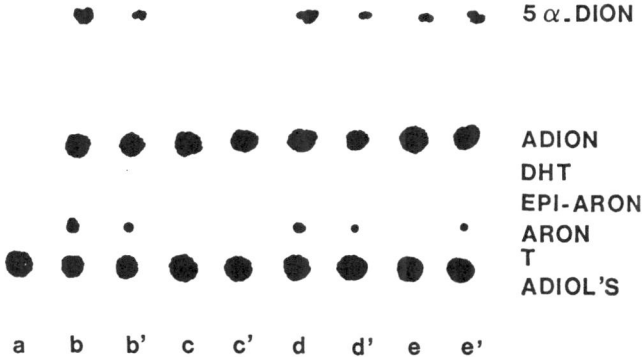

Figure 2 Autoradiograph of a chromatogram of the organosoluble metabolites of [³H]-testosterone. a: incubation without tissues (blank); b,b': incubation with human hair follicles; c, c': incubation with human hair follicles in the presence of progesterone (0.3 mmol/l); d,d': incubation with human hair follicles in the presence of cyproterone (0.3 mmol/l); e,e': incubation with human hair follicles in the presence of cyproterone acetate (0.3 mmol/l)

Scalp hair

Because it is not androgen-dependent, scalp hair differs from all other hair. However, androgens are paradoxically a prerequisite for the appearance of male-pattern baldness in subjects who are predisposed genetically.

Normal plucked scalp hair follicles have been examined for androgen metabolism. The follicles were incubated in a medium containing an NADPH-generating system and radioactive T. Using thin-layer chromatography and autoradiography, the metabolism was isolated and quantified. Figure 2 shows a typical autoradiograph.

Human scalp hair follicle cells have also been grown in culture. Epicult™ dishes[2] were used, which allow epithelial cells to be grown directly on a lens capsule. Most of the hair follicles placed on the capsule gave rise, within a week, to colonies of epithelial cells from the outer root sheath. The cells had stratified into several layers after 3 weeks, and were very similar to those of the freshly plucked follicles. About 10^7 keratinocytes were generated from a single hair follicle after trypsinizing and replating cells with 3T3 fibroblasts as feeders. Table 1 shows the androgen metabolism in cultured hair follicle keratinocytes compared with that of freshly isolated hair follicles (Table 2).

Table 1   Metabolism of testosterone-cultured hair follicle keratinocytes

amount (fmol ± SD) of the different metabolites per μg DNA	
5α-ADION	119 ± 51
ADION	561 ± 364
DHT	25 ± 14
epi-ARON	51 ± 13
ARON	473 ± 116
3α-ADIOL	43 ± 15
3β-ADIOL	6 ± 3
total amount of 5α-reduced metabolites	747 ± 186

Table 2   Metabolism of testosterone in freshly isolated hair follicles

amount (fmol ± SD) of the different metabolites per μg DNA	
5α-ADION	61 ± 12
ADION	324 ± 40
DHT	22 ± 10
epi-ARON	9 ± 4
ARON	29 ± 11
3α-ADIOL	9 ± 5
3β-ADIOL	0
total amount of 5α-reduced metabolites	138 ± 44

A MODEL FOR HAIR GROWTH STUDY: THE HAMSTER FLANK ORGAN

The flank organ is less developed on the female hamster than on the male. Its pigmentation is light, with only a few dark hairs. The size of the pigmented spot and the extent of hair regrowth were measured after local treatment with T or DHT. The pigmented spot reached its maximum size after 4 weeks of

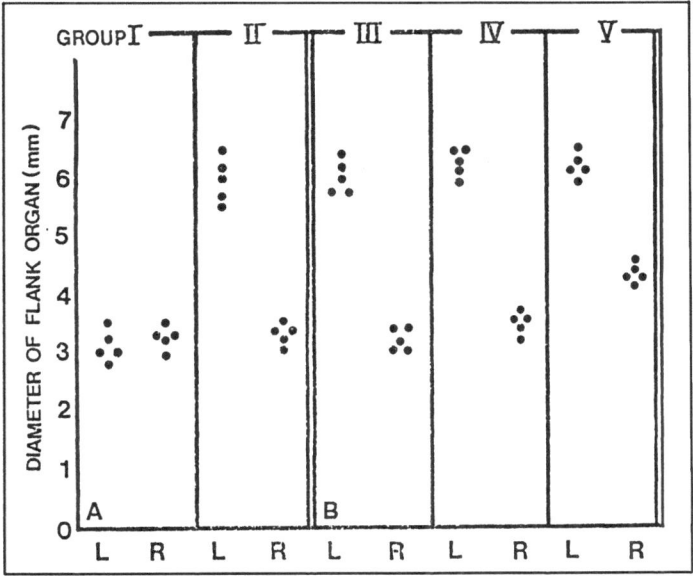

Figure 3 Visual assessment of the size of the pigmented spot of the left (L) and right (R, control) flank organs of female hamsters, after applications of different androgen mixtures

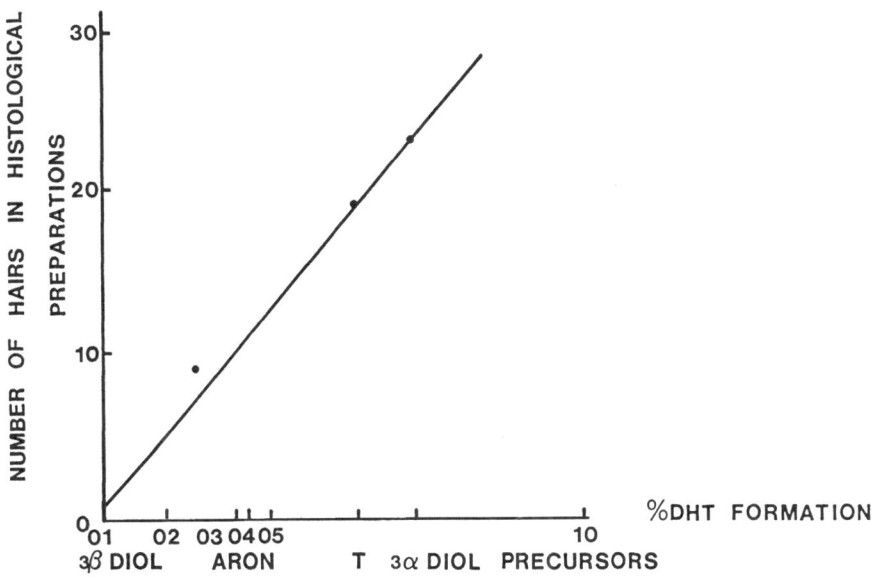

Figure 5 Relationship between the percentage of dihydrotestosterone formed from precursors and the numbers of hairs in the hamster flank organ

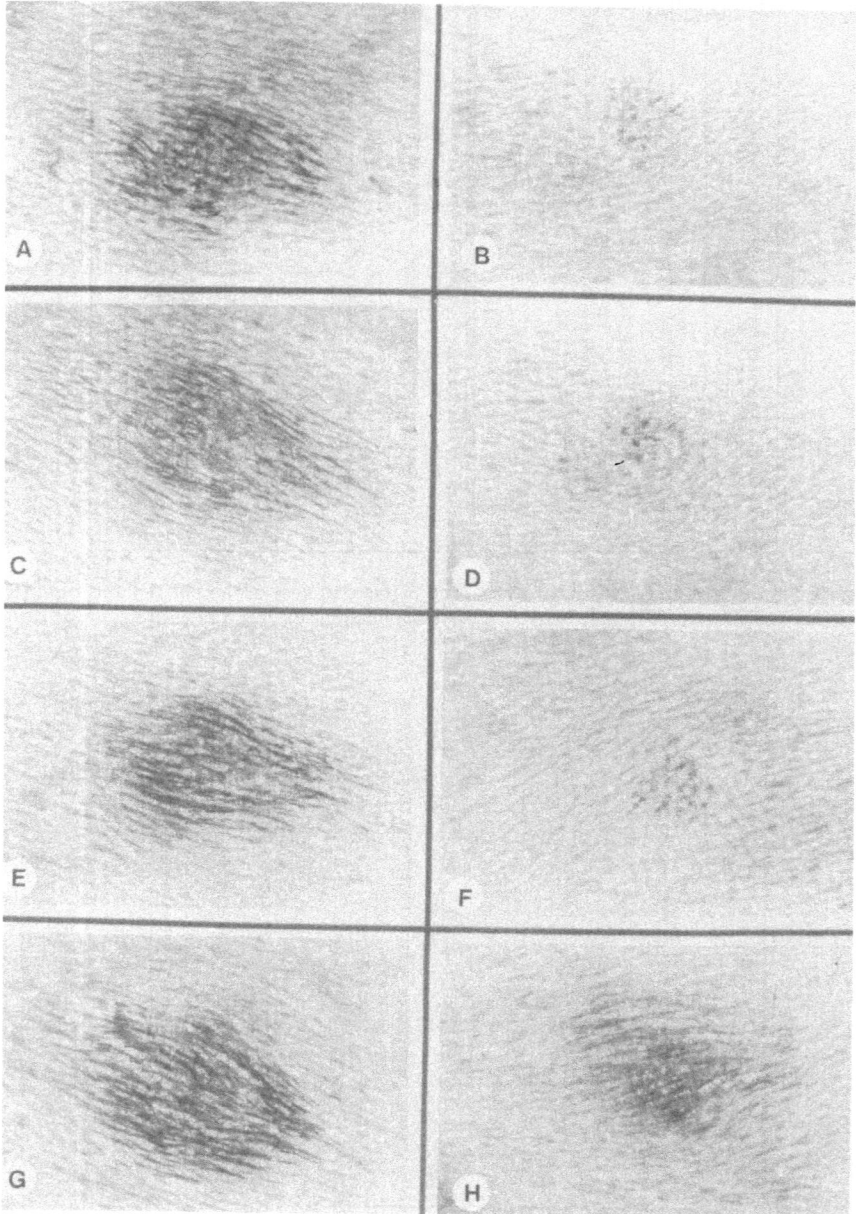

Figure 4 Magnification (x7) of a testosterone-stimulated female flank organ: its color is mainly produced by coarse dark hairs

treatment (Figure 3). The spot was photographed and an automatic image analyzer was used to quantify the formation of coarse dark hair. The spot was filled with more dark hairs after the application of DHT, corresponding to a concentration-dependent effect. DHT treatment induced the transformation of small light hairs into coarse dark hairs (Figure 4). In addition, there was a linear relationship between the percentage of DHT formed from precursors and the number of hairs in the histological preparations (Figure 5). Thus, the female hamster flank organ appears to be a useful model for quantifying androgen effects on hair growth.

CONCLUSION

Androgens induce the matrix cells of the pilosebaceous unit to produce terminal rather than vellus hairs. The length of time the terminal hairs remain in the anagen also appears to be increased by androgens. The larger mass of sexual hair in males than in females is caused by the added mass of terminal hair. As androgen levels increase, it would appear that an increasing proportion of pilosebaceous units are stimulated to develop terminal hair follicles, depending on the genetically determined sensitivity of the given area.

In view of the fact that androgen action requires the interaction of epithelial cells with mesenchymal cells[12], the presence of two-way reciprocal interaction between dermal and epithelial cells to promote hair growth suggests a system in which androgens may act at more than one site.

REFERENCES

1. Ebling FJG. Hair follicles and associated glands as androgen targets. *Clin Endocrinol Metab*, 15, 319–339, 1986
2. Vermorken AJM, Sultan Ch. The pilo-sebaceous unit: hormonal regulation in relation to cellular differentiation. *Dermatol Clin*, 1988 (in press)
3. Ebling FJG. The biology of hair. *Dermatol Clin*, 5, 467–481, 1987
4. Sultan Ch. Récepteurs hormonaux et peau. In *Biologie de la Peau*, (Thivolet J, Schmidt D, eds), pp. 111–126. Séminaire INSERM, vol. 148, 1987
5. Fazekas AG, Sandor T. Metabolism of androgen by isolated human hair follicles. *J Steroid Biochem*, 3, 485–492, 1972
6. Takayasu S, Adachi K. The conversion of testosterone to dihydrotestosterone by human hair follicles. *J Clin Endocrinol Metab*, 34, 1098–1101, 1972
7. Schweikert HU, Wilson JD. Regulation of human hair growth by steroid hormones. Testosterone metabolism in isolated hairs. *J Clin Endocrinol Metab*, 38, 811–819, 1974
8. Maudelonde T, Rosenfield RL, Schuler CF, Schwartz SA. Studies of androgen metabolism and action in cultured hair and skin cells. *J Steroid Biochem*, 24, 1053–1060, 1986
9. Vermorken AJM, Sultan Ch. The pilo-sebaceous unit in studies on hormone dependent differentiation in vivo and in vitro. *Current Probl Dermatol* 1988 (in press)
10. May JB, Hodgins MD. Distribution of androgen metabolizing enzymes in isolated tissue of human forehead and axillary skin. *J Endocrinol* 79, 29–36, 1978
11. Sultan Ch, Meynadier J, Jean R. Hirsutisme idiopathique de l'adolescente: étude physiopathologique in vitro. *Ann Pediat*, 34, 1–5, 1987

12.   Van Neste D, Sultan Ch, Descomps B. Exploration dynamique du follicule pileux, organe-cible des androgènes. *Nouv Dermatol*, **6**, 579–582, 1987

11

Effects of testosterone, dihydrotestosterone and estradiol on the growth behavior of cultured hair bulb papilla cells and root sheath fibroblasts

A Arai, K Katsuoka, F Kiesewetter, H Schell and
OP Hornstein
Department of Dermatology
University of Erlangen-Nürnberg
Federal Republic of Germany

ABSTRACT

Dermal papillae isolated from anagen hair bulbs of three healthy male subjects with normal hair pattern and fibroblasts derived from the mesenchymal root sheath of the same hair follicles were separately grown in culture. Both hair bulb papilla cells (PC) and root sheath fibroblasts (RSF) were subcultured in a medium containing two different doses of testosterone (30 and 300 ng/ml), dihydrotestosterone (30 or 300 ng/ml) or estradiol (1 and 10 ng/ml). The number of PC and RSF was counted every second day over two weeks. Growth rates of the PC and RSF were inhibited by doses of both testosterone and dihydrotestosterone. Especially the growth rates of PC were markedly lower than those of RSF at the higher doses. Estradiol was ineffective in both cell lines.

INTRODUCTION

Sex hormones are involved in both control of growth and cyclic activity of hair follicles. For example, in hirsutism excessive terminal hair growth is often due to increased androgen production or sensitivity of the hair follicles[1]. Hormonal responses are mediated via dermal papilla, which plays a fundamental role in induction, maintenance and regulation of hair growth[2,3]. The dermal hair papilla contains a peculiar population of fibroblast-like cells which are different in morphological and growth behaviour from fibroblasts of both papillary dermis and root sheath fibroblasts[4,5].

The 5-alpha-reductase activity/5-alpha-reduced-testosterone metabolites and estrogens have been suspected of being related to hair growth[6-8] and previously the 5-alpha-reductase and androgen receptors were demonstrated in dermal papilla cells as well as pubic skin fibroblasts[2,9,10]. Therefore it might be of great interest to study the effect of sex hormones on dermal papilla cells. The present study was designed to investigate the effect of testosterone, dihydrotestosterone and estradiol in physiological concentrations on the growth behavior of cultured human hair papilla cells compared to root sheath fibroblasts of identical hair follicles of the same male subjects.

MATERIAL AND METHOD

Isolation of dermal papilla cells (PC) and root sheath fibroblasts (RSF): scalp biopsy specimens (5 x 10 mm) were obtained from three healthy male volunteers aged 25 to 35 years, with informed consent. No male pattern alopecia or diseases of hair and scalp were noted. The specimens were immediately transferred into Dulbecco's modified Eagle medium (DMEM, Gibco, Karlsruhe, FRG). About 20 anagen hairs were meticulously dissected from adjacent connective tissue and transected above the base under a stereomicroscope (Zeiss, Wetzlar, FRG; magnification x 16). The portions thus obtained were immersed in Petri dishes containing DMEM, and the hair papillae were isolated according to Messenger's technique[5]. Simultaneously, fibroblasts were obtained from the anagen hair mesenchymal sheath of the same hair follicles.

Cell culture establishment and maintenance

Primary culture of both PC and RSF were set up as described previously[4]. After reaching confluency in primary cultures within approximately 5 weeks, both PC and RSF were subcultured using 0.25% trypsin and 0.02% EDTA solution (Gibco, Karlsruhe, FRG) to achieve single-cell suspensions. Petri dishes 35 mm in diameter were seeded with 3×10^4 cells for each dish. 588 dishes were prepared, 294 of each cell type, all in the third passage. Seven series of PC and RSF subcultures were achieved by seven kinds of medium (content see Table 1).

Table 1   Culture media tested

1.	2 ml DMEM[a] + 4% inactivated fetal calf serum (control medium: CM)
2.	CM + 30 ng/ml testosterone[b]
3.	CM + 300 ng/ml testosterone
4.	CM + 30 ng/ml dihydrotestosterone[c]
5.	CM + 300 ng/ml dihydrotestosterone
6.	CM + 1 ng/ml estradiol[d]
7.	CM + 10 ng/ml estradiol

[a] DMEM: Dulbecco's modified Eagle medium with penicillin (100 U/ml), streptomycin (100 ng/ml, L-glutamine (0.584 ng/ml) (all purchased from Gibco, Karlsruhe, FRG).
[b] Testosterone (Sigma Chemical, St Louis, USA)
[c] Dihydrotestosterone (Steraloids Inc., Wilton, USA)
[d] Estradiol (Sigma Chemical, St Louis, USA)

The medium was changed every third day and the growth behavior of PC and RSF was studied over a period of 14 days. The cell number was counted every second day using a hemocytometer.

RESULTS

Morphology

In subculture PC and RSF showed distinct morphological differences. PC were larger, flattened with cytoplasmic processes (Figure 1) whereas RSF were spindle-shaped with fewer but longer projections of the cell border (Figure 2). This difference in growth pattern was maintained for each dish throughout the duration of culture independent of testosterone, dihydrotestosterone or estradiol concentrations used.

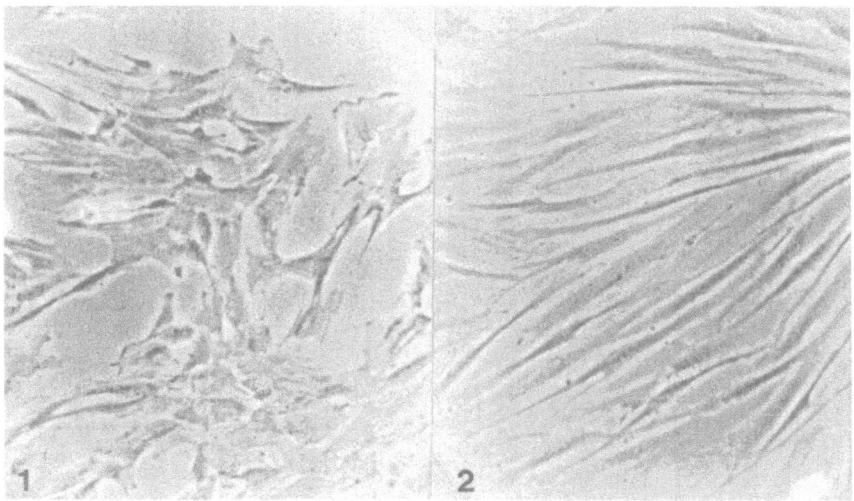

Figures 1 and 2   Morphology of papilla cells (**1**) and root sheath fibroblasts (**2**) in subculture after 8 days (third passage; phase contrast x 225)

Cell population growth

At the onset of the experiments there were approximately equal numbers of cells (3 x 10^4) from each source. Independently of culture media used the growth rates of PC were markedly slower than those of RSF. After 12 days in culture in control (Figures 3 and 4) the number of RSF was nearly double that of PC. Addition of testosterone and dihydrotestosterone inhibited the growth rate of PC as well as RSF. At the doses tested the inhibition of growth rate was found to be stronger in PC than in RSF, especially by the high concentrations of androgens tested. No distinct difference between the high con-

101

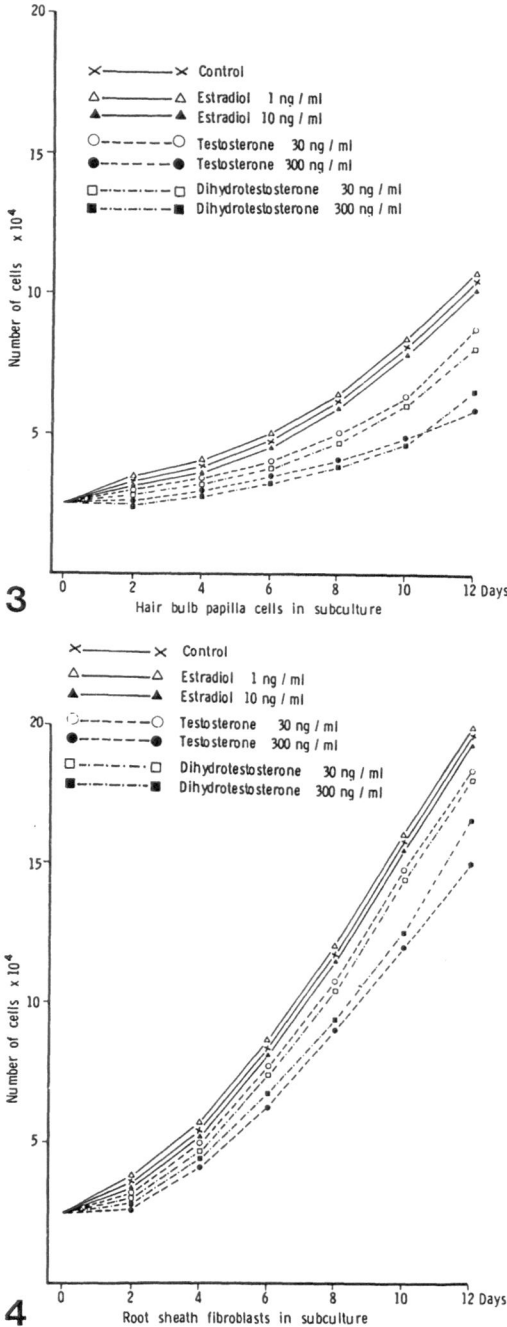

Figures 3 and 4 Growth curves of papilla cells (3) and root sheath fibroblasts (4) subcultured with different doses of testosterone, dihydrotestosterone and estradiol

centrations of testosterone or dihydrotestosterone on growth curves was noted. Compared to the cell number in control medium estradiol (Figures 3 and 4) was ineffective on both cell groups in both concentrations tested.

DISCUSSION

Previous studies demonstrated a distinct morphological difference of the dermal hair papilla cells (PC) compared to root sheath fibroblasts (RSF) when grown in culture[4, 11]. PC aggregated into clusters and therefore it was concluded that the aggregative behavior of cultured PC reflect the role of these cells in the hair cycle. This constringent behavior may prevent them from spreading into the surrounding mesenchymal tissue during telogen arrest of hair growth[4]. Neither testosterone, dihydrotestosterone nor estradiol inhibited this constringent behavior of the PC.

The growth rates of PC and RSF was influenced by testosterone and dihydrotestosterone, whereas the tested doses of estradiol were ineffective. The higher doses of testosterone and dihydrotestosterone especially inhibited the growth of PC and RSF *in vitro*, those of PC are remarkably reduced when compared to RSF. Additionally, the percentages of S-phase cells measured by DNA flow cytometry (see ref. 4) revealed values of PC and RSF when cultured with testosterone and dihydrotestosterone. We conclude that the slower growth rate of PC may reflect the physiological role of the PC in the development of androgenetic alopecia. These terminal hair follicles were transformed to vellus-like follicles, which in the latter stages become atrophic. The hair diameter, the hair density and the growth rate decrease[12]. The smaller hair diameter may be due to the growth inhibition of PC by androgens during early anagen stages of the hair follicles. Smaller dermal hair papillae consequently lead to reduced hair diameters, as previously demonstrated in a quantitative study of hair growth[13].

The cultivation of PC provides an interesting model to investigate the effects of hormonal and drug influence on dermal papilla cells which mediate the growth, cyclic activity, and induction of hair follicles[3].

REFERENCES

1. Kveolar JC, Gibson M, Krusinski PA. Hirsutism: evaluation and treatment. *Am Acad Dermatol*, **12**, 215–225, 1985
2. Eil C, Cutler GB, Loriaux DL. Androgen receptor characteristics in skin fibroblasts from hirsute women. *J Invest Dermatol*, **84**, 62–65, 1985
3. Messenger A. Isolement, culture et comportement in vitro des cellules proevenant de papilles de follcules pileux humains. *Nouv Dermatol* (Suppl. 1), 16–20, 1988
4. Katsuoka K, Schell H, Hornstein OP, Deinlein E, Wessel B. Comparative morphological and growth kinetics studies of human hair bulb papilla cells and root sheath fibroblasts in vitro. *Arch Dermatol Res*, **279**, 20–25, 1986
5. Messenger A. The culture of dermal papilla cells from human hair follicles. *Br J Dermatol*, **110**, 685–689, 1984
6. Bullough WS. Hormone and mitotic activity. *Vitam Horm*, **13**, 261–272, 1955

7. Kutenn F, Mowszowicz J, Schaison G, Mauvais-Jarvis P. Androgen production and skin metabolism in hirsutism. *J Endocrinal*, **75**, 83–91, 1977

8. Serafini P, Ablan F, Lobo RA. 5-reductase activity in the genital skin of hirsute women. *J Clin Endocrinal Metab*, **60**, 349–355, 1985

9. Maudelonde RL, Rosenfield CF, Schuler S, Schwartz A. Studies of androgen metabolism and action in cultured hair and skin cells. *J Steroid Biochem*, **24**, 1053–1060, 1986

10. Murad S, Hodgin M, Simpson N, Oliver R, Jahoda C. Androgen receptors and metabolism in cultured dermal papilla cells from human hair follicles. *Br J Dermatol*, **113**, 768, 1985

11. Katsuoka K, Schell H, Wessel B, Hornstein OP. Effects of epidermal growth factor, fibroblast growth factor, minoxidil, and hydrocortisone on growth kinetics in human hair bulb papilla cells and root sheath fibroblasts cultured in vitro. *Arch Dermatol Res*, **279**, 247–250, 1987

12. Runne U, Martin H. Veränderungen von Telogenrate, Haardichte, Haardurchmesser und Wachstumsgeschwindgkeit bei der androgenetischen Alopezie des Mannes. *Hautarzt*, **37**, 198–204, 1986

13. Ibrahim L, Wright E. A quantitative study of hair growth using mouse and rat vibrissal follicles. I. Dermal papilla volume determines hair volume. *J Embryol Exp Morphol*, **72**, 209–224, 1982

14. Oliver RF. The dermal papilla and the development and growth of hair. *J Soc Cosm Chem*, **22**, 741–754, 1971

12
Pharmacological aspects of hair follicle growth

H Uno
Wisconsin Regional Primate Research Center, University of
Wisconsin-Madison, Wisconsin, USA

ABSTRACT

The potent hypertrichotic effect of minoxidil opened a new field in both pharmacological study and clinical application of the drugs on hair growth. Topically applied minoxidil is effective for hair growth in the early stage of androgenetic alopecia and, to some extent, for the treatment of alopecia areata. Using the macaque model of androgenic alopecia, we studied sequential morphometric analysis (folliculogram) of the hair follicles after treatment with topical minoxidil as well as antiandrogen. Minoxidil also acts as a mitotic stimulator of the follicular cells in the secondary germ, follicular sheath, and bulbar matrix. Consequently, the vellus follicles in the bald scalp enlarge and transform to the terminal follicles. Minoxidil also induced a cyclic acceleration of rat hair follicles. The mechanism of this follicular growth will be discussed with the similar phenomenon caused by the activation of protein kinase C in the skin by phorbol ester. Topical applications of 4-MA (an inhibitor of 5α-reductase) on the bald scalp of macaques prevented the development of baldness during periadolescent age. Analysis of folliculograms revealed that the size and distribution pattern of cyclic follicles showed no change in 4-MA-treated scalps over 2 years, while the folliculograms of controls changed to a typical bald pattern. The drug also induced a substantial decrease of 5α-reductase activity in the scalp skin. These results strongly suggest that dihydrotestosterone is a potent androgen to trigger the regressive change in genetically linked hair follicles.

INTRODUCTION

Although androgens are the most potent hormones to stimulate hair growth, the hair follicles that respond to androgens are genetically determined and are distributed in particular body regions where they exhibit the dimorphotic patterns of secondary sexual hair growth. The hypertrichotic effect of minoxidil is more versatile than that of androgens, and the regressing vellus follicles in the bald scalp of androgenetic alopecia are also affected by minoxidil.

Nonetheless, the transformation of vellus to terminal follicles by these agents results in a thick growth of terminal hairs from fuzzy vellus hairs. However, androgens adversely affect scalp hair follicles in men having a trait for baldness. The postpubertal elevation of serum testosterone apparently triggers the development of baldness[1,2]. This is a result of a regressive diminution in size of the hair follicles from terminal to the vellus type. The mechanism of this dichotomous action of androgens on the hair follicles appears to involve different genetic expression of the follicular cells. Interestingly, antiandrogenic agents seem to block this phenomenon and show effects in both treatment of hirsutism and prevention of baldness[3-5].

During recent years, we have studied the sequential morphological changes of hair follicles in the bald scalp of stumptailed macaques (*Macaca arctoides*) after treatment with either topical minoxidil or antiandrogen.

Recently we have also studied the effect of topical minoxidil and phorbol ester on hair follicular growth in young rats. Our preliminary data suggest that an increased activity of protein kinase C being induced by topical application of phorbol ester (PMA) appears to involve stimulation of follicular germinal cell growth.

This paper will review the action of minoxidil and an antiandrogen (4-MA) on the cyclic dynamics and transformation of hair follicles in the scalp of stumptailed macaques, and will introduce preliminary data from studies on the activated protein kinase C and follicular growth in the rat.

HAIR FOLLICULAR GROWTH AND MINOXIDIL

The vellus follicles in bald stumptailed macaques

Histological study

Nearly 100% of postadolescent stumptailed macaques of both sexes develop frontal alopecia after 4 years of age. Hair follicles in the bald frontal scalp show regressed vellus follicles and the majority of them belong to the resting (telogen) phase. Naturally, hair follicles in the non-bald scalp of preadolescent animals are mainly terminal follicles and many of them are in the growing (anagen) phase[6].

Treatment with topical minoxidil (5% in a vehicle of propylene glycol, alcohol and water) on the bald scalp of adult stumptailed macaques induced a dramatic enlargement in size of the hair follicles after 3 months (Figure 1a and b). Morphometric analysis of the hair follicles (folliculogram) in biopsied skins between pre- and post-treatment stages showed remarkable differences. Minoxidil induced an acceleration of the cyclic growth of telogen follicles and simultaneously stimulated an enlargement in the size of early and mid (A3) and late (A5) anagen follicles (Figures 1c and d). These data obviously suggest that the major action of minoxidil is a stimulation of mitotic proliferation of the secondary germ in telogen follicles. It also suggests that cell proliferation occurs in the entire follicular structure resulting in an enlargement

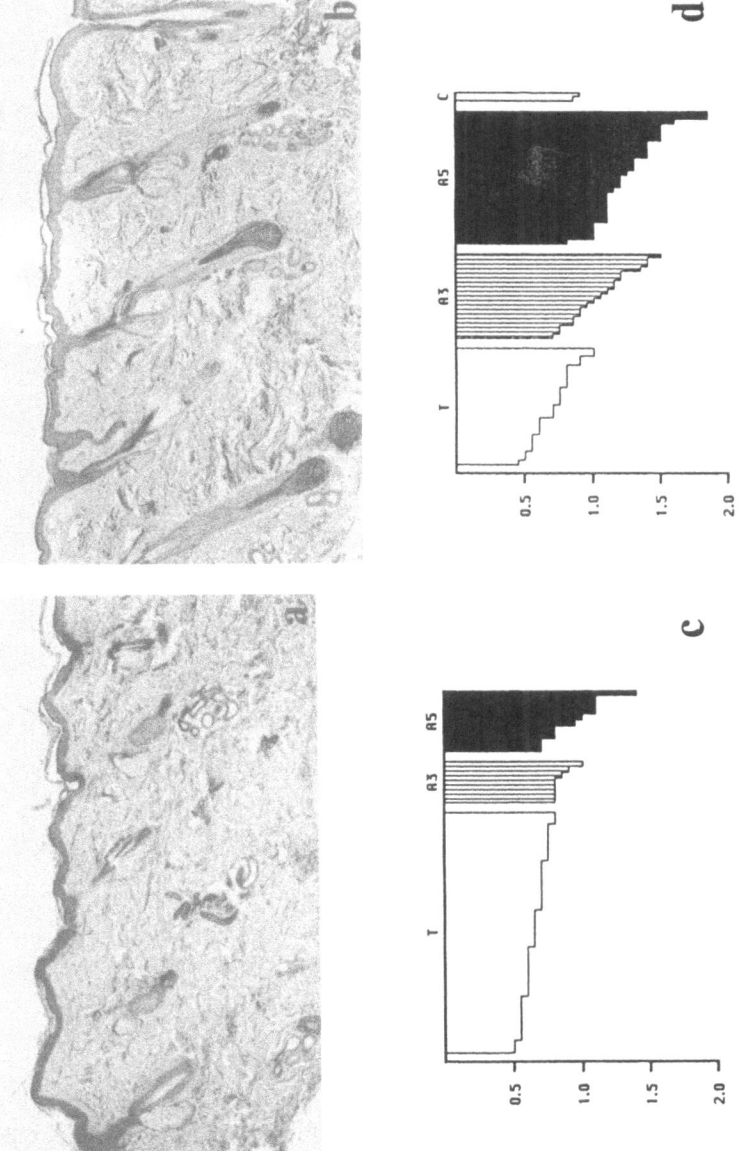

Figure 1 Microscopically, the bald scalp of pretreatment stage contains many vellus telogen follicles (**a**). Three months after treatment with minoxidil, markedly enlarged follicles show mostly growing anagen phase (**b**). The patterns of folliculograms show increased size and population of anagen follicles after treatment. Pretreatment (**c**). Three months after treatment (**d**). T: telogen, A3: early to mid-anagen, A5: late anagen (growing phase)

107

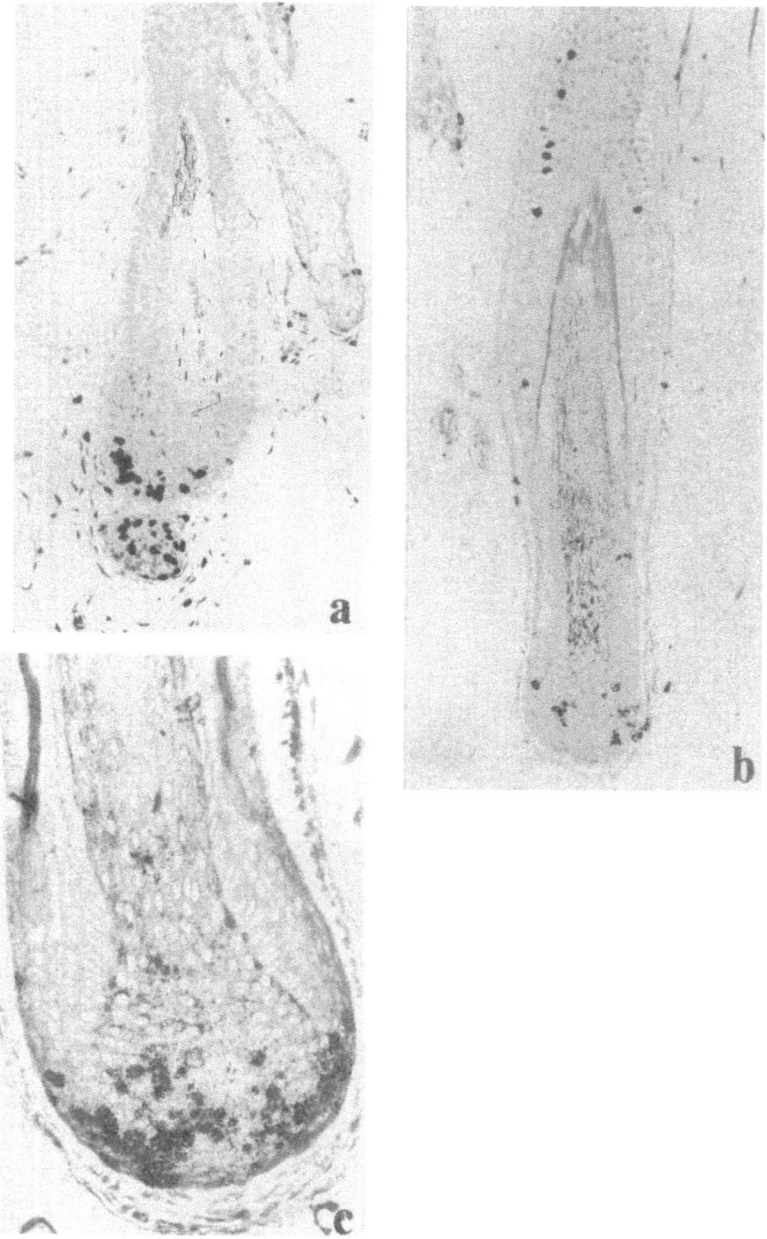

Figure 2 Autoradiographic pictures of [³H]thymidine showing many DNA synthesizing cells in the follicles and dermal papilla of early anagen follicles (**a**), in the outer root sheath (**b**) and bulbar matrix (**c**) of anagen follicles

of size in new anagen follicles. Subsequent treatment with minoxidil and analysis of the folliculogram revealed that new terminal anagen follicles appeared to have a much longer period of growth phase than that of the vellus anagen follicles; thus new hairs grow longer and thicker than the vellus hairs during the pretreatment stage. However, discontinuation of the treatment causes rather quick termination of the growth phase (about 1 month after withdrawal) and they turn into telogen follicles through catagenic involution[7].

DNA synthesis of follicular cells

In vitro uptake of [^{3}H]thymidine was examined in the scalp skin of both minoxidil- and vehicle-treated cases by means of autoradiography[7]. The hair follicles in the skin of minoxidil treated cases showed markedly increased numbers of DNA-synthesizing cells compared with those in vehicle-treated cases. This occurred in the follicles of all cyclic phases, telogen to early, mid, and late anagen phases (Figure 2). Surprisingly, DNA synthesizing cells were found in the entire follicular structure from the upper and lower follicular sheath and bulb portion including the perifollicular connective tissue cells. An increased number of such premitotic cells was seen most strikingly in the germinal cell group and dermal papilla cells in the early anagen follicles (Figure 2a) as well as the outer root sheath of the anagen follicles (Figure 2b). Thus the whole structure of the vellus follicle becomes enlarged through a cyclic remodeling process and transforms to a terminal follicle. Minoxidil not only induces hyperplastic enlargement of remodeling anagen follicles, but also stimulates continuous cell proliferation in the bulbar matrix of the anagen follicles (Figure 2c). Withdrawal of the treatment appears to halt the mitotic potential in the bulbar cells of the anagen follicles and thus terminates the anagen phase. The potential for cell proliferation is also present in the dermal mesenchymal cells, particularly in the perifollicular sheath (Figures 3a and b). An interaction of mesenchymal–epithelial cells appears to be indispensable to grow the secondary germ to complete a remodeling of the follicular structure, as well as leading to maintenance of both the structural and functional integrity of the anagen follicles. Although there is no doubt that minoxidil induces mitotic proliferation of the follicular cells, clarification of direct or indirect action on the hair follicle is still needed. Since minoxidil is a potent peripheral vasodilator, continuous topical application of minoxidil will probably cause a longstanding vasodilatory condition of the cutaneous microcirculatory beds. Indeed, another vasodilatory agent, diazoxide, is also known to have a hypertrichotic effect[8–10]. Additional research is necessary to elucidate such basic mechanisms for follicular growth.

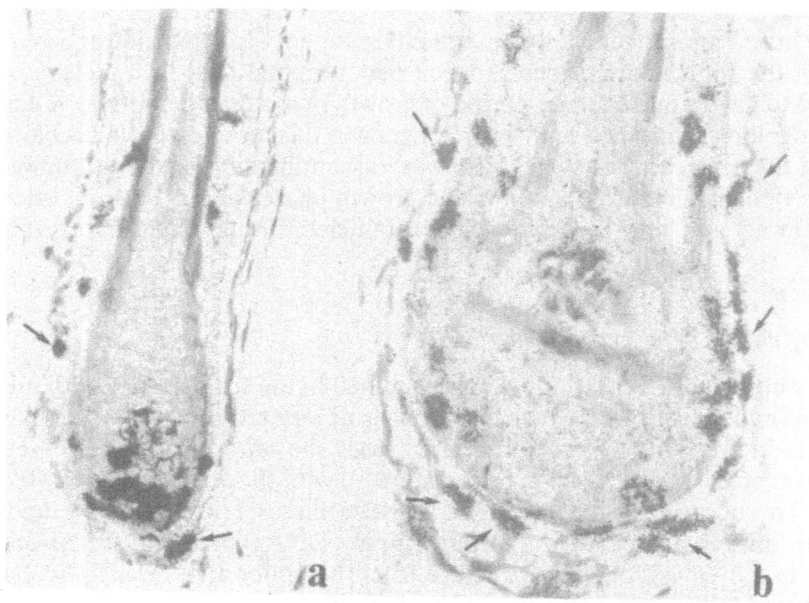

Figure 3 Autoradiographic pictures of [³H]thymidine of the mid-anagen phase showing DNA synthesizing cells in both follicular bulb and perifollicular connective tissue sheath (**a** and **b**, arrows)

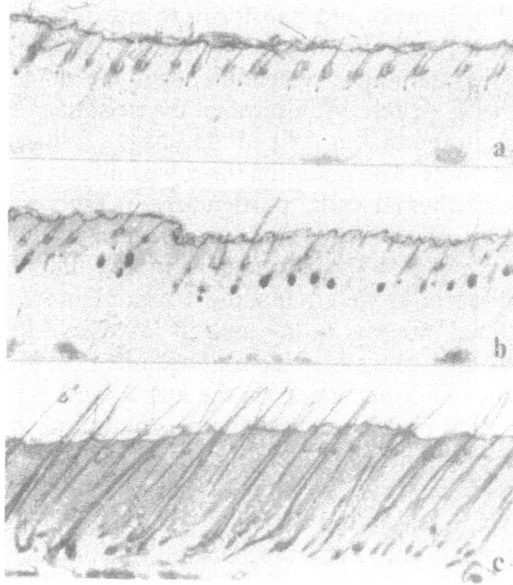

Figure 4 Microphotographs of the hair follicles, stained with histochemical method of alkaline phosphatase, in the back skin of rat. (**a**) telogen, 22 days, (**b**) mid-anagen, 27 days, and (**c**) late (growing) anagen phase, 47 days

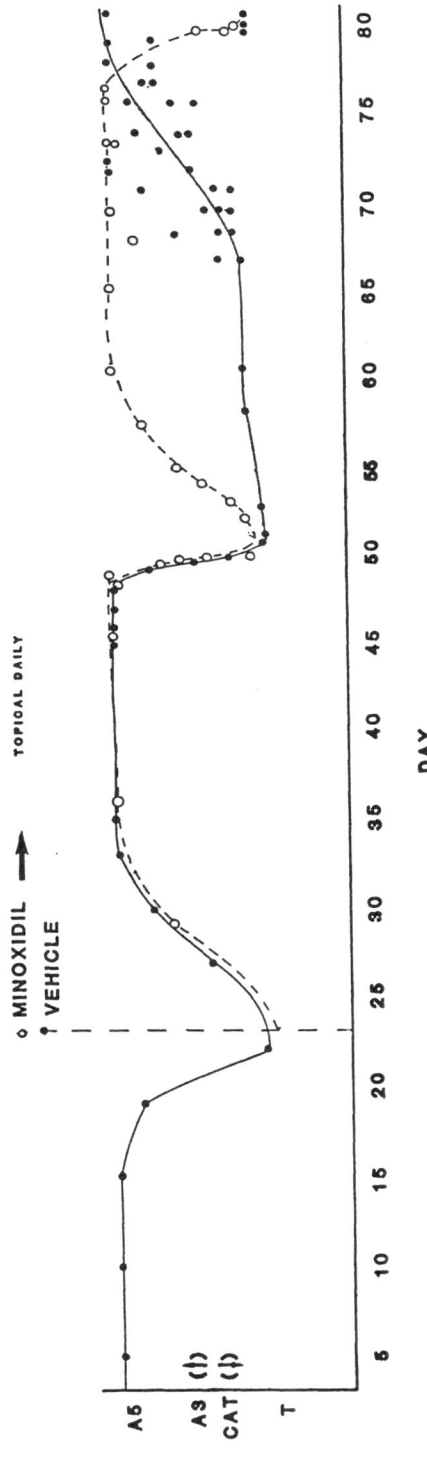

Figure 5 Topical minoxidil (5%) and vehicle applied daily from 23 to 80 days. The interval of the 2nd anagen phase was the same in both groups but the 2nd telogen phase in the treated group was extremely short and quickly entered the anagen (A3) phase. The 2nd telogen phase of control group lasted nearly 70 days. The interval of the 3rd anagen phase of the treated group was almost the same with the 2nd phase. T: telogen (Figure 4a), A3: mid-anagen (Figure 4b), A5: late anagen (Figure 4c)

111

Hair follicular cycles in adolescent rats

Histological studies

The hair follicles on the back of juvenile rats (Sprague-Dawley) exhibit synchronized cyclic turnover (Figure 4). At weaning (22–23 days), the follicles enter the first postnatal telogen phase (Figure 5). Subsequently, the follicles quickly grow and enter into the second growth anagen phase at around 30 days of age. This growth phase continues until 50 days. At 50–52 days of age the follicles enter the catagen phase. Usually all of the follicles enter the second telogen phase and then stay in the telogen phase from 53 days to nearly 70 days of age. The age and sexual variation of the cyclic phase in individual animals is 2–3 days in the first telogen, second anagen and second telogen phases. However the individual variation becomes much greater after 80 days of age. The variation of each individual follicle on the back skin is almost negligible until 80 days of age, though a few follicles always show some delay or advancement of the phases.

Effect of topical minoxidil on the cyclic dynamics.

Daily topical minoxidil (5% in the same vehicle) was applied on the shaved back of rats after weaning (23 days). The control group received the vehicle alone. Skin biopsies (6 mm punch) were performed every 3–5 days in the different advancing age groups (at least 6 consecutive biopsies on the same animal).

The results revealed a dramatic effect of minoxidil on cyclic dynamics of the follicles during the second telogen phase, from 50 to 60 days of age (Figure 5). While all of the follicles in the vehicle-treated group remained in the telogen phase for up to 70 days, the telogen follicles in the minoxidil-treated group began to grow at 53 days. At 55 days, all of the follicles developed to the mid-anagen phase (A3) when the secondary germ formed the primordial bulb structure in the skin of the minoxidil-treated group. At approximately 60 days all follicles developed to the anagen phase (A5). It is obvious that minoxidil neither prolonged the growth (anagen) phase nor induced an enlargement of follicular size[11]. The epidermis and other cutaneous structures were not affected by either minoxidil or the vehicle treatment.

Similar to the above-described study with bald stumptailed macaques, minoxidil stimulated proliferation of the secondary germ cells in the telogen follicles in the adolescent rat skin. However, we also noticed that the terminal follicles in rat skin have genetically coded programs for the interval of growth (anagen) period as well as the size of the follicle. Under these physiological conditions the drug only produced a premature onset of the anagen phase in terms of an acceleration of cyclic progression of the telogen phase. This experimental system may be a good model to examine the effect of drugs on hair growth. Indeed, our preliminary data from the study of phorbol ester showed remarkable effects in accelerating follicular cyclic progression and increased activity of calcium- and phospholipid-dependent protein kinase C activity in the skin of adolescent rats after topical application of PMA (approximately 40 μg/0.2 ml dimethylsulfoxide, twice a week, for 2 weeks). It is conceivable that this tumor-promoting agent, known as a specific binder of protein kinase C, stimulates germinal cell proliferation in the telogen follicle. The activity of protein kinase C, which is known as an enzyme that stimulates cell mitosis, will be a good marker for the effect of drugs on follicular growth[12].

PROPHYLACTIC EFFECT OF AN ANTIANDROGEN (4-MA) ON THE DEVELOPMENT OF BALDNESS IN STUMPTAILED MACAQUES

Four male and two female adolescent stumptailed macaques were divided into two groups. The first group (two male and one female) was treated daily with 0.5 ml of 4-MA (*N,N*-diethyl-4-methyl-3-oxo-4-aza-5α-androstane-17β-carboxamide) solutions (14 mg/ml dimethylsulfoxide) for 27 months[4]. The other group received 0.5 ml dimethylsulfoxide alone. To assess the rate of hair growth, a defined area of the frontal scalp was shaved every 2 months, and the hair was weighed. Skin biopsies (6 mm punch) were obtained before and after 27 months of 4-MA applications. The skin samples were used for both folliculogram analysis and assay of steroid 5α-reductase. Serum levels of testosterone and dihydrotestosterone were measured every 2 to 4 months throughout the study.

The animals treated with 4-MA had significantly greater weight of shaved hair than control animals throughout the study. The seasonal enhancement of hair growth rate between March and May was well maintained in the 4-MA animals, while the rate for control animals dropped markedly during the second spring. Toward the end of the study the mean weight of hair from the two groups showed nearly a 3-fold difference. Analysis of folliculograms in the pre- and post-treatment stages clearly showed the difference between 4-MA and control animals. The patterns of folliculograms in the treated group showed essentially the same distribution and size of cyclic follicles, whereas the control animals showed a marked increase of resting follicles, and the follicles became much smaller after 27 months (Figure 6). The results of both the hair weight and folliculogram analyses showed that 4-MA apparently prevented the regressive changes of frontal hair follicles during the critical period of developing baldness. The 5α-reductase activity in the skin samples taken at 27 months showed that the control group had significantly greater activity than the 4-MA group. Interestingly, topical application of 4-MA induced no systemic effect in serum concentration of testosterone and dihydrotestosterone. Since dihydrotestosterone is known as an active and potent androgen for hair follicle, prostate and seminal vesicles, th conversion of circulating testosterone in the target organs plays a major role in androgenic action. Thus an inhibition of 5α-reductase activity in the local

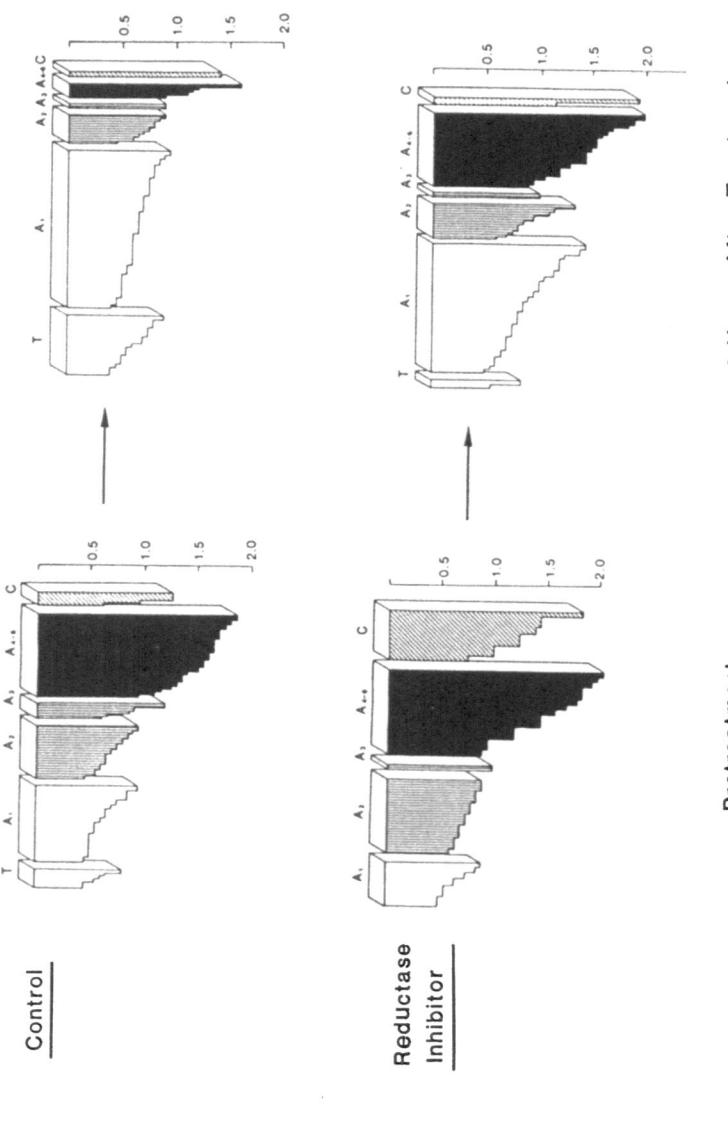

Figure 6 Folliculograms of controls and the animals treated with 5α-reductase inhibitor. The patterns in the pretreatment stage of both control and treatment cases show typical non-bald type containing many early (A1), mid (A2-3), and late (A4-6) anagen follicles. This pattern and the size of the follicles were maintained for over 2 years of treatment while control case changes to the typical bald type (decreasing the size and populations of mid and late anagen follicles) (see ref. 5)

environment reduces the production of dihydrotestosterone from testosterone. In this case, topical application of 4-MA appears to reduce the level of dihydrotestosterone in the hair follicles. Thus, it can prevent the androgen mediated regressive change of the hair follicles in the hereditarily balding stumptailed macaque.

COMMENT

The cyclic remodeling of the hair follicles is a unique activity in postnatal mammalian skin. This repeated process of degeneration and regeneration of the follicular structure is comparable to the cyclic change of the endometrium. Both are influenced by steroid sex hormones. However the structural and functional complexity is far greater in hair follicles than in endometrial tissues. The germinal reserve cells remaining in the base of the telogen follicle are usually unidentifiable. This group of cells appears to translocate from the bulbar matrix of the anagen follicles to the base of telogen follicles through the involution process of the lower follicular sheath during the catagen phase. The dermal papilla cells in anagen follicles follow the same process as the follicular cells. In the vicinity of the telogen follicle those cells become almost invisible. These two heterogenetic groups of reserve cells (epithelial and mesenchymal) have great potential for induction and proliferative reconstruction of a follicular structure. The actual triggering mechanism that induces the constructive process of the hair follicle remains unknown. However, minoxidil apparently stimulates this process: it accelerates anagen induction from the telogen (resting) phase. In addition, it induces an increased rate of DNA synthesis in both the follicular epithelium and the mesenchymal dermal papilla cells. Minoxidil also stimulates the proliferation of the reserve cells in the entire follicular structure, including the upper and lower follicular sheath during the early to mid-anagen phase. While the secondary germ proliferates and forms a new bulb as well as a new lower follicular sheath, the reserve cells in the upper follicular sheath also join in the construction. Together with the increased rate of cell proliferation a new anagen follicle becomes much larger than it was in the previous cycle. However, an enlargement of the follicular size through the cycle process is most obvious in the vellus follicles. Using rat skin, we found that minoxidil stimulated a premature onset of anagen induction in the telogen follicles. Interestingly, a similar phenomenon can be produced by phorbol ester, which binds and activates calcium- and phospholipid-dependent protein kinase C, an enzyme known as a stimulator of cell mitosis. Further study of this enzyme system will elucidate the action of minoxidil on follicular growth and determine whether it acts directly on the hair follicular cells or indirectly due to the vasodilatory condition of the skin. Contrary to stimulation of growth, androgens induce a regression of scalp terminal follicles in bald-trait men and the stumptailed macaques. The mechanism of this action is much debated. However, topical application of an inhibitor of 5α-reduc-

115

tase can prevent the balding process at least during the critical age period in the macaque model. We found that this drug induced a local reduction of 5α reductase activity,but it produced no significant systemic effect on the levels of systemic androgens. The results of the present study strongly support the hypothesis that dihydrotestosterone is a potent androgen that triggers the regression of genetically linked hair follicles. Experimental results, using the macaque model, will provide a new scope for the study of different genic expressions of steroid receptors and their intracellular roles in cell growth.

REFERENCES

1.   Hamilton JB. Male hormone stimulation is prerequisite and an incitant in common baldness. *Am J Anat*, 71, 451–480, 1942
2.   Frieden IJ, Price VH. Androgenetic alopecia. In *Pathogenesis of Skin Disease* (Thiers BH, Dobson RL, eds), pp. 41–55. New York: Churchill Livingstone, 1986
3.   Ebling FJ, Thomas AK, Cooke ID. Effect of cyproterone acetate on hair growth, sebaceous secretion and endocrine parameters in a hirsute subject. *Br J Dermatol*, 97, 371, 1977
4.   Rittmaster RS, Uno H, Povar ML, Mellin TN, Loriaux DL. The effect of 4-MA, a 5α-reductase inhibitor, on the development of baldness in the stumptailed macaque. *J Clin Endocrinol Metab*, 65, 188–193, 1987
5.   Uno H. Biology of hair growth. *Semin Reprod Endocrinol,* **4, 131–141, 1986**
6.   Uno H. Stumptailed macaques as a model of male-pattern baldness. In *Models in Dermatology*. (Maibach HI, Lowe NJ, eds), pp 159–169. Basel: Karger, 1987
7.   Uno H, Cappas A, Brigham P. Action of topical minoxidil in the bald stump-tailed macaque. *J Am Acad Dermatol*, 16, 657–668, 1987
8.   Baker L, Kaye R, Root AW, Prasad ALN. Diazoxide treatment of idiopathic hypoglycemia of infancy. *J Pediat*, 71, 494–505, 1967
9.   Burton JL, Schutt WH, Caldwell IW. Hypertrichosis due to diazoxide. *Br J Dermatol*, 93, 707–711, 1975
10. Meier A, Weidmann P, Gluck Z, Keusch G, Grimm M, Minder I, Reubi FC. Vergleich von oralem Diazoxid und Minoxidil bei therapieresistenter Hypertonie. *Klin Wochenschr*, 58, 681–687, 1980
11. Schroeder B, Uno H. Unpublished data
12. Rozengurt E, Rodriguez-Pena A, Coombs M, Sinnett-Smith J. Diacylglycerol stimulates DNA synthesis and cell division in mouse 3T3 cells: Role of Ca^{2+}-sensitive phospholipid-dependent protein kinase. *Cell Biol*, 81, 5748–5752, 1984

13
Human hair follicle grafts onto nude mice: morphological study

D Van Neste*, G Warnier**, M Thulliez***, F Van Hoof[§]
*Department of Dermatology, **Ludwig Institute for Cancer Research (Brussels Branch), ***Dermatology Practice Group and [§]International Institute of Cellular and Molecular Pathology, Catholic University of Louvain, Brussels, Belgium

ABSTRACT

In recent years, genetically immunodeficient animals have been widely used for xenograft experiments, mainly in the field of cancer research. Heterologous skin, including human skin, has been grown away from the donor after grafting on congenitally athymic nude mice. Normal human skin and diseased skin processes have been studied in this model. In this paper we report preliminary data on morphological aspects of skin appendageal behavior and especially hair follicle growth in a number of skin specimens grafted onto nude mice.

Skin specimens

* Pigmented naevi with or without clinically visible growing hairs were taken from four patients during minor surgical interventions; the following sites were involved: scalp ($n = 1$), face ($n = 1$), back ($n = 1$) or leg ($n = 1$). With the exception of a dysplastic naevus from the back, all pertained to dermal–epidermal types.

* Two 3 mm punch grafts, from a zone of short regrowing hairs, were taken from the scalp of a female patient with trichotillomania.

* Male pattern baldness specimens consisted of 3 mm punches ($n = 16$), taken from a male patient during a scalp punch grafting session.

Full-thickness skin grafting

Classically, we used grafting of the skin specimens on an open graft bed. For smaller samples like a single or a small group of follicles we used the subcutaneous implantation. Grafted human skin was sampled 2 months later. Light and electron microscopy were used to control the differentiation of follicular and interfollicular epidermis.

As a first step in the development process of a clinically relevant model for human balding scalp, we felt that grafting both normal and balding follicles and evaluating their behavior after transplantation onto nude mice would be a reasonable approach.

Our preliminary observations indicate that around 30% of full-thickness grafts containing human hair follicles were functionally active for a period of 2 months after grafting on the nude mouse. When examined microscopically the complete human hair follicular structure is maintained, including the sebaceous glands which, however, became extremely atrophic. Further improvements of the grafting technique by preparing the graft bed and its vascular supply could be promising in the very near future for full-thickness grafting. This would provide an alternative approach to the evaluation of the pharmacology of hair growth. We believe that having at our disposal a set of normal and/or hypotrophic human hair follicles growing on recipient mice for performing precisely controlled experiments will be most valuable in terms of clinical–pharmacological trials and of *in vivo* human hair growth regulation studies.

INTRODUCTION

In recent years, genetically immunodeficient animals have been widely used for xenograft experiments, mainly in the field of cancer research. Heterologous skin, including human skin, has been grown away of the donor after grafting on congenitally athymic nude mice (for a review see references 1 and 2). Normal human skin maintains its morphologic characteristics[3,4] after grafting. Furthermore, *in vitro* cultured epidermal cells re-express a number of differentiation markers and re-form an epidermal type epithelium after transplantation to nude mice[5,6]. Diseased skin processes can also be studied in this model: successful transplantation of lamellar ichthyosis or psoriatic skin[7,8] maintaining pathological characteristics or their re-expression after grafting of 'apparently undifferentiated' *in vitro* cultured epidermal cells (i.e. lamellar ichthyosis[9,10]) and healing of wounded human epidermis[11,12] are but a few examples of novel experimental approaches using the nude mouse model.

More recently, Horne *et al.*[13] proposed to use this system for further defining host-dependence or genetically determined factors in alopecia. Indeed the bald DEBR rat skin regrows hair after transplantation onto nude mice, illustrating, by the way, that systemic host-related factors are important for the determination of hair growth, or in this case follicular growth/arrest. A similar technique was used by Gilhar and Krueger[14] in experimental studies grafting alopecia areata punch biopsies from human subjects onto nude mice. Finally, *in vitro* reconstruction of mouse-hairy-skin-equivalents and their successful grafting on the nude mouse has also been reported[15].

In this paper we report preliminary data on the morphological aspects of skin appendageal behavior, and especially hair follicle growth, in a number of skin specimens grafted on to the nude mice.

MATERIAL AND METHODS

Grafting procedure

Specific pathogen-free congenitally athymic nude mice (Balb/c nu/nu: Dr B Sordat, ISREC, Epalinges, CH) aged 4–6 weeks, were housed in a clean high-pressure limited-access room under continuous laminar flow (ESI-Cachan, France). Autoclaved cages, cage tops and cage filters were used. Irradiated wooden bedding chips, water and mouse chow were delivered ad libitum from sterile containers. Animals to be grafted were anesthetized with ether, and a piece of skin, adapted to the graft bed, was tailored according to the size of the human skin graft. This graft was usually less than 1 cm in diameter. The site chosen for grafting was usually the lateral aspect of the back.

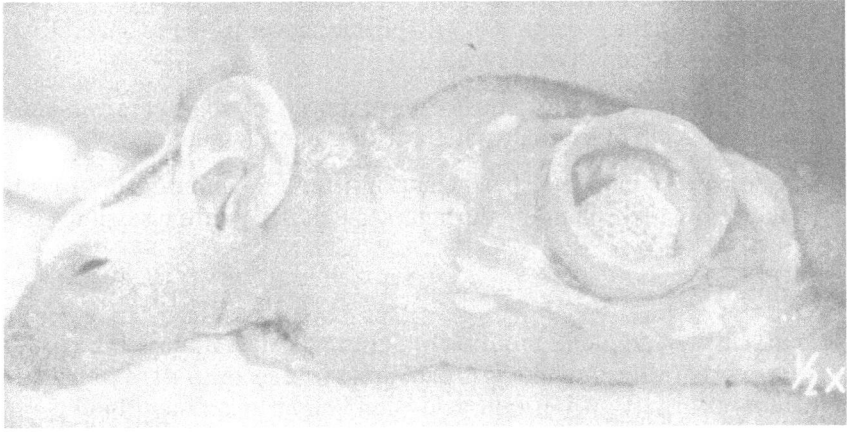

Figure 1 Dressing of freshly grafted human skin onto nude mouse. After grafting of the human skin specimen the grafted site is covered with hydrocolloid adhesive dressing. The bottom of a syringe is fixed onto nude skin with instant glue

Two grafting techniques were used:

(a) The most usual technique of air-exposed skin grafts was used for the largest skin specimens. After a series of preliminary trials we adopted the following dressing procedure: the full-thickness skin specimen was fitted into the prepared graft site, the mouse skin covering slightly the human specimen (1–2 mm) in order to improve the graft take. The grafts were fixed in position with sterile hydrocolloid dressings (Duoderm®, Convatec-Squibb, Brussels). The grafted site was finally protected from mechanical damage by a home-made protecting device as shown in Figure 1. Graft site protection was obtained by fixing the bottom of a 5 ml syringe on the skin surface of the mice with instant glue. The site was inspected every second day, and when possible the protection was left in place over a period of 10 days.

(b) The subcutaneous graft technique has also been used for smaller specimens (usually less than 2 mm in diameter containing a single or a pair of isolated hair follicles). The specimens were inserted into a space created by blunt dissection in a plane inferior to the panniculus carnosus. From the caudal incisional site the skin specimen was placed into a more cephalic position close to the costal grid.

Human skin specimens

* Pigmented naevi with or without clinically visible growing hairs were taken from four patients during minor surgical interventions; the following sites were involved: scalp ($n = 1$), face ($n = 1$), back ($n = 1$) or leg ($n = 1$). With the exception of a dysplastic naevus from the back, all were of the dermal–epidermal type.

* Two 3 mm punch grafts, from a zone of short regrowing hairs, were taken from the scalp of a female patient with trichotillomania.

* Male pattern baldness specimens consisted of 3 mm punches ($n = 16$), taken from a male patient during a scalp punch grafting session.

Skin sampling

Human skin was sampled 2 months after grafting. After Bouin's fluid fixation and classical paraffin embedding procedure, serial sections were stained with hemalum-eosin-saffron, periodic acid Schiff, and rhodamine toluidine blue, according to Hanau et al.[16]. In pigmented naevi pigment was silver-stained by Fontana-Masson's method (Laboratory of Professor JM Lachapelle, Louvain University). Small skin specimens were also fixed in glutaraldehyde (2% in 0.1 mol/l Na cacodylate buffer, pH 7.4) post-fixed in 1% osmium tetroxide and included in Spurr resin. Semi-thin and thin sections were made with a Reichert ultratome and stained either with toluidine blue or with methylene blue. Ultrathin sections were stained with both uranyl acetate and lead citrate, and examined with a Philips EM301 microscope.

RESULTS

Our preliminary observations indicate that around 30% of full-thickness grafts containing functionally active human hair follicles can be maintained on the nude mouse for at least 2 months. This period of time was selected before starting the experiments, as it is known that nude mice undergo a wasting process after the age of 3 months.

When examined macroscopically and microscopically (Figure 2) the interadnexial epidermal structures are preserved and complete terminal differentiation proceeds. There is complete keratinization and persistence of melanization, especially in the case of grafted naevus, where melanin detection ends sharply at the margin of the graft (Figure 2d). In the dermal aspects of the naevus there is persistence of dermal pigmentation, which is also limited to the original human skin specimen and does not extend into the mouse tissues.

The light microscopy and electron microscopy of the epidermal differentiation steps and of the naevus-type melanization are shown 2 months after grafting (Figure 2c,d). In a dysplastic naevus the overall dysplastic aspect was not maintained, and there was a marked epidermal atrophy, however, pigment synthesis was still present 2 months after grafting.

Hair growth proceeds when human skin is grafted onto nude mice (Figures 2a,b and 3), and the presence of functionally active human hair follicular structures, including sebaceous glands, is demonstrated microscopically (Figures 3–6). As compared with the original size in the human adult skin, the latter, however, became extremely atrophic with a mono- or bilayer of poorly differentiated or undifferentiated basal sebocytes almost completely embedded in the outer root sheath (Figures 3 and 4).

Figure 2 Macroscopic aspects and epidermal structures in a human naevus (2 months after grafting onto nude mouse).
(a) Immersion photography of epidermal side (magnification x2). There is persistence of naevus-type pigmentation in most of the specimen. The presence of an actively growing hair follicle is shown. Clearcut differences exist between human and mouse epidermal surface patterns.
(b) Dermal side of the same specimen as in Figure 2a (magnification x2). By reclining the grafted skin the presence of two hair roots is recognized.
(c) Electron microscopy of epidermal differentiation (magnification c1: x4938; c2: x12,060). All stages of terminal epidermal differentiation are identified and the presence of numerous desmosomes is illustrated at higher magnification.
(d) Naevus-type pigmentation persists 2 months after grafting (d1: light microscopy: Fontana Masson stain, magnification x15; d2: electron microscopy of the dermal epidermal junction, magnification x18,050). Melanin detection ends sharply at the margin of the graft (arrow) in both epidermal and dermal aspects. Electron microscopy shows the presence of tightly packed melanosomes at the level of the basal layers.

121

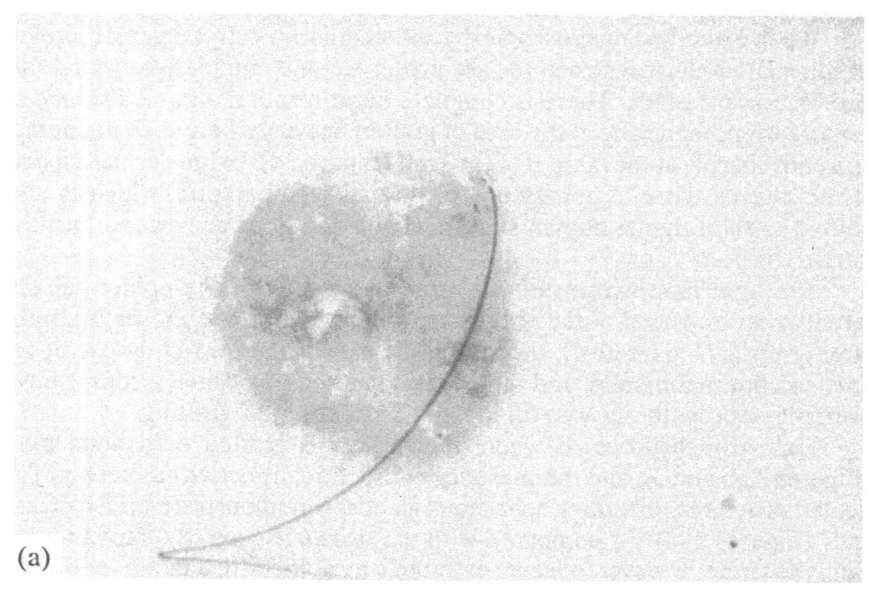

(a)

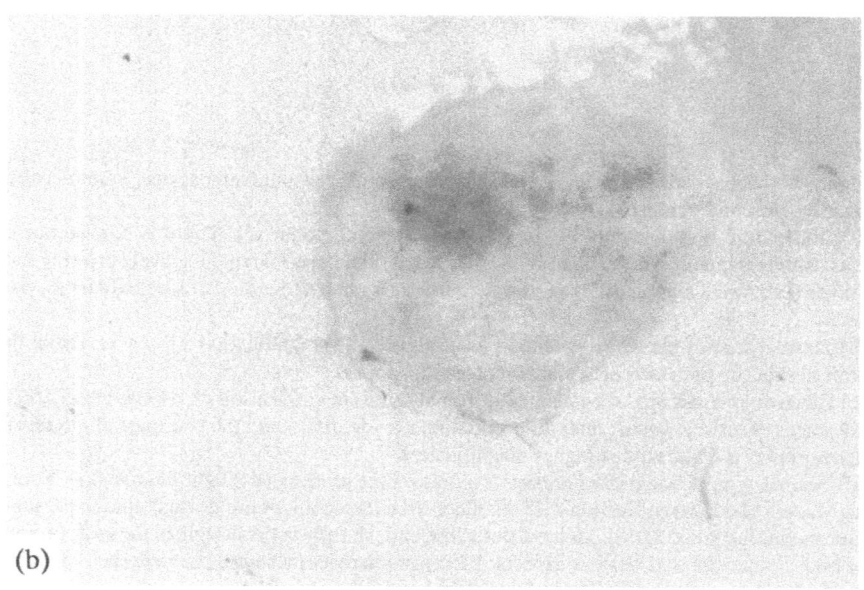

(b)

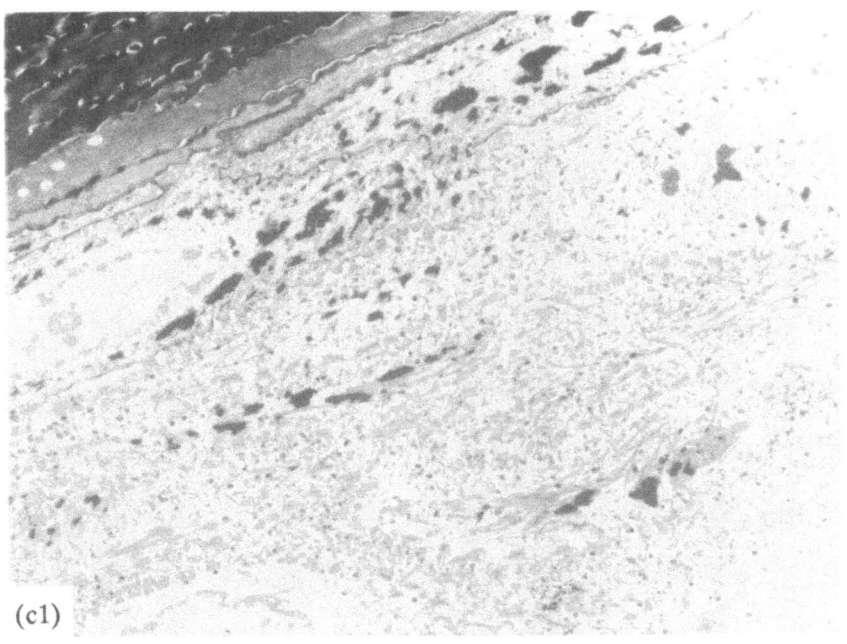

(c1)

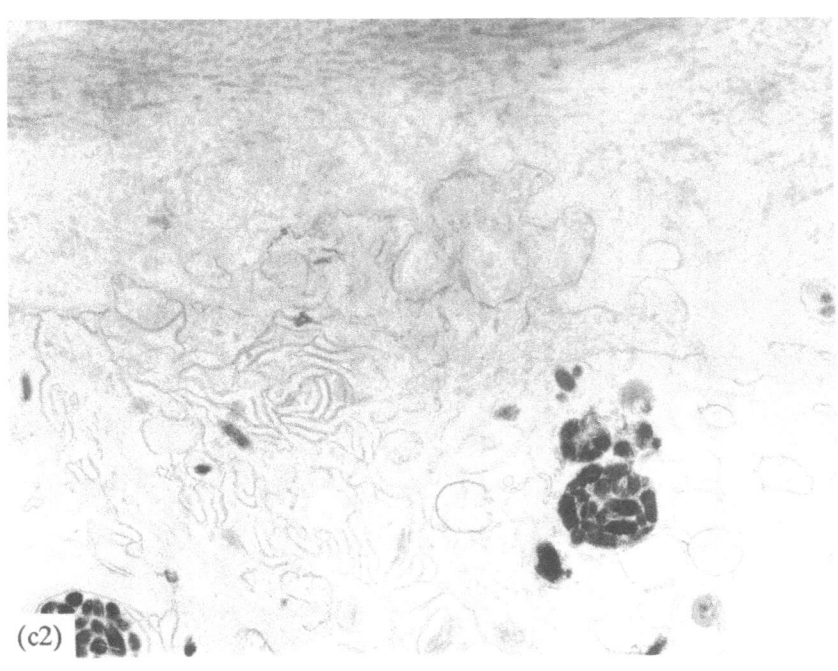

(c2)

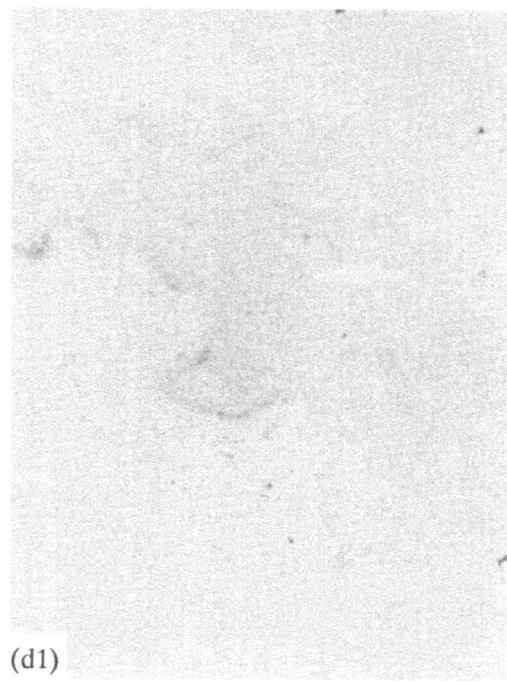

(d1)

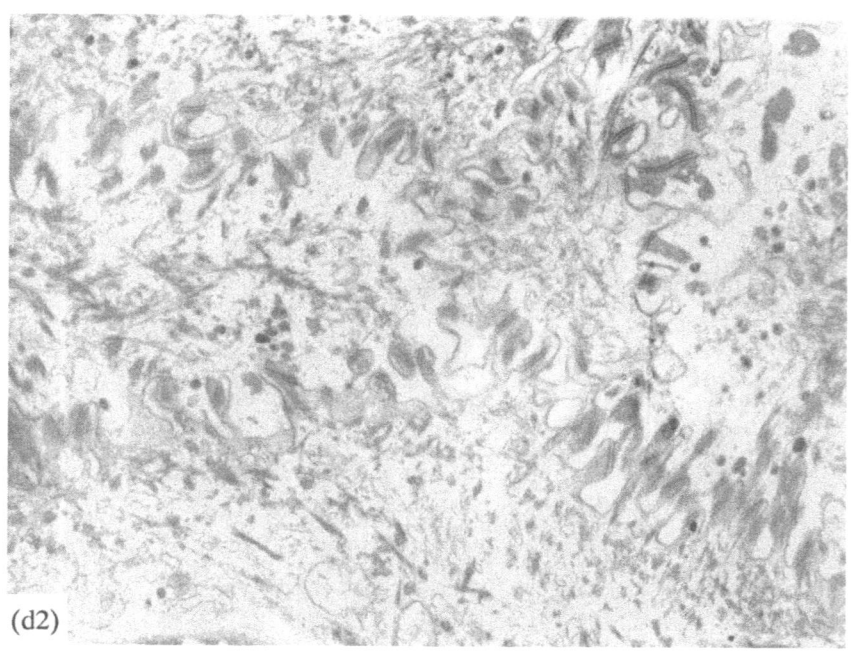

(d2)

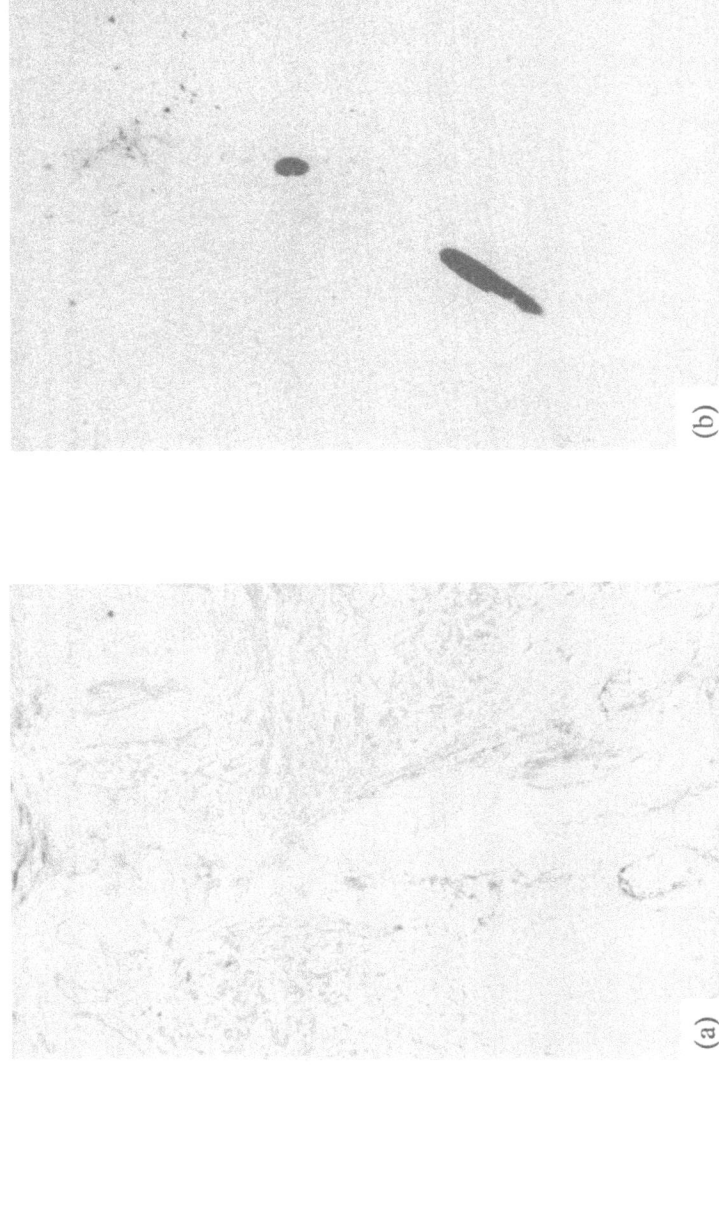

Figure 3 Hair infundibular structure in a human nevus 2 months after grafting onto nude mouse (3a: PAS stain; 3b: Fontana Masson's stain; magnification x14). Serial sections through the acroinfudibulum of the grafted human hair follicle from the naevus shown in Figure 2a clearly illustrate that all components of the upper hair follicle are present, including active pigment synthesis (3b). As compared with the original size in the human adult skin, the sebaceous glands are, however, atrophic with a mono- or bilayer of poorly differentiated sebocytes.

125

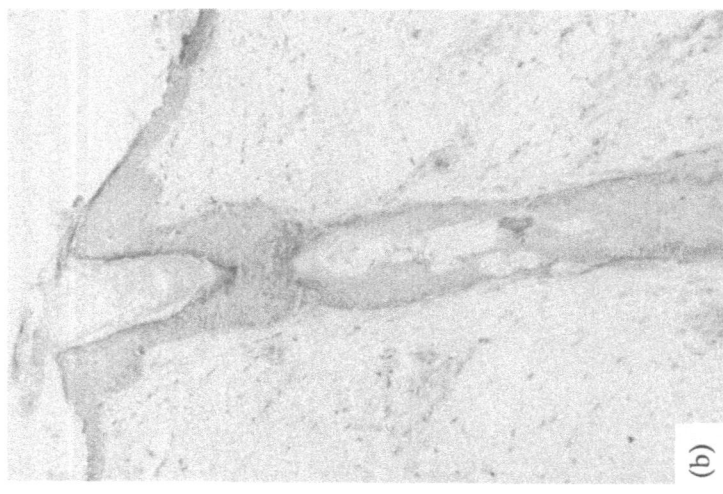

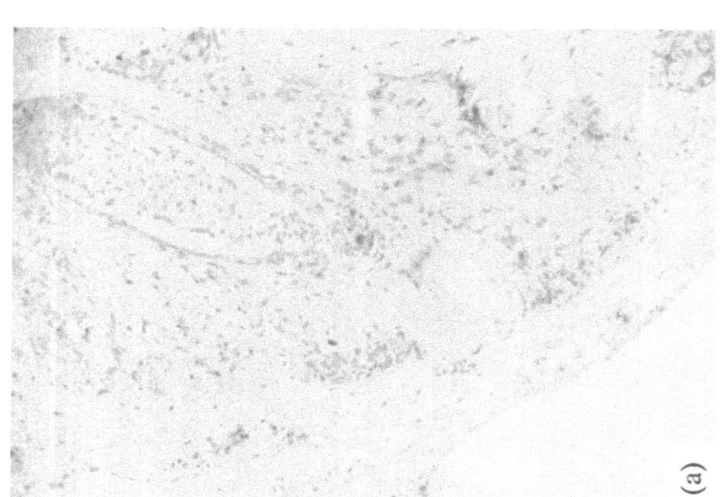

Figure 4 Hair follicle growth in human scalp grafted onto nude mice (human scalp, two months after grafting; rhodamine-toluidine blue stain; magnification x14). The presence of functionally active human hair follicular structures is shown in 4a. Early anagen starts from the undifferentiated epithelial column and dermal papilla is enclosed in the downward-progressing follicular bud (light arrow). The sebaceous gland (in 4b as in Figure 3) is barely recognizable. It is almost reduced to a small number of clear cells embedded in the outer root sheath.

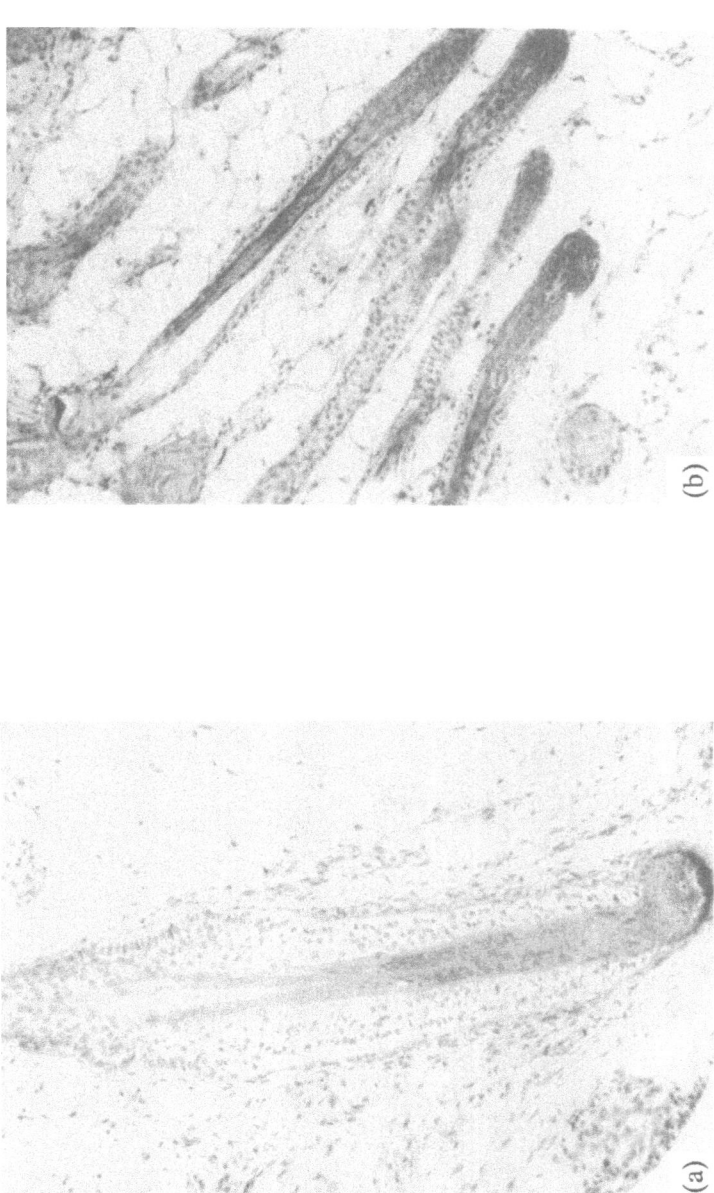

Figure 5 Comparative aspects of deep follicular structures of grafted human scalp (5a) and nude mouse skin (5b) (HES stain, magnification x14). The overall aspect of human and mouse hair follicles is easily distinguished. The human follicle is broader and longer than mouse follicles. The multi-layered outer root sheath is almost completely surrounded by dense dermal connective tissue. The thickness of mouse dermis being much less than human dermis, the shorter and smaller mouse follicles are already protruding in hypodermis, as compared with the dermal location of grafted human follicles at the same depth from the epidermal surface.

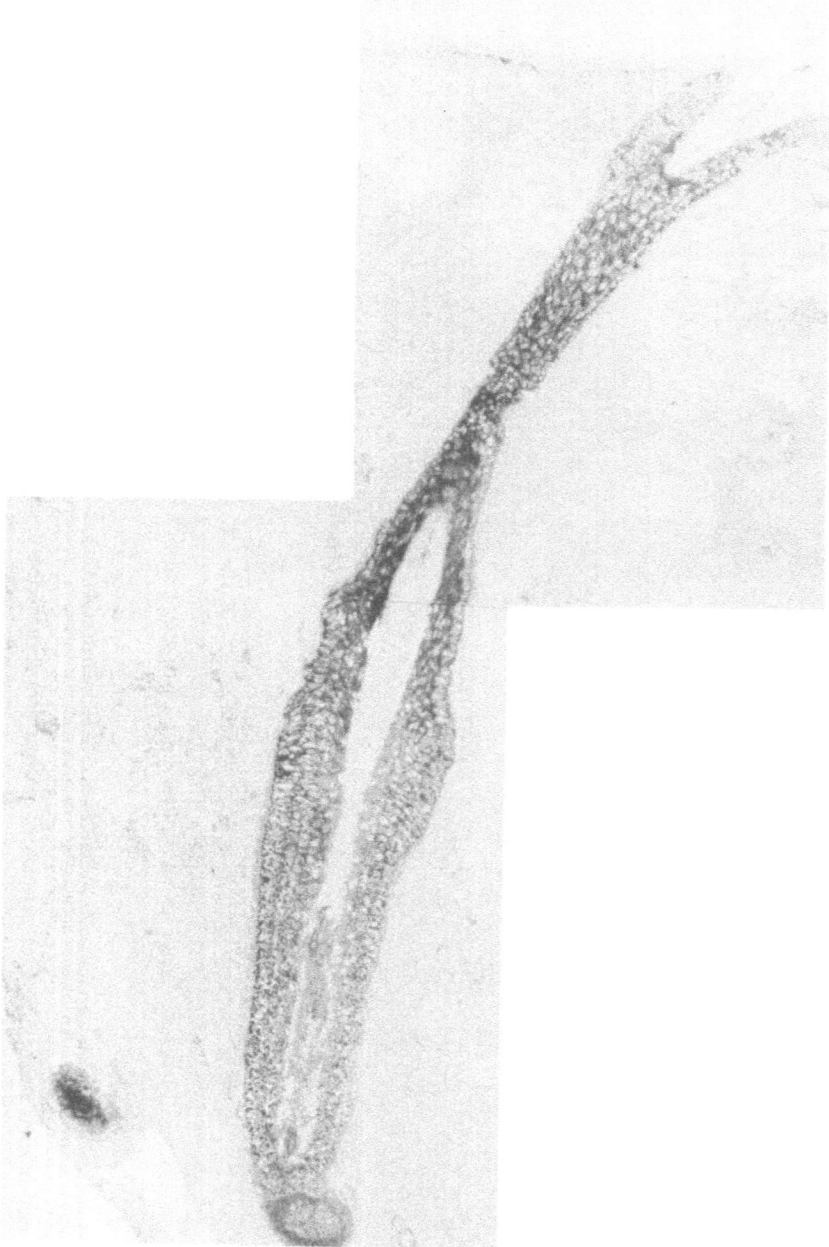

Figure 6 Longitudinal section through grafted human hair follicle (PAS stain, magnification x15). The PAS-positive basement membranes and connective tissue sheath, as well as the glycogen-rich outer root sheath, are shown. This is in sharp contrast with the interadnexial epidermis where glycogen granules are barely visible.

DISCUSSION

There are conflicting results in the literature concerning the maintenance of adnexial structure and/or function in grafted human skin on the nude-mouse model. Indeed Petersen *et al.*[17], reported that human sebaceous glands of facial skin responded to stimulation by androgens after grafting onto the nude mouse. Interestingly the grafted skin retains donor-responsive features such as response to protein kinase C activator TPA[18,19]. This property could further be exploited in experiments according to the observations reported by Uno (this volume, Chapter 12). As could be expected from the present knowledge of the biological role played by the dermal papilla in the induction of hair growth, Rygaard[4] reported that hair loss is the usual feature after removal of deep dermis and hypodermis from the human skin before grafting; some arrector muscles, eccrine sweat glands and deeper sweat ducts are, however, preserved. Barr *et al.*[20] noted the presence of epithelium, sebaceous glands and sweat glands at the transplantation site of malignant melanomas less than 1 mm thickness. In their review, Black and Jederberg[2] anticipated that adnexial structures, including nails, would require study. Results recently published in the literature, as well as our own studies, confirm this statement. Our results indicate that there is a future for this model in the field of investigating pathophysiology of male-pattern baldness and follicular response to hormonal stimulation/inhibition.

Horne *et al.*[13] recently reported an animal model for alopecia areata. The strain of hairless rats (DEBR) is characterized by growing an apparently normal first coat of hair, after birth, and then becoming progressively hairless. During morphological examination of skin biopsies the authors noted the presence of a dense peri- and intra-follicular lymphocytic infiltrate. This reaction pattern is much like the observations in alopecia areata. When full-thickness macroscopically hairless DEBR skin was grafted onto the flank of nude mice the authors observed hair regrowth within 2 weeks. This observation argues for a genetically inherited pathogenesis depending upon host-related factors, namely autoimmune related processes inhibiting follicular maturation. The inhibitory signals appear to be no longer available when the skin evolves in an immunologically neutral environment. It is also necessary to mention at this stage that similar experiments by Gilhar and Krueger[14] showed hair regrowth in scalp biopsies from balding patches of patients with alopecia areata grafted onto nude mice. In such a system they were also able to demonstrate that hair regrowth was stimulated in alopecia areata grafts after 78 days of oral intake of cyclosporin by graft-bearing mice. Finally, in a recent paper by Rogers *et al.*[15], maintenance of the mouse hair follicle function was demonstrated by transferring *in vitro* cultured follicles along with fibroblasts to prepared skin sites in nude mouse recipients. The authors report that after 2–3 weeks of grafting (either cultured or freshly biopsied follicles), grafted sites contained densely haired skin.

As a first step in the development process of a clinically relevant model for human balding, we tried to graft both normal and balding follicles and to evaluate their behaviour after transplantation onto the nude mice. Indeed, actually available *in vitro* models seem to reflect poorly the clinical situation, as well as the biochemical aspects. Jones *et al.*[21] recently reported that synthesis of high sulfur proteins was markedly reduced after 3 days *in vitro* culture of plucked human hair follicles. Awaiting further improvements of such *in vitro* models (see Messenger, this volume, paper 7) we think that having at our disposal complete normal or hypotrophic hair follicles is most valuable for performing precisely controlled experiments relating to *in vivo* hair growth regulation.

Our preliminary observations indicate that human hair follicles can be maintained on the nude mouse, providing a useful approach to the evaluation of the pharmacology of hair growth. Further improvements of grafting technique, such as the use of 2 mm punch grafts, as proposed by Gilhar and Krueger[7], or even smaller minigrafts, or by preparing the graft bed and its vascular supply, could be promising in the very near future.

ACKNOWLEDGEMENTS

The excellent technical assistance of Mrs MA Douniau and A Stefanovic and the electron microscopy by Mrs Thahn-Müller are acknowledged.

REFERENCES

1. Briggaman RA. Localization of the defect in skin diseases analyzed in the human skin graft–nude mouse model. *Cur Prob Dermatol*, **10**, 115–123, 1980
2. Black KE, Jederberg WW. Athymic nude mice and human skin grafting. In *Models in Dermatology*, vol. 1 (Maibach H, Lowe N, eds), pp. 228–239. Basel: Karger, 1985
3. Manning DD, Reed ND, Shaffer CF. Maintenance of skin xenografts of widely divergent phylogenetic origin on congenitally athymic (nude) mice. *J Exp Med*, **138**, 488–494, 1973
4. Rygaard J. Skin grafts in nude mice. 3. Fate of grafts from man and donors of others taxonomic classes. *Acta Pathol Microbiol Scand Sect A*, **82**, 105–112, 1974
5. Banks-Schlegel S, Green H. Formation of epidermis by serially cultivated human epidermal cells transplanted as an epithelium to athymic mice. *Transplantation*, **29**, 308–313, 1980
6. Worst PKM, Mackenzie IC, Fusenig NE. Reformation of organized epidermal structure by transplantation of suspensions and cultures of epidermal and dermal cells. *Cell Tissue Res*, **225**, 65–77, 1982
7. Krueger GG, Manning DD, Malouf J, Ogden B. Long-term maintenance of psoriatic human skin on congenitally athymic (nude) mice. *J Invest Dermatol*, **64**, 307–312, 1975
8. Haftek M, Ortonne JP, Staquet MJ, Viac J, Thivolet J. Normal and psoriatic skin grafts on 'nude' mice: morphological and immunochemical studies. *J Invest Dermatol*, **76**, 48–52, 1981
9. Haftek M, Zambruno G, Reano A, Faure M, Thivolet J. Cultivated pathological keratinocytes from Darrier's disease, lamellar ichthyosis and ichthyosis vulgaris are in-

sufficiently differentiated to express disease-characteristic features. *J Invest Dermatol*, **89**, 341, 1987

10. Joubaud A, Haftek M, Zambruno G, Faure M, Thivolet J. Re-expression of lamellar ichthyosis after grafting of epidermal sheets obtained by pathological keratinocyte culture to 'nude' mice. *J Invest Dermatol*, **89**, 340, 1987

11. Dermarchez M, Sengel P, Prunieras M. Wound healing of human skin transplanted onto the nude mouse. *Devel Biol*, **113**, 90–96, 1986

12. Dermarchez M, Desbas C, Prunieras M. Wound healing of human skin transplanted onto the nude mouse. *Br J Dermatol*, **113**, Suppl. 28, 177–182, 1985

13. Horne KA, Jahoda CAB, Johnson BE, Michie HJ, Oliver RF. An animal model for alopecia. *J Invest Dermatol*, **89**, 316, 1987

14. Gilhar A, Krueger GG. Hair growth in scalp grafts from patients with alopecia areata and alopecia universalis grafted onto nude mice. *Arch Dermatol*, **123**, 44–50, 1987

15. Rogers G, Martinet N, Steinert P, Wynn P, Roop D, Kilkenny A, Morgan D, Yuspa SH. Cultivation of murine hair follicles as organoids in a collagen matrix. *J Invest Dermatol*, **89**, 369–379, 1987

16. Hanau D, Marchand B, Grosshans E. La rhodamine B: un marqueur de la kératinisation folliculaire. *Ann Dermatol Vénéréol (Paris)*, **107**, 997–1004, 1980

17. Petersen MJ, Zone JJ, Krueger GG. Development of a nude mouse model to study human sebaceous gland physiology and pathophysiology. *J Clin Invest*, **74**, 1358–1365, 1984

18. Krueger GG, Chambers D, Shelby J. Epidermal proliferation of nude mice skin, pig skin and pig skin grafts: failure of nude mouse skin to respond to tumor promoter, 12-O-tetradecanoyl phorbol 13-acetate. *J Exp Med*, **152**, 1329–1339, 1980

19. Krueger GG, Shelby J. Biology of human skin transplanted to the nude mouse. I. Response to agents which modify epidermal proliferation. *J Invest Dermatol*, **76**, 506–510, 1981

20. Barr LH, Gartside RL, Goldman LI. The biology of malignant melanoma. Preliminary findings in the nude mouse. *Arch Surg*, **114**, 221–224, 1979

21. Jones LN, Fowler KJ, Marshall RC, Ackland ML. Studies of developing human hair shaft cells *in vitro*. *J Invest Dermatol*, **90**, 58–64, 1988

14

On the behavior of dye ions in an isotachophoresis boundary: application to the mitosis mechanism

K Uyttendaele
Laboratory for Dermatology, Sint Lucas Kliniek
Sint Lucaslaan, 8320 Brugge 4 Belgium

ABSTRACT

The behavior of dye molecules introduced between the leading and terminating electrolyte of isotachophoresis systems is described. Islands of dye molecules are formed which attract each other in the direction of lines formed between the different islands. In cationic isotachophoresis systems differences are observed in the patterns formed by the dyes, depending on the type of dye and on the type of leading ion used. A magnetic property of the atoms in an electric field can explain the features. The application of this magnetic property of molecules into an electric field lead us to propose a new theory explaining the mechanism of mitosis.

INTRODUCTION

When a small amount of dye ion with an intermediate mobility is introduced between the leading and terminating electrolyte in an isotachophoresis system, the concentration of this dye will be adapted to the concentration of the leading ion. This results in a very concentrated dye layer. We describe a series of phenomena which occur in this dye layer.

EXPERIMENTAL CONDITIONS

In anionic isotachophoresis systems, chloride, phosphate and sulfate are used as leading electrolyte, generally at 0.01 mol/l. Tris (hydroxymethyl) amino-methane (Tris) imidazole or aniline are used as cations in the leading electrolytes, with pH values of respectively 7.6 and 4.5. We use 0.8 ml of dye at 0.0001 mol/l concentration dissolved in terminator or leader. The terminator electrolyte is Tris 0.03 mol/l, glycine 0.03 mol/l. The dyes bromophenol blue, rose bengal and acid red 4 are used. The isotachophoresis apparatus is as described earlier[1]. In cationic isotachophoresis systems we use as leading electrolyte the acetate of sodium, potassium, rubidium, cesium, magnesium, calcium, zinc, cadmium, barium, thallium, lead, ammonium, cobalt or nickel, all at 0.01 mol/l concentration. Acetic acid is added to 0.02 mol/l concentration. As terminator we used glycine 0.03 mol/l, acetic acid 0.01 mol/l in all the experiments. In one experiment we used 4 morpholine ethane sulfonic acid (MES) 0.01 mol/l β-alanine 0.01 mol/l as terminator to demonstrate the influence of the terminator on the behavior of the dye molecules. We used crystal violet, ethyl violet, pararosaniline base, neutral red and a mixture of crystal violet and neutral red dyes. The current is as described[1].

RESULTS: DESCRIPTION OF THE ANIONIC ISOTACHOPHORESIS EXPERIMENTS

Results of experiments with Tris as cation in the leading electrolyte

Experimental conditions: leading ion in the beaker; Tris 0.015 mol/l, orthophosphoric acid 0.01 mol/l; Tris 0.03 mol/l, glycine 0.03 mol/l, current 14 mA. A few minutes after switching on the current a very sharp dye layer is formed as a consequence of the adaptation of the concentration of the dye to the concentration of the leading ion. In the two-dimensional dye layer which is formed on top of the shorter branch of the column a few dark points of the bromophenol blue appear in which the dye becomes concentrated.

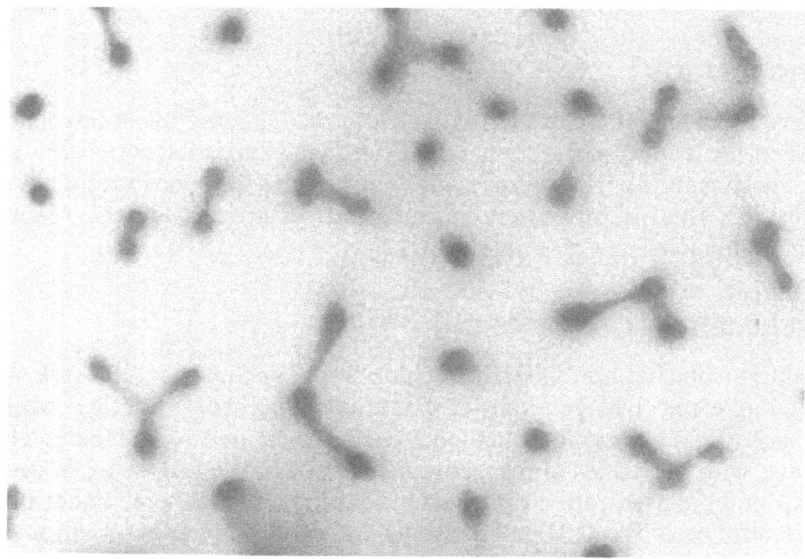

Figure 1 Bromophenol blue is concentrated in islands or points in a Tris 0.015 mol/l, phosphoric acid 0.01 mol/l, Tris 0.03 mol/l, glycine 0.03 mol/l system. The points are attracted to one another in the direction of the lines formed between the points

Seconds later a few hundreds of these points can be observed over the whole surface of the column. As the dark points appear, the zones surrounding the points discolor. As soon as the points are present, connections are formed between neighboring points. Those connections can be seen as a line of bromophenol blue between two points. A few seconds later again, three or four points are interconnected by such color lines. Then the interconnected points migrate to each other and fuse into one large point (Figure 1). If these experiments are repeated at higher current intensity, the lines between the

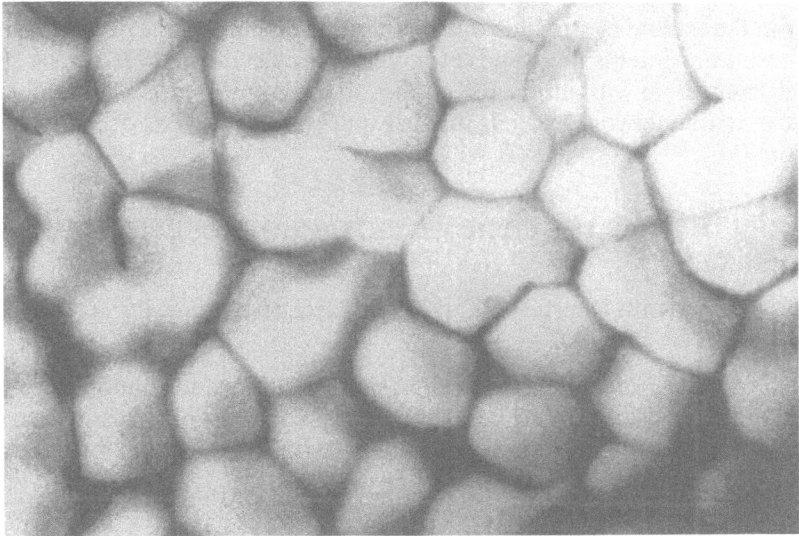

Figure 2 At higher field strength in the leading zone, a complete network of bromophenol blue is formed

different points will be more pronounced (Figure 2). There are now many more connections between the different points. The interconnections have the form of a network. With hydrochloric acid or sulfuric acid as the leading ion similar results are obtained. Larger points occur only in experiments with sulfate as leading ion and bromophenol blue as the dye. If rose bengal or acid red 4 are used as the dye, again similar results are obtained. The meshes of the networks have approximately the same dimension in experiments with chloride, phosphate or sulfate as leading ion.

Results of experiments with imidazole as cation

In the imidazole 0.015 mol/l, orthophosphoric acid 0.01 mol/l, Tris 0.03 mol/l, glycine 0.03 mol/l system at 14 mA, the networks of bromophenol blue appear immediately after the formation of the concentrated dye layer.

The meshes of the network are smaller than the meshes described in the experiments with Tris as cation, but larger than meshes in experiments with aniline as cation.

Results of experiments with aniline as cation

In an aniline 0.03 mol/l, sulfuric acid 0.01 mol/l, Tris 0.03 mol/l, glycine 0.03 mol/l system very regularly constructed networks are formed. The meshes of the network are very small and they appear first in the vicinity of the wall of the column. The networks in this system are much more stable than in the aniline hydrochloric acid or aniline orthophosphoric acid system. In these experiments thousands of points of bromophenol blue can be seen, much more than with imidazole or Tris as the counter ion. The number of meshes in the network exceeds that in experiments with Tris or imidazole as cation.

DESCRIPTION OF THE CATIONIC ISOTACHOPHORESIS EXPERIMENTS

Experiments with Na, K, Rb, Cs, Tl and NH3 as leading ion, crystal violet as dye

When sodium, potassium, rubidium, cesium, thallium and ammonia are used as leading ion, disks are formed. Their center contains much less dye so that they look empty (Figure 3). In experiments with these leading ions, the spe-

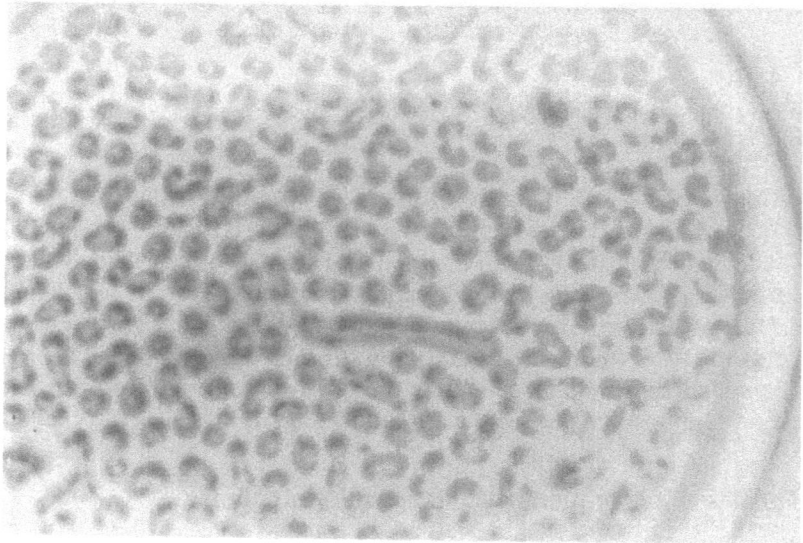

Figure 3 Repulsion of the dye crystal violet by the cesium ion. Formation of circles of crystal violet and formation of uncolored lines

cific result is the formation of a double dye line of crystal violet, in such a way that there is a less concentrated zone in the middle of the dye spot. These double dye lines are visible during the formation of the networks (Figure 4). The phenomena are much more visible when atoms with a large number of electrons in group IA of the Mendeleiev table are used than the small sodium ion.

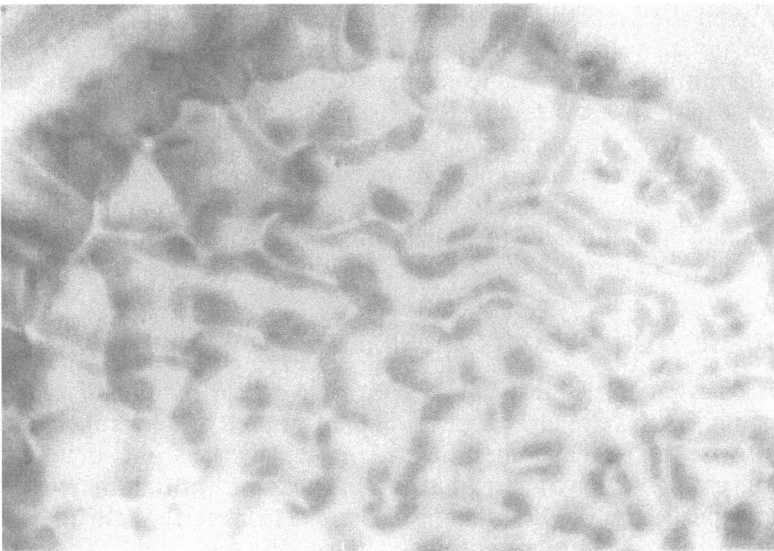

Figure 4 Crystal violet network in an experiment with ammonia 0.01 mol/l as leading ion and glycine 0.03 mol/l, acetic acid 0.01 mol/l pH 4 as terminator. The specific properties of ammonia are demonstrated by the uncolored spaces in the middle of the dye lines

In experiments with ammonia 0.01 mol/l acetic acid, 0.03 mol/l as leading electrolyte and β-alanine 0.03 mol/l MES, 0.01 mol/l pH 5.3 as terminator, big meshes are observed in the network of crystal violet. Here too uncolored lines are formed in the dye layer. The meshes of the network are larger than in the experiments with glycine as the terminator ion. The bigger meshes in these experiments can be related to the higher pH in the terminator zone, or to the use of another anion in the terminator.

Experiments with cations Mg, Ca, Zn, Cd, Ba, Pb, Co, Ni as leading ion

Here too the dye molecule is crystal violet. The same anion and the same terminator are used as in the previous experiments. The leading ions are magnesium, calcium, zinc, cadmium, barium, lead, cobalt and nickel. In all these experiments after the formation of a concentrated dye layer and increasing the current to 40 mA, islands of dye and attraction between the islands, as described in anionic systems, appear.

Experiments with other dye molecules and ammonia as leading ion

In experiments with neutral red dye it was not possible to show the presence of lines with a less concentrated space in the middle of the dye line. On the other hand the patterns formed by pararosaniline base and crystal violet, molecules with a similar structure are fairly similar. There are differences in the behavior between crystal violet and neutral red. We are able to separate a mixture of the dye molecules crystal violet and neutral red in the isotachophoresis boundary by using ammonia as leading ion. This can be realized in the experimental conditions, leading ion in the glass column, dye dissolved in leading ion. The neutral red substance appears in the middle as a single line, around this neutral red there is an uncolored space and around this space the crystal violet dye can be seen.

DISCUSSION OF ANIONIC EXPERIMENTS

In our experimental conditions, one can observe the formation of a very thin and homogeneous dye layer, which will be disrupted by a hydrogen ion or a cation. We propose a hypothesis in order to explain these phenomena, summarized as follows. If we accept that an atom in an electric field acquires magnetic properties by the orientation of the electrons in the outside electric field, we can then consider the isotachophoresis boundary with the dye molecules as a layer of identical magnets arranged one next to the other in a dynamic equilibrium. The Zeeman phenomenon and the Stark phenomenon prove that these orientations of electrons in a magnetic and an electric field really exist. The magnetic hydrogen ion which touches a magnetic dye molecule will disturb this equilibrium by forming a bigger magnet, for instance a complex between a hydrogen ion and a dye molecule or a complex of two dye molecules or a complex between a dye molecule and a leading ion. This bigger magnet will now attract the smaller magnets from the surroundings. By this mechanism the islands can be formed; they need the isotachophoresis conditions, these islands have magnetic properties and attract each other, and this explains all the phenomena. This hypothesis can also explain all our observations in cationic systems.

DISCUSSION OF CATIONIC EXPERIMENTS AND APPLICATION TO THE MITOSIS

If we accept that the electrons change their orbits in the electric field it will be the most external orbits that will be changed in the first place. It is now observed that the NH_4^+ ion and the elements with an unpaired number of electrons in the outermost orbit provoke other phenomena as atoms with a paired number of electrons. The NH_4^+ ion is composed of five atoms with an unpaired number of electrons in the outermost orbit. We observe that the elements from group IA and IIIA of the Mendeleiev table and the ammonia ion provoke the same phenomena. We also observe that the described phenomena caused by elements from groups II, IV and VIII are identical to each other, and finally we see an opposition between the two types of phenomena in the experiments. We also observe in group IA that the phenomena are more easily visible with cesium than with potassium or sodium as leading ion. We can explain this as follows. The hydrogen ion or anion in the neighborhood of the dye layer can touch a leading ion as well as a dye molecule, and then we have the formation of a leading ion complex. If the magnetic moment of this leading ion is in the same sense as the magnetic moment of the dye molecule then we have attraction between the dye molecules and the leading ion and formation of islands composed of both ions. If the magnetic moment of the leading ion is opposed to the magnetic moment of the dye we have magnetic push-off from the dye and a colorless space in the place of the leading ion, the dye molecules then concentrate at a distance from the leading ions. Differences between elements from group I can be explained by differences in the orbits when the elements have more electrons.

These same principles can be applied to explain the differences between the dye molecules. Dye molecules with many atoms of carbon (group IVA) and less atoms of nitrogen (group VA), such as crystal violet or pararosaniline or ethyl violet, behave differently in the neighborhood of ammonia than, for instance, neutral red, which contains relatively more nitrogen. From our results we can suppose that hydrogen and nitrogen have very similar properties and carbon and oxygen are also very similar.

In our opinion these observations, and the hypotheses formulated in this paper, are of importance in explaining movements of macromolecules in the cell under the influence of electric currents especially in relation to the mitosis[1-3]. Also the physical magnetic differences described between potassium and calcium can be of importance for the movement of the chromosomes. In the prophase we will have magnetization of the atoms of the chromosomes. As a result of this, the chromosomes become large magnets and attract each other. In metaphase and anaphase we have a push-off of the chromosomes.

The different membrane pumps can have also a function in the formation of chromosome clusters. We defend the possibility that calcium pumps are responsible for the formation of the chromosomes before the prophase, and in fact stimulate the concentration of the DNA molecule. A magnetic interaction between the calcium ion and DNA will be on the basis of this mechanism. On the other hand the unrolling of a chromosome can be caused by potassium pumps. We know that calcium and potassium have an opposite magnetic effect on the movement of some molecules.

REFERENCES

1. Uyttendaele K (ed.). Mitosis as magnetophoresis, an application to the magnetic fields of the ions. *Laboratory for Dermatology*, Moerstraat 62, Brugge, Belgium, pp. 4–19, 1983
2. Uyttendaele K. Mitosis as magnetophoresis. *Acta Biol Hung*, **37**, 14, 1986
3. Uyttendaele K. Mitosis as magnetophoresis. *Arch Biol (Brux)*, **94**, 511, 1986
4. Everaerts FM, Beckers JL, Verheggen Th PEM. Isotachophoresis. *Journal of Chromatography Library*, Vol. 6. Amsterdam; Elsevier, 1976

Part II
Diagnostic Methods

15

Dynamic exploration of hair growth: critical review of methods available and their usefulness in the clinical trial protocol

D Van Neste
Skinterface
9 rue du Sondart
B-7500 Tournai, Belgium

ABSTRACT

Various methods are available for exploring human hair follicle activity. The aim of this review is to provide the reader with theoretical information on each method, some guidelines about how each test should be performed practically and, when available, data on the reliability of the method. For practical purposes, methods will be separated into three main sections according to the relative trauma and/or damage inflicted to the patient, i.e.:

* invasive,

* semi invasive, and

* non-invasive methods.

Many dimensions and variations characterize the problem of hair growth evaluation (variations according to site, time, physical aspects, biology, etc.). It is to be hoped that standardization of the evaluation techniques of alopecia will further improve the evaluation of the severity of alopecia, as well as the influence of drug administration on the dynamics of the disease process.

INTRODUCTION

Various methods are available for exploring human hair follicle activity. Validity and reproducibility of each of those methods has not always been clearly established. Indeed, they were usually developed in order to answer a specific question of basic interest to the hair growth investigator. The application of the method to the clinical trial protocol that eventually follows is usually restricted to the inventor or his laboratory and no 'ready to use' method is available to the practitioner or the clinical laboratory. The advent of drugs which, during clinical trials, showed to be actively inducing hair regrowth encourages the development of reliable methods which must be easy to use in the clinic. The problem of hair growth evaluation in health and disease covers many aspects, and one has to take into account important parameters such as feasibility in the clinical office and acceptance by the patient whose main concern is usually the cosmetic aspect. This will substantially influence the compliance of the patient to the clinical trial protocol.

The aim of this review is to provide the reader with theoretical information on each method, some guidelines about how each test should be performed practically and, when available, data on the reliability of the method. At this stage one must be aware that the latter aspect is difficult to achieve, because, there are no 'golden standards' available for considering a given zone as being at risk for developing alopecia, so as to be able to establish prognostic criteria, and if so, the timespan necessary to validate such tests requires a large study involving a cohort of patients and volunteers over a period of many years. With this in mind, this paper considers methods for evaluating hair growth. For practical purposes we shall separate them into three main sections according to the relative trauma and/or damage inflicted to the patient, i.e.: invasive, semi-invasive, and non-invasive methods.

INVASIVE METHODS

Taking scalp biopsies is considered to be an invasive method. Local anesthesia is necessary for taking the biopsy, and the definitive removal of a piece of scalp results in absence of hair growth on that site. Hence information about a given group of hair follicles by performing scalp biopsies cannot be repeatedly gathered. This makes it almost impossible to conduct a time-course study of changes in hair growth. Therefore if scalp biopsies are to be used in a clinical trial protocol they should be sufficiently representative of the area under consideration so as to provide statistically reliable information about its overall behavior; good examples are male-pattern baldness and alopecia areata. Up to now such methods are the only ones available for extracting the deepest parts of the hair follicle. Microdissection allows performance of more basic studies on the biological behavior of the cells constitutive of the hair follicle. After separating the hair matrix from the dermal papilla. Results obtained with such methods are discussed in greater detail in other papers published in this volume (see papers 7 and 12).

The dynamic constituent of the hair growth process can be inferred from a scalp biopsy. For this purpose there are two main methods of cutting scalp specimens, i.e. parallel to the scalp surface and vertically along the slant of the follicles. The preselection of the plane of sectioning is of prime importance because two different views of the follicle are displayed.

Sections parallel to the scalp surface

Quantitative data on the deep follicular structure by the so-called 'horizontal sectioning method' have been published by Van Scott and Ekel[1]. Indeed, by serial sectioning it is possible to reach the level of the hair bulb. Then qualitative and quantitative observations can be made. Qualitatively, the action of the dermal papilla upon the overlying epithelial structures can be appreciated by examining serial sections through the hair bulb, for example in cases of uncombable hair syndrome. It is known that the dermal papilla defines the shape of the inner root sheath (Henle's layer) as it terminally differentiates; then by passive complementation the less differentiated cells (i.e. cortex and cuticle) gradually move upwards into a rigid funnel[2], where the hair shaft acquires its final, usually circular, section; in the case of the uncombable hair syndrome we found that the shape of the dermal papilla was irregular, and that the inner root sheath was triangular[3]. From this we concluded that the dermal papilla not only regulates the size, but also modulates the shape of the shaft. More sophisticated measurements allow quantitative evaluation of the volumes of the matrix and dermal papilla[1]. As shown in studies in animals (see Messenger, paper 7 of this volume), the dermal papilla controls the epithelial differentiation process. We performed a comparative study of the dermal–epithelial interacting volumes in a case of the trichorhinophalangeal (TRP) syndrome[4] and attempted a computer-assisted three-dimensional reconstruction of the papilla–matrix complexes in comparison with an age- and sex-matched control[5]. By comparing our volumetric data with those published by Van Scott and Ekel[1] who studied male-pattern baldness, it was suggested that hypotrophic follicles in the TRP syndrome are characterized by atrophic hair bulbs, but that the dermal atrophy was even more pronounced than in male-pattern baldness. The endresult of this imbalance is a decreased hair shaft diameter, even though the epithelial volume is less atrophic than the dermal papilla. This supports the idea that the volume of the dermal papilla plays an active and leading role in conditioning the pattern of epithelial differentiation in the formation of the shaft. As in the model of the animal vibrissal follicles[6], it could be that a constant relationship exists between the volume of the dermal papilla and the volume of the growing hair shaft. Our study focused on the interacting dermal papilla–epithelium complex, and we did not make any correlation with the diameters of hairs produced by individual follicles; hence it seems premature to conclude that a similar relationship has been demonstrated for human follicles, but up to now, qualitative and quantitative studies seem to support the view that dermal papillae play a significant role by modulating both shape and size of the hair shafts.

The serial sectioning method is, however, time-consuming and the information is rather of limited clinical interest. However, as it serves primarily to improve our understanding of the basic biology of a pathological process, we think that it could be worthwhile conducting some more detailed studies in order to generate clinically relevant data; for example as to the hypothetical action of minoxidil on the dermal papilla[7]. Indeed, in order to get easier access to some relevant information about hair growth patterns, Headington[8] published a method which consists in transversely cutting the scalp

145

specimen at the level of the sebaceous duct opening into the follicle or just below this level. By this method it is possible to observe, in a single section, a representative sample of follicles (60–80 terminal hairs in a 6 mm punch biopsy; 40–60 in the case of alopecia according to the calculations of James and Rushton[9]) and to define parameters of growth such as growth phase, diameter of the shaft, number of follicular units, etc. These quantitative data helped to answer some questions concerning the mechanism of action of minoxidil in male-pattern baldness. Indeed, Headington[8] showed that there is no evidence for development of new hair follicles in patients treated with minoxidil, but that the pre-existing atrophic, follicular structures with shortened anagen growth phase grew into larger functional units with normal structure but prolonged anagen phase. These data fit in well with data obtained with the vertical sectioning method, which will be discussed below. The author states that 'there are no observable dysplastic or atypical changes in the follicular germinal epithelium during or after application of minoxidil' and concludes that 'the most probable site of action of minoxidil is on the specialized mesenchymal cells of the follicular dermal papilla'. However, as mentioned earlier, no precise measurements on the dermal papilla volume or its cellular and extracellular components were performed so as to support this mechanism of action.

As stated by Barth[10] in his comments on the Headington method, it could be difficult to estimate reliably the number and diameter of vellus hairs, as the specimen is cut below the level of the matrix of such atrophic follicles. This must be taken into consideration when negative results are reported in diameters of growing hairs and numbers of hair follicles per unit area under treatment with minoxidil; this is contrary to results obtained with the alternative sectioning method, which will be discussed in greater detail in the next section.

Vertical sections and folliculogram studies

The alternative sectioning method for analysis of hair growth patterns is to cut the specimen along the slant of the hair shafts as they merge from the scalp surface. The observation of the hair follicles on thick sections allows definition of growth stage in various categories, and allows measurement of the depth of individual hair bulbs, as well as the diameter of the hair shaft. These quantitative parameters are presented as a graph, a 'folliculogram'. In experimental studies about the balding process in the stumptailed macaque it was shown by Montagna and Uno (reviewed by Uno[11]) that folliculograms appeared to have a similar pattern to those observed in male-pattern baldness of humans. This method has been used to evaluate experimentally the mechanism of action of minoxidil[12] and of antiandrogens in this animal model (see Uno, paper 12 in this volume). The effect of minoxidil seems to prolong the duration of the new anagen phase, allowing the follicle to grow deeper into the scalp tissue and to produce thicker hairs. In the rat model it

146

was shown to initiate early anagen regrowth after telogen effluvium, but did not prolong the genetically predetermined length of the second anagen hair growth phase. This demonstrates that the process of waves of synchronous hair growth in rat only partly reflects the process of hair growth inhibition and/or arrest observed in male-pattern baldness, and that the mechanism of action of minoxidil in this model is to initiate more rapidly normal hair regrowth from telogen follicles. If the invasive methods bring about relevant data in terms of quantification of hair growth/hair growth arrest the main drawback is that the sampling cannot be indefinitely repeated. Therefore the information must be considered as isolated shots for any given site on the scalp.

Some problems in relation with regional variation may arise when selecting the site for repeated sampling. Therefore less invasive methods have been developed.

SEMI-INVASIVE METHODS

Semi-invasive methods consist essentially in pulling a small group of hairs briskly out of the scalp without biopsy. By extracting them at once along the direction of hair growth hair roots are well preserved, and after their classification into anagen, catagen and telogen it is possible to determine a ratio between growing and resting hairs; a technique better known as trichogram[13–16]. It must be remembered that early anagen follicles cannot be identified, as the hair shaft is just merging from the scalp surface. The same also holds true for anagen stages 4 and 5 as at those stages the hair shaft is still inaccessible from the scalp surface and cannot be taken into account in the trichogram. Finally, in balding scalps it is not easy (and in most cases it is impossible) to remove all hairs from a given area. So in the presence of a chronic balding process, with hypotrophic follicles and short vellus hairs, the classical trichogram technique can give rise to false negative data, and it should no longer be considered a valid method for evaluation of hair regrowth in the clinical trial protocol. In more acute situations, however, long hair shafts are still present, and in such cases the trichogram helps to differentiate between anagen and telogen effluvium. Myers and Hamilton[17] suggested measurement of the mean regeneration time, by monitoring during a given period of time the site from which hairs were pulled out in order to measure the time needed to regrow hairs. For obvious reasons this method, which is not easily used in the clinic, has been used in only one instance. As stated abovee, under physiological conditions the classical trichogram gives a quite reasonable approximation of reality; the data are, however, expressed in relative terms and further detailed quantification is needed. For this purpose other methods, such as defining the density of implantation and the diameter of the hair shafts[18], sampling by total epilation of a given zone[19] and definition of the density of implantation[20] are to be taken into account. These methods have been used for demonstrating the effect of antiandrogen administration in female-pattern baldness[21,22] and should be more widely included in future clinical trial protocols for hair growth evaluation. These parameters are indeed of primary importance in time-course evaluation of the intensity of the balding process or, on the contrary, to evaluate the response to treatment in chronic progressive disease states. In a recent exchange of letters it appears that counting hairs on the scalp of a patient in the office could give rise to extremely wide variations from time to time, and between observers, and that the method cannot be considered as entirely reliable[9,23,24]. Indeed in cases of male-pattern baldness there are good reasons to believe that clinical assessment of numbers and diameters of hairs is a hard job to do *in vivo*, and that a large fraction of atrophic hair follicles producing short vellus hairs are ignored with the classical extraction method; it could

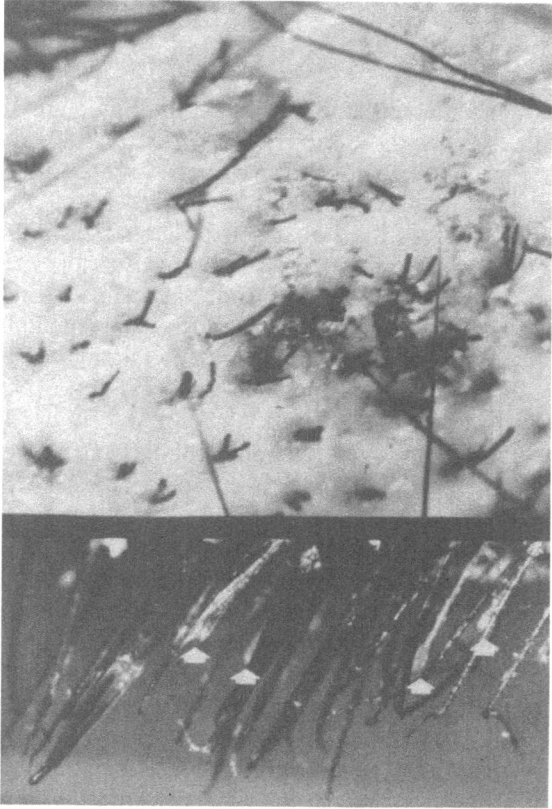

Figure 1 Total semi-invasive extraction of hair follicles: normal scalp of male pattern baldness. Top: face view of the scalp before extraction (magnification x2); below: lateral view of the extracted hair roots (magnification x2). A majority of anagen follicles is present. Telogen hairs are shorter and somewhat more brilliant (less pigment and absence of sheaths; white arrows)

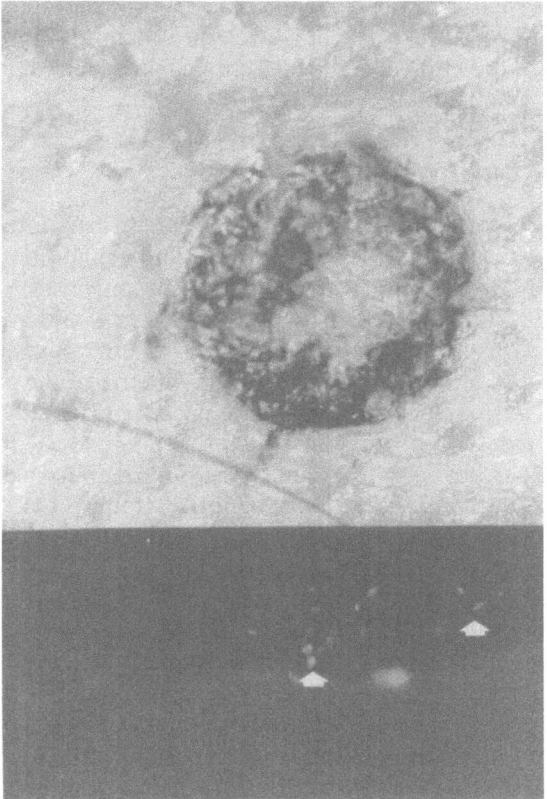

Figure 2 Total semi-invasive extraction of hair follicles: balding scalp of male pattern baldness. Top: face view of the bald scalp before extraction (magnification x2); below: lateral view of the extracted hair roots from the central area shown in a (marked area; magnification x2). A few atrophic telogen hairs are even shorter and thinner as compared to those shown in Figure 1

be that a minor but still significant fraction is being neglected with the so-called 'total epilation technique' (personal unpublished data). Therefore it would seem advisable to develop more appropriate sampling procedures. In a number of preliminary attempts based on the principle of the wax epilation technique we were able to obtain total samples of a given bald spot, but in hairy areas of the scalp total epilation 'en bloc' proved to be painful, and in a series of preliminary experiments reproducibility was not satisfactory. Interestingly, the pictures obtained by this method in a number of samples gave a view of the scalp as if it was 'transparent', and this could be of interest to adapt to the folliculogram technique which was mentioned earlier (Figures 1 and 2). Indeed the extraction force needed for epilating atrophic hairs (most of which are in telogen) is quite low compared to an estimated force of 65 g necessary for extracting a single anagen hair[25]. Some methods derived from the principle of differential extraction forces are currently being tested in the laboratory and in the clinic, but further studies are needed before a ready-to-use diagnostic set could be developed.

NON-INVASIVE METHODS

The least invasive method, i.e. clinical assessment, is currently used most of the time in clinical practice. Taking a history and evaluation of the overall pattern of alopecia, is sufficient for classification purposes in the vast majority of cases. So is it that 'pattern alopecia in males'[26] and in 'females'[27], as well as 'female-pattern baldness in males'[28], have been reported. The severity scales are useful for defining the various grades of the balding process. It must be emphasized here that these classifications were originally proposed for evaluating the presence of long hair patterns, and proved to be useful in evaluating the degree of alopecia. The question is then to quantify what the patient wants us to treat, i.e. the alopecia. Some attempts have been made to analyze macroscopic topography with computer-assisted image analysis of pictures giving an overall view of the scalp. For a detailed discussion of the mathematical aspects of the problem we refer the readers to the papers published by Gibbons and Fiedler-Weiss[29] and Gibbons et al.[30]. At the present time our opinion is that macrotopographic analysis of the clinical patterns, even if computer evaluation is used, gives more a qualitative appreciation of the hair pattern than a real quantification of alopecia. The use of a semi-quantitative evaluation procedure based on the analysis of the overall pattern of alopecia was unable to objectivate any hair growth-promoting effect of polysorbate 60[31].

Linear growth evaluation has been performed by repeated shaving and weighing[32] and by isolating hairs in microcalibrated capillary tubes, which were repeatedly photographed[33]. These methods are refined but cumbersome, and one example of the application of this method is given in an experimental study with an animal model, but we have some doubt as to their feasibility in the dermatology clinic[34].

One of the most recently developed non-invasive methods is known as the 'phototrichogram'[35,36]. The combination of this method with computer-assisted image analysis is still a matter of debate, and must be critically studied. Some investigators[29,30] reviewed some of the mathematical aspects that could be applied to this method. We (see paper 16 in this volume) and others used the computer-assisted methodology in relation with close-up photography[37,38].

In a prospective study of proxigraphic photography we came to the conclusion that the best method would be a fully automated analysis procedure of hairs on a given site[39]. Some problems arise with variability during the preparation of the site to be photographed and it is not excluded that during the preparation of the area for picture taking, i.e. while cutting hairs and shav-

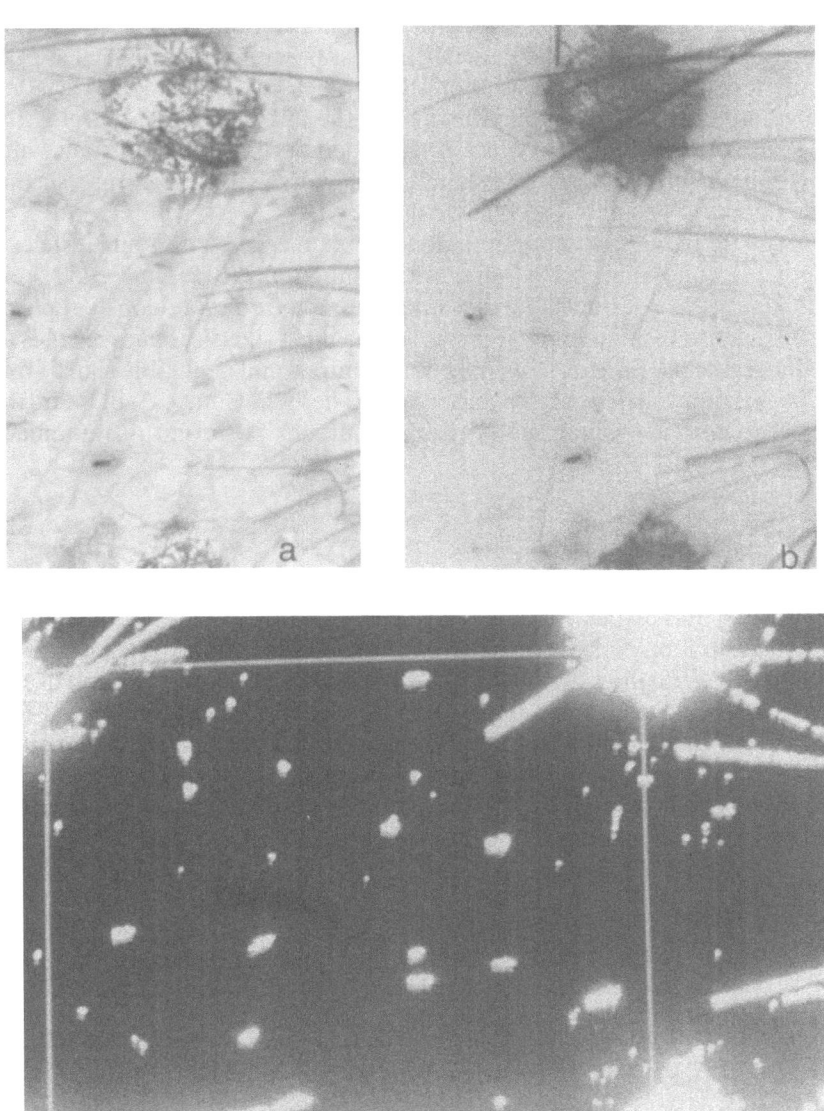

Figure 3 Phototrichogram evaluation. (a) Scalp photography without preparation; (b) scalp immersion photography of the same site at the same point in time; (c) computer-generated binary picture of the same zone

ing of the scalp, some hairs at least could be removed. Indeed, by examining the proximal endings of specimens of cut hairs we occasionally identified telogen bulbs, and in one instance, out of several hundred hairs examined, an anagen hair bulb. This illustrates that some error, most probably of no sig-

151

nificance, can be generated during the preparation of the scalp; we advise cutting and sampling the hairs with the least possible traction. Some other parameters (such as variations of density along a given hair shaft, variations of pigmentation, errors in parallax due to the angle between merging hair and scalp, the depth of field which is small and becomes of importance after a given period of growth), are significant factors to be taken into account when quantitative analysis is being considered.

A more detailed discussion of this problem is given by Van Neste *et al.* (paper 16), concerning scalp immersion photography (SIP). Indeed, it seems to us that SIP constitutes a further improvement of the previously reported phototrichogram techniques (Figure 3). The most significant advantages are a reduction of the third dimension, better contrast and negligible signals from the background such as scales and sebum. These advantages will be further subject to critical evaluation in order to routinely perform fully automated CAIA.

CONCLUSION

Because of their many dimensions (site, time, physical aspects, biology, mathematical aspects associated with image analysis) the problems related to hair growth evaluation address themselves to a multidisciplinary team capable of coping with difficulties arising from each of the facets. Some of those aspects have been reviewed in this paper, and more details can be obtained from reading the papers cited in the reference list. It is to be hoped that standardization of the evaluation techniques of alopecia will further improve the evaluation of the severity of alopecia, as well as the influence of drug administration on the dynamics of the disease process.

REFERENCES

1. Van Scott EJ, Ekel TM. Geometric relationship between the matrix of the hair bulb and its dermal papilla in normal and alopecic scalp. *J Invest Dermatol*, **31**, 281–287, 1958
2. Chase HB. The behavior of pigment cells and epithelial cells in the hair follicle. In *The Biology of Hair Growth* (Montagna W, Ellis RA, eds), pp. 229–237. New York: Academic Press, 1958
3. Van Neste D, Armijo-Subieta F, Tennstedt D, Mrena E, Marchal G, Lachapelle JM, Gengoux P, Dumont M, Decroix J. The uncombable hair syndrome: four non-familial cases of pili trianguli et canaliculi. *Arch Dermatol Res*, **217**, 223–227, 1981
4. Van Neste D, Dumortier M. Tricho-rhino-phalangeal syndrome. Disturbed geometric relationships between hair matrix and dermal papilla in scalp hair bulbs. *Dermatologica*, **165**, 16–23, 1982
5. Van Neste D, Thievenaz H, Dumortier JL, Dumortier M. Spatial relationships of the matrix–papilla unit of the hair bulb: a computer-assisted representation in 3 dimensions. *Ann Dermatol Vénéréol*, **113**, 767–771, 1986
6. Ibrahim L, Wright EA. A quantitative study of hair growth using mouse and rat vibrissal follicles. 1. Dermal papilla volume determines hair volume. *J Embryol Exp Morphol*, **72**, 209–224, 1982

7. Headington JT. Hair follicle biology and topical minoxidil: possible mechanism of action. *Dermatologica*, **175**, suppl. 2 19–22, 1987
8. Headington JT. Transverse microscopic anatomy of the human scalp: a basis for a morphometric approach to disorders of the hair follicle. *Arch Dermatol*, **120**, 449–456, 1984
9. James KC, Rushton DH. Evaluation technics for male pattern baldness. *J Am Acad Dermatol*, **14**, 849–850, 1986
10. Barth JH. Measurement of hair growth. *Clin Exp Dermatol*, **11**, 127–138, 1986
11. Uno, H. Stumptailed macaques as a model of male-pattern baldness. In *Models in Dermatology* (Maibach HI, Lowe NJ, eds), pp. 159–169. Basel: Karger, 1987
12. Uno H, Cappas A, Schlagel C. Cyclic dynamics of hair follicles and the effect of minoxidil on the bald scalps of stumptailed macaques. *Am J Dermatopathol*, **7**, 283–297, 1985
13. Van Scott EJ, Reinertson RP, Stein Muller R. The growing hair roots of the human scalp and morphological changes therein following amethopterine therapy. *J Invest Dermatol*, **29**, 197–204, 1957
14. Kligman AM. Pathologic dynamics of human hair loss. *Arch Dermatol*, **83**, 175–195, 1961
15. Barman JM, Pecoraro V, Astore I. Method, technic and computations in the study of the trophic state of the human scalp hair. *J Invest Dermatol*, **42**, 421–425, 1964
16. Barman JM, Astore I, Pecoraro V. The normal trichogram of the adult. *J Invest Dermatol*, **44**, 233–236, 1965
17. Myers RJ, Hamilton JB. Regeneration and rate of growth of hair in man. *Ann NY Acad Sci*, **53**, 562–568, 1951
18. Runne U, Martin H. Veränderungen von Telogenrate, Haardichte, Haardurchmesser und Wachstumsgeschwindigkeit bei der androgenetischen Alopezie des Mannes. *Hautarzt*, **37**, 198–204, 1986
19. Peereboom-Wynia JDR. Hair root characteristics of the human scalp hairs in health and disease. Thesis, 1982
20. Rushton H, James KC, Mortimer CH. The unit area trichogram in the assessment of androgen-dependent alopecia. *Br J Dermatol*, **109**, 429–437, 1983
21. Van der Willigen AH, Peereboom-Wynia JDR, Van Joost Th, Stolz E. A preliminary study of the effect of 11 alpha-hydroxyprogesterone on the hair growth in men suffering from androgenetic alopecia. *Acta Derm Venereol (Stockh)*, **67**, 82–85, 1985
22. Mortimer CH, Rushton H, James KC. Effective medical treatment for common baldness in woman. *Clin Exp Dermatol*, **9**, 342–350, 1984
23. Olsen EA, Pinnell SR, Weiner MS, DeLong E. Topical minoxidil in early male pattern baldness. *J Am Acad Dermatol*, **13**, 185–192, 1985
24. Olsen EA, Pinnell SR, Weiner MS, DeLong E. Evaluation technics for male pattern baldness. *J Am Acad Dermatol*, **14**, 850–851, 1985
25. Tsuda K. Study on the extractive properties of human head hair. *J Kyoto Prefecture Medical University*, **61**, 936–940, 1957
26. Hamilton JB. Patterned long hair in man; types and incidence. *Ann NY Acad Sci*, **53**, 708–714, 1951
27. Ludwig E. Classification of the types of androgenetic alopecia (common baldness) occurring in the female sex. *Br J Dermatol*, **97**, 247–254, 1977
28. Kuhlwein A. Androgene Alopezie vom weiblichen Typ beim man. *Z Hautkr*, **60**, 576–578, 1985
29. Gibbons RD, Fiedler-Weiss VC. Computer-aided quantification of scalp hair. *Dermatol Clin*, **4**, 627–640, 1986
30. Gibbons RD, Fiedler-Weiss VC, West DP, Lapin G. Quantification of scalp hair: a computer-aided methodology. *J Invest Dermatol*, **86**, 78–82, 1986
31. Groverman HD, Ganiats T, Klauber MR. Lack of efficacy of Polysorbate 60 in the treatment of male pattern baldness. *Arch Intern Med*, **145**, 1454–1458, 1985

32. Hamilton JB. Age, sex, and genetic factors in the regulation of hair growth in man: a comparison of caucasian and japanese populations. In *The Biology of Hair Growth* (Montagna W, Ellis RA, eds), pp. 399–433. New York: Academic Press, 1958

33. Saitoh M, Uzuka M, Sakamoto M. Human hair cycle. *J Invest Dermatol*, **54**, 65–81, 1970

34. Rittmaster RS, Uno H, Povar ML, Mellin TN, Loriaux DL. The effect of 4-MA, a 5 alpha-reductase inhibitor, on the development of baldness in the stumptailed macaque. *J Clin Endocrinol Metab*, **65**, 188–193, 1987

35. Courtois M, Giland S, Grollier JF. A contribution to the study of the growth and shedding of hair. In *Capelli e Medecina Estetica – Hair and Aesthetic Medicine* (Montagna W, Serri F, Bartoletti L, Celleno L, Morganti F, Secchi, GF, eds) pp. 43–53. Salus Internazionale, 1984

36. Bouhanna P. The phototrichogram: a technique for the objective evaluation of the diagnosis and course of diffuse alopecias. In *Capelli e Medecina Estetica – Hair and Aesthetic Medicine* (Montagna W, Serri F, Bartoletti L, Celleno L, Morganti F, Secchi, GF, eds) pp. 277–280. Salus Internazionale, 1984

37. Pelfini C, Calligaro A. Some notes on the evaluation of hair growth by means of morphometric computerized analysis. *J Appl Cosmetol*, **4**, 67–76, 1986

38. Guarrera M, Ciulla MP. A quantitative evaluation of hair loss: the phototrichogram. *J Appl Cosmetol*, **4**, 61–66, 1986

39. Van Neste D, De Coster W. Scalp immersion proxigraphy (SIP): a novel approach for hair growth evaluation by computer assisted image analysis. *Bioeng Skin*, (in press)

16

Phototrichogram analysis: technical aspects and problems in relation to automated quantitative evaluation of hair growth by computer-assisted image analysis

D Van Neste*, M Dumortier* and W De Coster**
*Skinterface, Tournai and **CEBAN, Rijksuniversiteit Gent, Gent, Belgium

ABSTRACT

Non-invasive methods are particularly suited for evaluation of the dynamics of hair growth and/or hair growth arrest. In particular, the duration of the growth phase of each individual follicle cannot be repeatedly estimated by invasive methods, i.e. skin biopsies which give an 'irreversible snapshot' of a dynamic process.

Computer-assisted image analysis (CAIA) is available, and high-quality pictures are prerequisite to the automated data treatment procedure. In this paper, we compare figures obtained from shaved scalp areas (96 mm^2, taken twice at a 48 h interval) with three photographic methods and evaluate their relative interest in relation with automatic CAIA. Slides were taken under standardized enlargement (x3) and lighting (Medical Nikkor®, Nikon). The three methods are as follows: (0) without preparation, (1) immersion photography with mineral oil or (2) with application of a glass slide without immersion.

All figures were subjected to the following procedure: a preselected window of each image is automatically scanned (IBAS II, Kontron, FRG) and binary pictures obtained with a given threshold value (pixels of hair density ($h\partial$) $\neq$ scalp density); hair growth is estimated as: ([area of $h\partial$ 48 h after shaving – area of $h\partial$ immediately after shaving]/area of scanned window).

Our results are based on the observation of 50 pictures. By visual examination, a better contrast between hair and scalp was obtained by immersion photography. The latter also reduced the third dimension. Blurred pictures were generated by method (2) and data from method (0) were obscured by the presence of squames and sebum.

By automated CAIA, however, the number of discrete zones with $h\partial$ is extremely variable due to the presence of segments of varying density within a single hair. As a rule, an artificially high number of hair segments were recorded.

In order to reduce such artefacts, further improvements of software are necessary. This will also help to prevent the potential bias introduced by the observer during interactive selection of 'hair' and 'non-hair' zones in a given picture.

INTRODUCTION

Non-invasive methods are particularly well suited for evaluation of the dynamics of hair growth and/or hair growth arrest. In particular, the growth phase of individual follicles cannot be repeatedly estimated by invasive methods (for a review of this topic see Van Neste, paper 15 in this volume). Repeated picture-taking of a preselected zone of the scalp and evaluation of the percentage of growing and resting hairs has been named 'phototrichogram'[1,2].

Computer-assisted image analysis (CAIA) is now available for experimental purposes. Some of the technical, essentially mathematical problems have been discussed for pictures giving an overall view of the scalp[3,4] (distance ± 1 m). Close-up photography without preparation has already been used for computer-assisted phototrichogram analysis (see Pelfini, paper 23 in this volume, and refs 5 and 6). However, some technical problems which will be illustrated and discussed below, still make it necessary to 'improve' interactively the original pictures (i.e. the observer has to select in the recorded picture which hairs will be taken into account for image analysis and which hairs will be discarded). As with any other observers' intervention, there is a risk of introducing a bias in the evaluation procedure. In this case the CAIA method originally proposed to improve the objective measurement of hair growth would fail to achieve its goal, especially in the field of product development and clinical trials.

In this paper we discuss standardized picture-taking, and we tested three photographic methods in order to evaluate feasibility of automatic CAIA in the field of hair growth investigation. We show that 'scalp immersion photography' or 'SIP' seems to substantially improve the quality of contrast between hair and scalp. This is especially appreciated in the presence of dandruff, a condition that occurs frequently in association with pattern baldness. Quantitative analysis is possible but the automated procedure needs further improvement of imaging and analysis methods.

MATERIAL AND METHODS

Patients and pictures

Five subjects (four males and one female) with pattern baldness were included in this study; 24 x 36 mm slides were taken from shaved scalp areas (two per individual, 96 mm², at a 48 h interval) with three different photographic methods in order to evaluate their relative interest in relation to automatic CAIA.

Slides were taken under standardized enlargement (x3) and lighting (Medical Nikkor, Nikon)

(0) without preparation,

(1) with immersion (mineral oil on glass slide), or

(2) with a glass slide (without mineral oil).

Computer-assisted image analysis

All figures were subjected to the following procedure (IBAS II, Kontron, FRG; the basic principles of which are illustrated schematically in Figure 1.):

1. recording of the image (Figure 2a and 2b)

2. contrast enhancement (Figure 3a and 3b)

3. binary pictures are produced with predetermined threshold value, i.e. (pixels of hair density ($h\partial$) ≠ scalp density ($s\partial$))

4. preselected window for measurement (Figures 2b, 3a, 4)

5. automatic elimination of hairs crossing the frame of the window (Figure 4)

6. automatic scanning and

7. hair growth estimation: ([area% of $h\partial$ 48 h after shaving – area% of $h\partial$ immediately after shaving]/area% of scanned window) x 100.

Steps 1 and 2 of the CAIA procedure are illustrated in Figures 2 and 3 for photographic method (0) and (1) (i.e. without preparation or SIP (*a* and *b* respectively)). Step 5 is illustrated in Figure 4 and shows the binary image after processing of the recorded picture shown in Figure 1b.

Hair diameter measurement

Two observers (DM, VND) independently measured hair shaft diameters in a sample of hairs cut from an area to be photographed. A light microscope equipped with a lateral drawing objective was used and measurements were calibrated with a 200 x 0.01 mm ruler (Leitz, Wetzlar, FRG). The photographs taken from that zone were scanned with CAIA and the frequency distributions of diameters of the individually measured hairs were recorded.

157

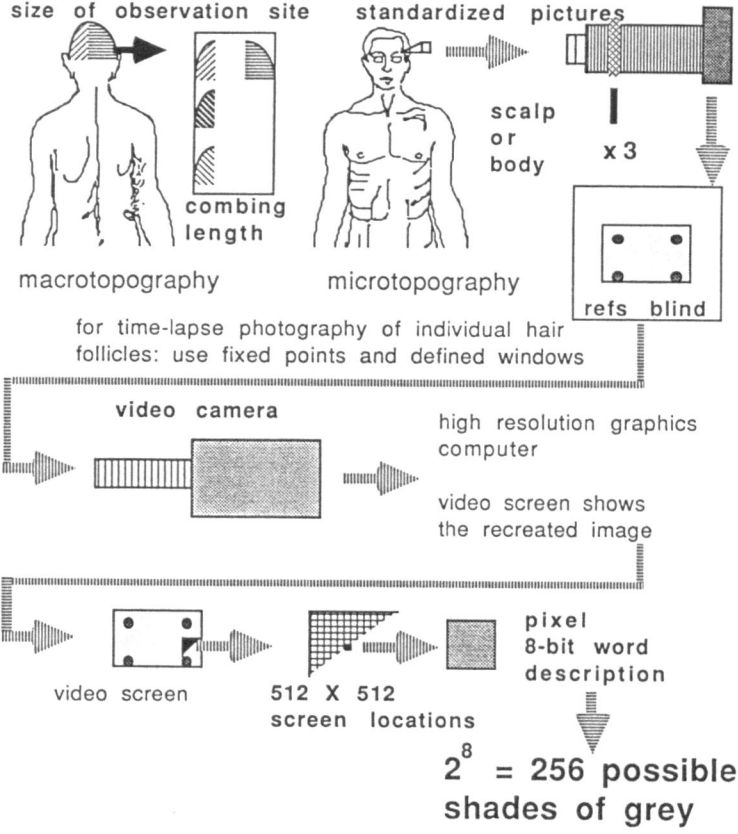

Figure 1 Phototrichogram: Picture-taking and computer-assisted image analysis. After selecting a shaved and marked zone on the scalp (8 mm x 12 mm) pictures are taken under standardized lighting and enlargement. The same procedure is repeated 48 h later. The pictures are taken to the laboratory for CAIA (IBAS II, Kontron, FRG) with the following steps: (1) recording of the image, (2) contrast enhancement, (3) binary pictures, predetermined threshold value, (pixels of hair density ($h\partial$) $\neq$ scalp density ($s\partial$)), (4) preselected window for measurement, (5) automatic elimination of hairs crossing the frame, (6) automatic scanning and, (7) hair growth estimation

RESULTS

Our results are based on the observation of 50 pictures.

By visual examination, and after recording of the original pictures with the video camera (step 1), a better contrast between hair and scalp was obtained by scalp immersion photography (compare Figures 2a,b and 3a,b). SIP

158

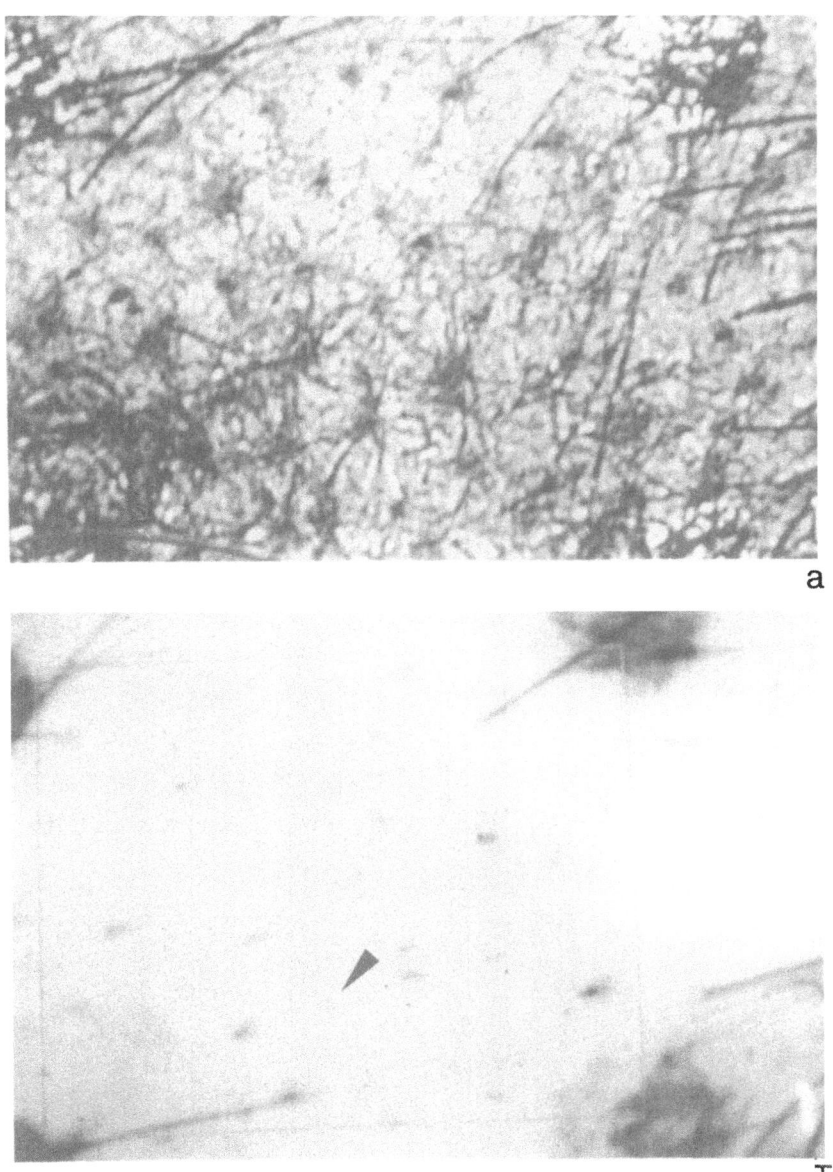

Figure 2 Pictures taken under standardized enlargement (x3) and lighting (Medical Nikkor®, Nikon) with method (0) without preparation (Figure 2a) and method (1) with immersion (Figure 2b). Recording of the pictures reproduced on the high-resolution video screen show marked differences. Hairs are easily identified in (b) because the scalp background is reduced to nothing. Arrowhead relates to comment of Figure 4

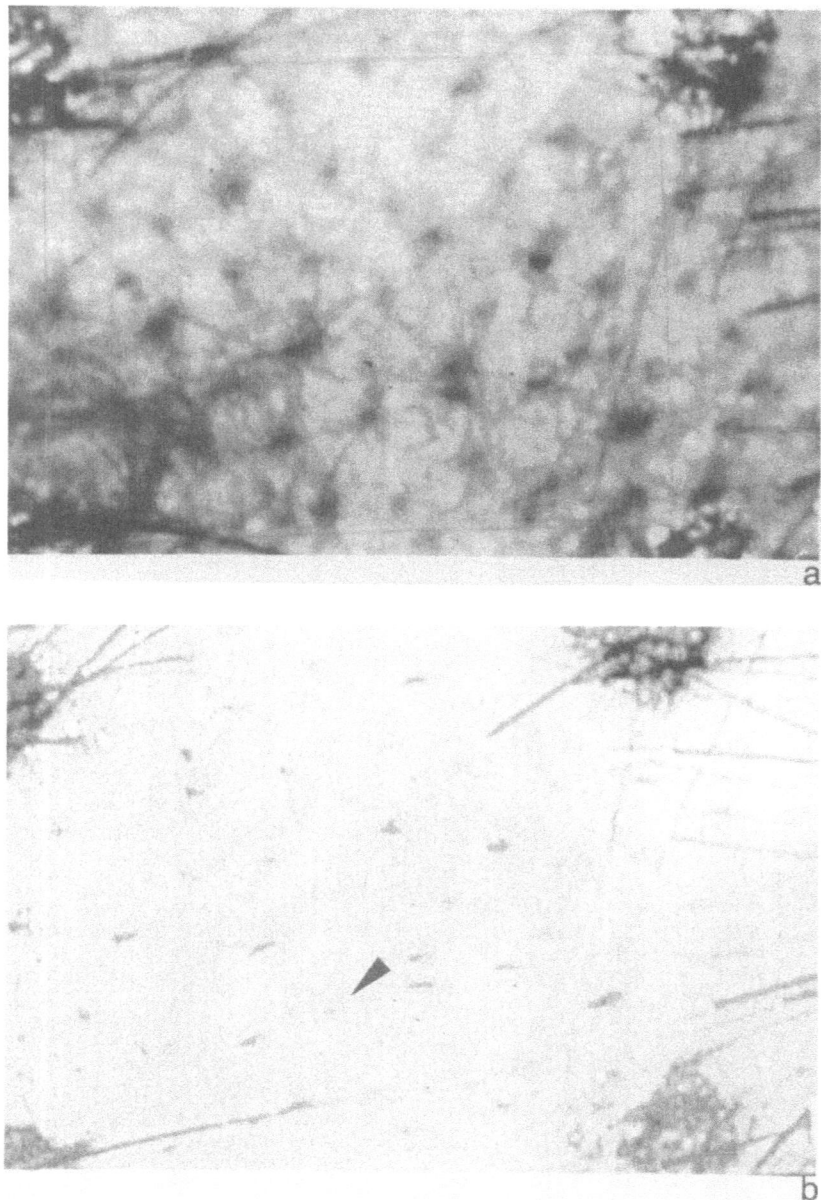

Figure 3 Contrast enhancement step of the CAIA method (step 2 in Figure 1). Pictures shown in Figures 2a and 2b obtained with photographic methods (0) and (1) are shown after contrast enhancement in *a* and *b* respectively. Arrowhead relates to comment on Figure 4

also reduced the third dimension. This is of little importance on freshly shaved areas but becomes significant after a period of time during which hair growth proceeds (48 h in our study). Blurred pictures were generated by method (2) and data from method (0) were obscured by the presence of squames and sebum (see for example Figures 2a and 3a).

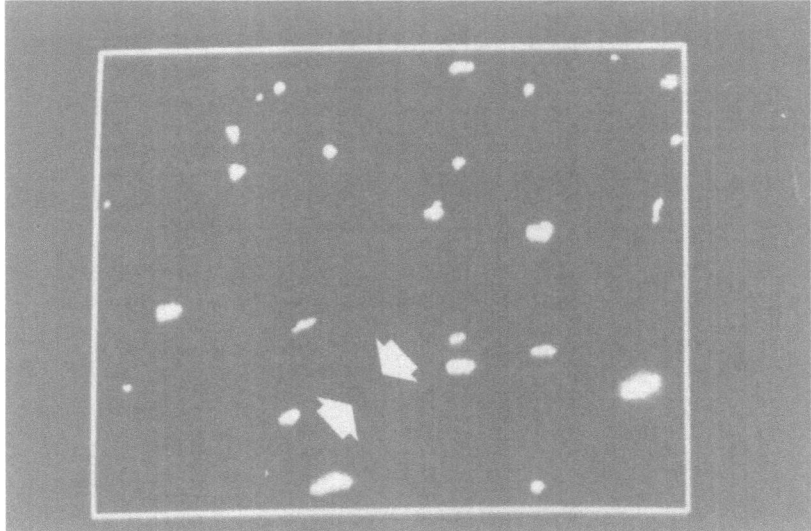

Figure 4 Binary picture of Figure 1b after elimination of the hairs which crossed the preselected window. Some hairs are not identified by automated CAIA: the white arrows in this Figure show the presumptive location of one of the 'vanishing' hairs, which is marked by a black arrowhead in Figures 2b and 3b. Needless to say that it is almost impossible to identify that hair, as well as others, in Figure 2a. After contrast enhancement (Figure 3a) it is shown to be obscured by the density of the follicular ostium

Some of the problems of binary thresholding which are related to the distinction between hair and scalp background are illustrated in Figure 5.

The number of discrete zones with $h\vartheta$ is variable, due to the presence of segments of varying density within single hair (see also steps 1–7 of the CAIA procedure).When the frames of the $h\vartheta$ zones as they show up after CAIA are put on the original picture (Figure 6) some differences are observed: some hairs are unidentified (large arrowhead in Figure 6) and some hairs are viewed as a series of individual segments (five small arrows in Figure 6) As a rule, a variable but usually artificially high number of hair segments were recorded. It must also be stated at this stage that a number of hairs (small and/or less pigmented, especially at t_0, immediately after shaving) are not recognized as such by the automated CAIA procedure. Such 'vanishing' hairs are shown in Figures 2b, 3b, and 6. Even though clearly visible in Figure 2b

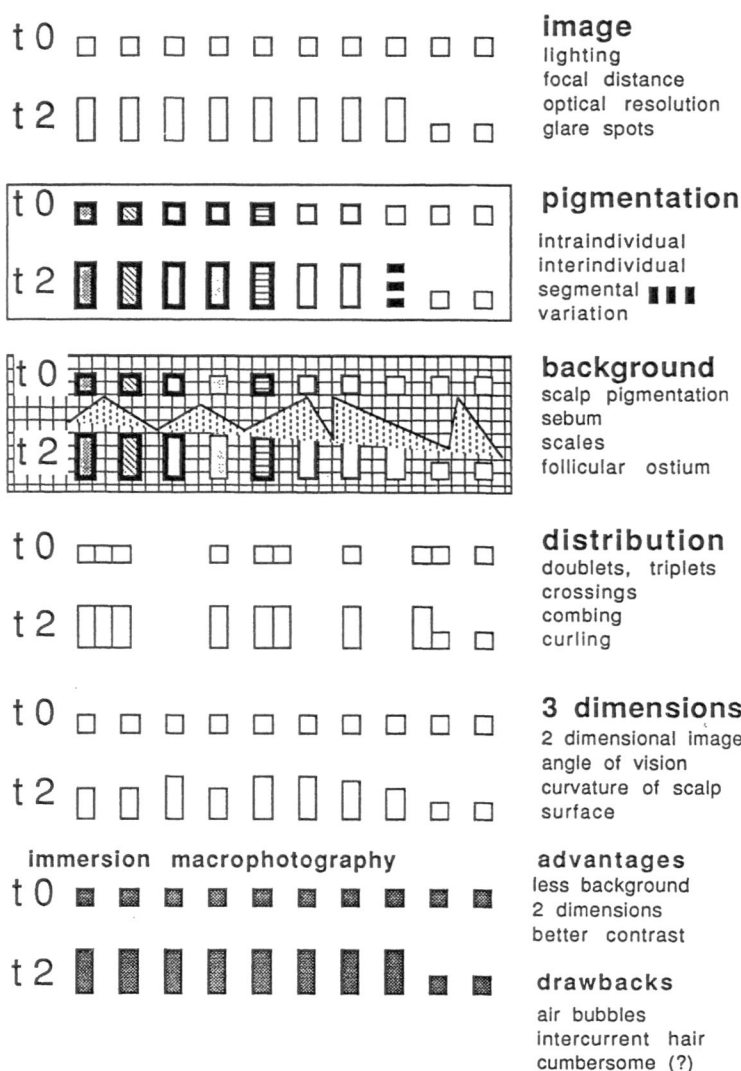

Figure 5 Some of the problems of automated CAIA of phototrichogram. As stated in the text, evaluation of dynamics of hair growth needs comparative analysis of two pictures taken at different times (in our case 48 h). Some of the problems of quantification of hair growth seem to be overcome by scalp immersion photography

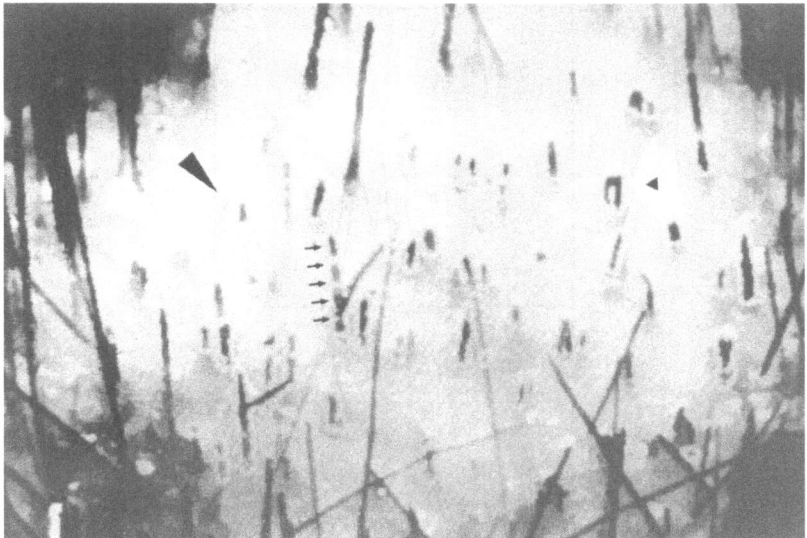

Figure 6 Overlay of CAIA estimated hair zones on the originally recorded picture. There are some 'vanishing' hairs (black arrowhead), segmented hairs (five small arrows) and 'extra-large' hairs (white arrow with triangle) as a result of 'doublets'. These artefacts make automated determination of numbers of hair on the spot quite unreliable

(arrowhead), contrast enhancement seems to reduce density (3b) and the end result is 'vanishing' hair after binary thresholding as shown in 4 (white arrows). Hence, automatic CAIA determination of scalp hair density, as well as of individual hair length, cannot yet be considered a reliable method.

A correlative study between hair diameter measurement by conventional microscopic techniques and with CAIA was made. As shown in Figure 7 (top) there was an excellent correlation of the distribution curves obtained by observers 1 and 2. The same comment can be made for correlation of the absolute data (original pixel data + 5, horizontal arrows) obtained with CAIA after shifting (Figure 7, middle) and data recorded with light microscope measurements (Figure 7, bottom).

Hence it is possible to estimate hair diameters reliably by CAIA. As extra-large hairs (arrowheads in Figure 7 middle show, doublets and triplets as pointed out by the white arrow and triangle in Figure 8) are easily identified because their diameter is two or three times the mean diameter of the sample; their values can be transformed by simple division. With this exception in mind, it can be shown that shifting of the distribution curve of the CAIA data fits well with the microscopic data made by two independent observers.

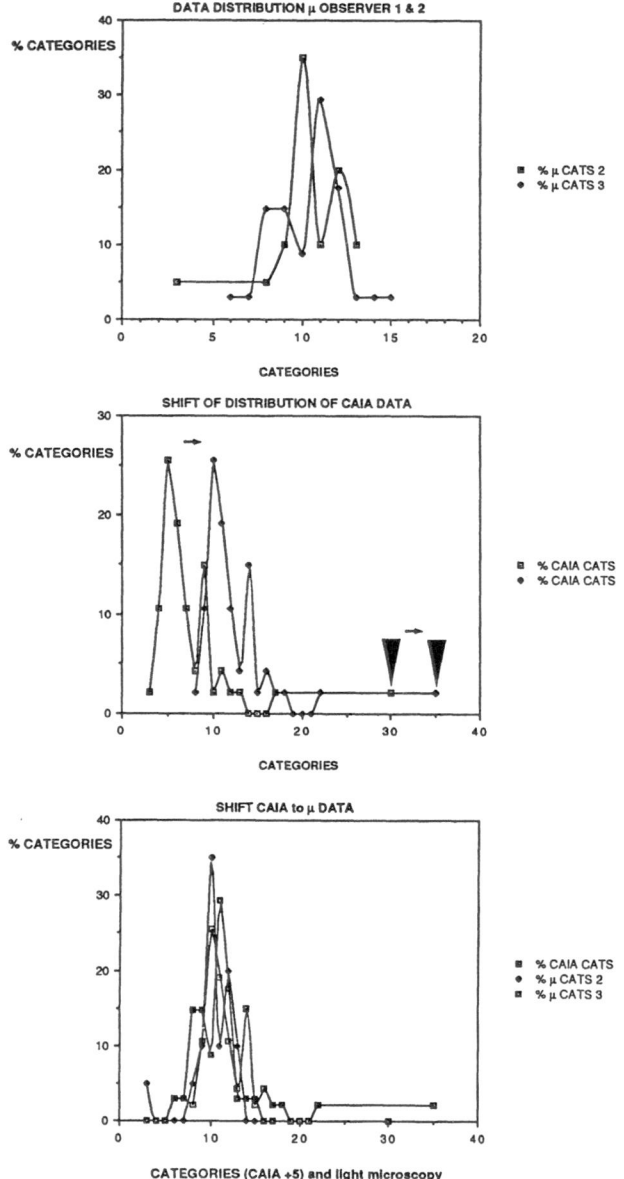

Figure 7 Hair diameter measurements. Top: frequency distribution curves of hair diameters in a sample of hairs cut from an area to be photographed (two observers). Middle: the photographs were scanned with CAIA and the individual diameters of the measured hairs were recorded. Extra-large hairs (doublets (white arrow and triangle in Figure 7) and triplets (vertical arrowheads)) are easily identified. Bottom: after shifting of the distribution curve of the CAIA data (horizontal arrows in middle picture) the distribution curve fits well with the one obtained by microscopic observation (bottom)

DISCUSSION

In this study, we confirm the impression gained from preliminary studies, performed during the past two years, that scalp immersion photography, i.e. SIP constitutes a further improvement of the previously reported phototrichogram techniques[1,2,5,6]. We attempted to appreciate the effect of SIP such as reducing the third dimension, increasing contrast and decreasing the background from scales and sebum, in order to perform automated CAIA.

By quantitative image analysis, variability of hair density and length estimation according to the picture technique, sites and individuals, is partly due to artefacts, and it is problematical whether automated CAIA quantification is actually readily available for clinical use and evaluation of hair growth. However, when hair diameters are to be evaluated it seems, from our present preliminary experiment, that CAIA gives quite reliable data.

In order to reduce the artefacts mentioned above, further improvements in photographic method and software are necessary. This will essentially help to prevent the potential bias introduced by the observer during interactive selection of 'hair' and 'non-hair' zones in a given picture.

REFERENCES

1. Courtois M, Giland S, Grollier JF. A contribution to the study of the growth and shedding of hair. In *Capelli e Medecina Estetica – Hair and Aesthetic Medicine*. (Montagna W, Serri F, Bartoletti L, Celleno L, Morganti F, Secchi, GF, eds), pp. 43–53. Salus Internazionale, 1984
2. Bouhanna P. The phototrichogram: a technique for the objective evaluation of the diagnosis and course of diffuse alopecias. In *Capelli e Medecina Estetica – Hair and Aesthetic Medicine*. (Montagna W, Serri F, Bartoletti L, Celleno L, Morganti F, Secchi, GF, eds), pp. 277–280. Salus Internazionale, 1984
3. Gibbons RD, Fiedler-Weiss VC. Computer-aided quantification of scalp hair. *Dermatol Clin*, 4, 627–640, 1986
4. Gibbons RD, Fiedler-Weiss VC, West DP, Lapin G. Quantification of scalp hair: a computer-aided methodology. *J Invest Dermatol*, 86, 78–82, 1986
5. Guarrera M, Ciulla MP. A quantitative evaluation of hair loss: the phototrichogram. *J Appl Cosmetol*, 4, 61–66, 1986
6. Pelfini C, Calligaro A. Some notes on the evaluation of hair growth by means of morphometric computerized analysis. *J Appl Cosmetol*, 4, 67–76, 1986

17
PIXE microanalysis in green hair

KH Kurz*, HF Merk*, GK Steigleder*, M Höfert** and B Gonsior**
*Universitäts-Hautklinik, Köln and **Institut für Experimentalphysik III, Ruhr-Universität, Bochum, Federal Republic of Germany

ABSTRACT

PIXE microanalysis, a special X-ray fluorescence technique (PIXE = proton-induced X-ray emission), allows the determination of trace elements, such as copper and zinc, down to a level of 1 ppm. By means of this method cryo-sections of the hair shafts of a 25-year-old female patient suffering from the green hair syndrome were measured. The distribution of Cu, Zn, Ca and S in a 10 μm disk perpendicular to the hair axis could be evaluated. Our results showed a high content of Cu and Zn at the hair shaft periphery, whereas the center of the hair shaft was free of copper. Total concentration was: Cu 6638 ppm, Zn 1353 ppm, Ca 3004 ppm and S 43,788 ppm.

All other elements with an atomic number $Z \geq 14$ were in normal range. After topical treatment with an aqueous solution of 1.5% 1-hydroxyethyl diphosphonic acid, the copper content was found markedly decreased in the periphery of the hair with 684 ppm. Zn and Ca were decreased too with 562 ppm and 867 ppm respectively, whereas the concentration of sulfur was nearly unaffected with 37,186 ppm. Our results show that in opposite to alternative methods, PIXE is able to detect and quantify trace elements in different areas of the hair shaft and as such, it is a most sensitive method to control therapeutic effects.

INTRODUCTION

PIXE microanalysis, a special X-ray fluorescence technique (PIXE = proton-induced X-ray emission), enables the determination of trace elements, such as copper and zinc, down to a level of 1 ppm. Using this method cryosections of the hair shafts of a patient suffering from the green hair syndrome were measured. The distribution of Cu, Zn, Ca and S in a 10 μm disk perpendicular to the hair axis could be evaluated before and after treatment.

MATERIAL AND METHOD

Case report

The 25-year-old female patient observed a green discoloration of the scalp hair for two months. Green scalp hairs were plucked from the occipital region (Figure 1) and cut carefully 1 cm distal from the hair follicle, where the green coloration appeared to be highest.

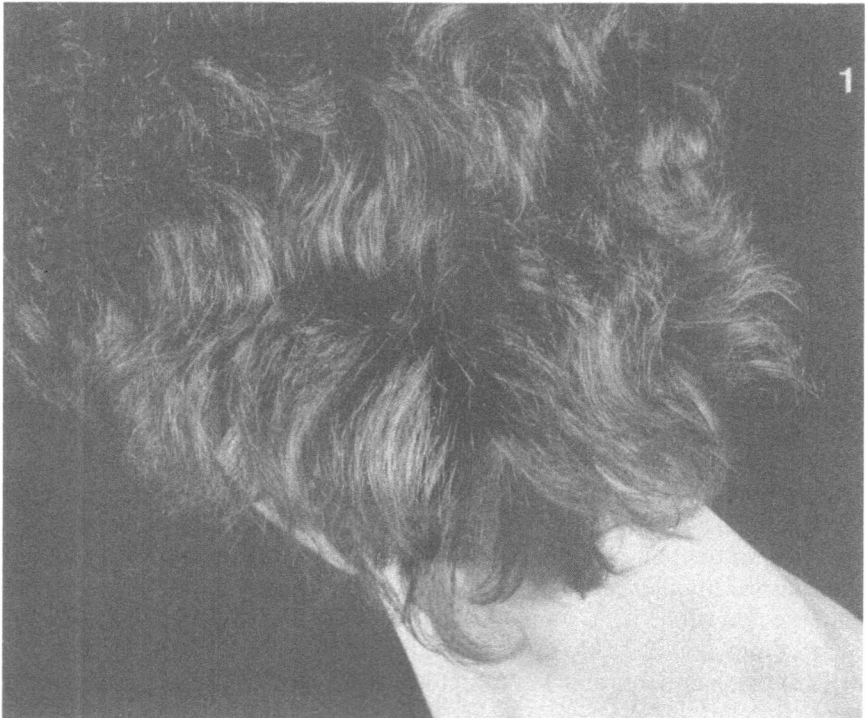

Figure 1   Patient with green hair. Note discoloration of the hair tips

Hair processing

The hairs were put in water (50 μl) and deep-frozen with liquid nitrogen at –196 °C. Cryosections of 10 μm thickness were cut perpendicular to the hair axis at a temperature of –20 °C. The sections were fixed as thin (< 0.5 μm) Formvar foils without any supplement and then completely dried at a temperature of –20 °C. The PIXE method, in combination with the Bochum proton microprobe, was used for determination of the elemental distributions. The analyses were accomplished using a lateral resolution of 5 x 5 μm^2, a beam current of 1 nA, and a proton energy of 3 MeV. The Bochum proton

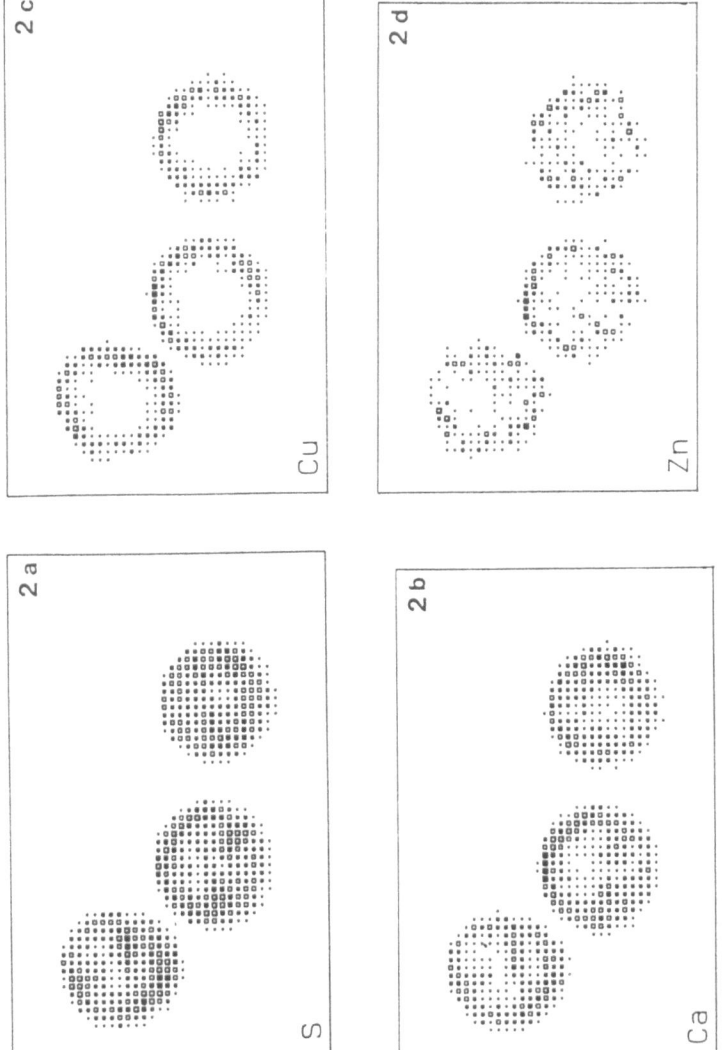

Figure 2 The distribution of S, Ca, Cu and Zn in 10 μm hair disks cut perpendicular to the hair shaft before washing with a copper resolving substance is given

microprobe is equipped with a magnetic scanner and a PPD 11/44/CAMAC data handling system.

RESULTS

The distribution of S, Ca, Cu and Zn in 10 μm hair disks cut perpendicular to the hair shaft before washing with a copper resolving substance is given in Figure 2a–d.

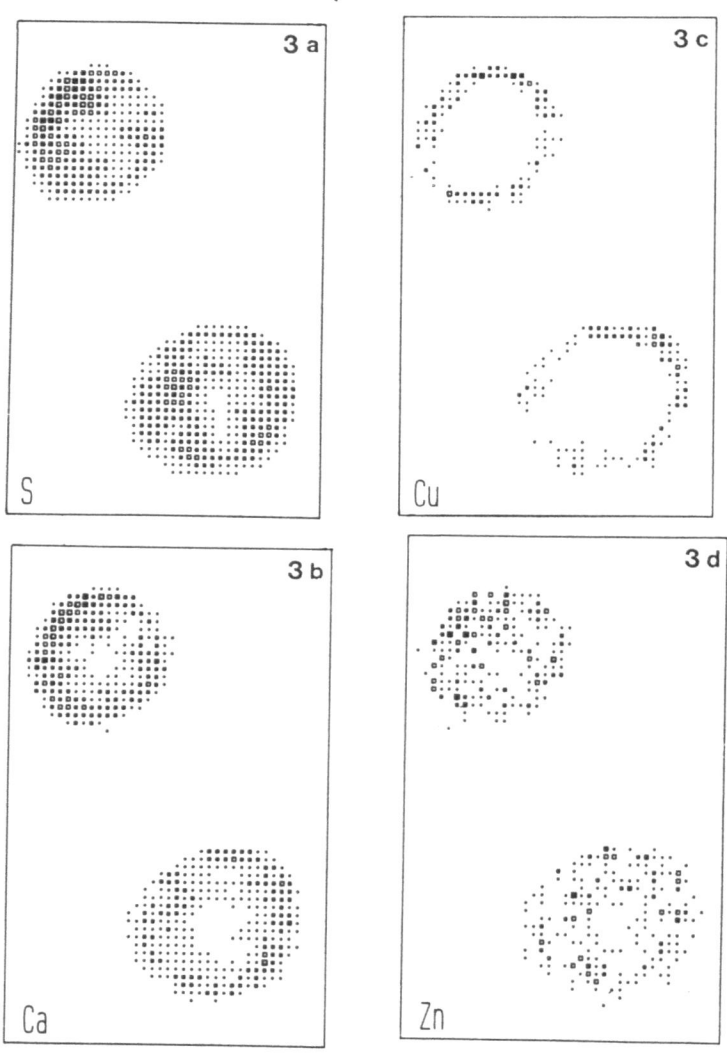

Figure 3 As compared with data shown in Figure 2, the copper (Cu, 3c) content was found markedly decreased in the periphery of the hair shaft after treatment. Zn and Ca were decreased too, however there was no significant change in the concentration of sulfur

There is a high content of Cu and Zn at the hair shaft periphery; however the center of the hair shaft is free of copper. After topical treatment with an aqueous solution of 1.5% 1-hydroxyethyl diphosphonic acid (Fa. Henkel, Düsseldorf, West Germany) (Figure 3a–d), the copper content was found markedly decreased in the periphery of the hair shaft. Zn and Ca were also decreased; however, there was no significant change in the concentration of sulfur.

Total concentration of the measured elements before and after topical treatment are presented in Table 1. All other elements with an atomic number $Z > 14$ are in normal range.

Table 1 Elemental concentrations in ppm dry weight before and after topical treatment

Element	Before	After
S	43,788	37,180
Ca	3,004	867
Cu	6,638	684
Zn	1,353	562

CONCLUSIONS

A major advantage of the proton-induced X-ray emission (PIXE) – used here – is its high sensitivity (e.g. copper down to a level of 1 ppm) compared with other methods such as the scanning transmission electron microscope. Furthermore, it enables one to determine trace elements in different areas of the hair shaft. Therefore therapeutic effects are very effectively controlled, and this may also help to differentiate between endogenous or exogenous sources of increased trace elements in hairs.

REFERENCES

1. Bischof W, Höfert M, Raith B, Wilde HR, Gonsior B, Enderer K. Trace element analysis of biological samples by means of proton microprobe. In *Trace Element-Analytical Chemistry in Medical Biology*, vol. 2(12) (Brätter P, Schramel P, eds), pp. 1053–1061. Berlin, New York: Walter de Gruyter, 1984
2. Kurz KH, Steigleder GK, Bischof W, Gonsior B. PIXE analysis in different stages of psoriatic skin. *J Invest Dermatol*, **88**, 223–226, 1987

18
Office diagnosis of pathological changes of hair cuticular cell pattern

D Van Neste[*], **Y Houbion**[**]
[*]Department of Dermatology, Catholic University of Louvain, Brussels, Belgium and [**]Electron Microscopy Unit, Facultés Notre-Dame-de-la-Paix, Namur, Belgium

ABSTRACT

A rapid and reliable method for obtaining hair surface replicas has recently been described. Besides ease of use in the clinical office, detailed figures of hair cuticular cell pattern are obtained with an excellent resolution at the level of the light microscope as compared with scanning electron microscopy.

In this paper we present comparative pictures of the hair surface obtained with the light microscope (LM) and the scanning electron microscope (SEM) in normal hair shafts, and in typical cases of hair dysplasias such as monilethrix, trichothiodystrophy, or hairs taken from a patient with trichorhinophalangeal syndrome.

As the pictures in LM are more or less identical to SEM, we conclude that the generation of hair surface replicas is an easy technique that can be used in the office for the study of alterations occurring at the distal edges of the cuticular cells of the hair shaft. Such changes are induced at early stages in some hair dysplasias, but in other syndromes which affect hair growth they are absent. In monilethrix there are dramatic changes of cuticular cell arrangements at both nodal and internodal segments.

INTRODUCTION

Weathering of the human hair shaft[1] is no different from any other process of chronologic aging of textile fibers, metals, etc. The main characteristic with hair is that the process goes on for the period of time that separates the merging of the hair tip at the scalp surface from the end of the anagen phase, i.e. about three years, unless it is cut during the growth phase of the follicle. During that time, hairs are subject to various kinds of injuries: physical manipulations such as friction, brushing, exposure to sunlight; chemical insults from environment (water, swimming pool, dust, etc.) and from cosmetic mismanagement (bleaching, detergents, etc.). Under certain circumstances, for example in the case of hair dysplasias, there might be a constitutional fragility of the shaft and premature weathering occurs. In this paper we present some comparative figures of hair shaft alterations as they appear with the hair surface replica technique and with scanning electron microscopy.

MATERIAL AND METHODS

Hair samples were taken from a patient with normal hair, and the following dysplasias: monilethrix, trichothiodystrophy[2], and trichorhinophalangeal syndrome[3]. The shafts were subjected to the replica technique as initially described by Van Neste[4]. Briefly, hairs are dipped in a drop of cyanoacrylate glue (Eurecryl®, Schering Chimie Industrielle, Rungis, France) and after a few seconds they are gently pressed onto glass slides. After polymerization (usually within less than 30 s) the hair shafts were gently removed. The casts left on the glass slide were then examined with a light microscope (Figures 1–3). Comparative light microscopy (LM) and scanning electron microscopy (SEM) pictures (LM on the right, SEM on the left) of some hair dysplasias are shown in Figures 4–7.

RESULTS

For monilethrix (Figures 4 and 5), trichothiodystrophy (Figure 6), and trichorhinophalangeal syndrome (Figure 7) we observed almost identical scale patterns, whatever the observation technique, or normal and pathological aspect of the hair surface. The overall correlation between the aspects observed with the light microscope and those obtained with SEM can be described as being excellent.

Changes of cuticular cell patterns along the hair shaft were observed in monilethrix (nodal and internodal) and TTD hairs, but TRP hairs showed a normal pattern.

DISCUSSION

The method described in this paper gives a detailed figure of hair cuticular cell pattern with an excellent resolution at the level of the light microscope[4]. Casting is very easily performed in the clinic or in the office. Hence information can be rapidly (less than 1 min) generated as to the hair surface pattern, as well in normal environmental-induced damage or in cases of hair dysplasias[5].

The comparative pictures obtained with light microscopy and scanning electron microscopy in normal hair shafts and in monilethrix, TTD or TRP syndrome showed that there is an almost perfect correlation between the aspects observed with the light microscope and those obtained with SEM. This confirms our previous correlative study in normal or environmental-induced hair damage[5] and the image resolution seems to be in the same order of magnitude as the celluloid imprint method recommended by Schell et al.[6]. In this

174

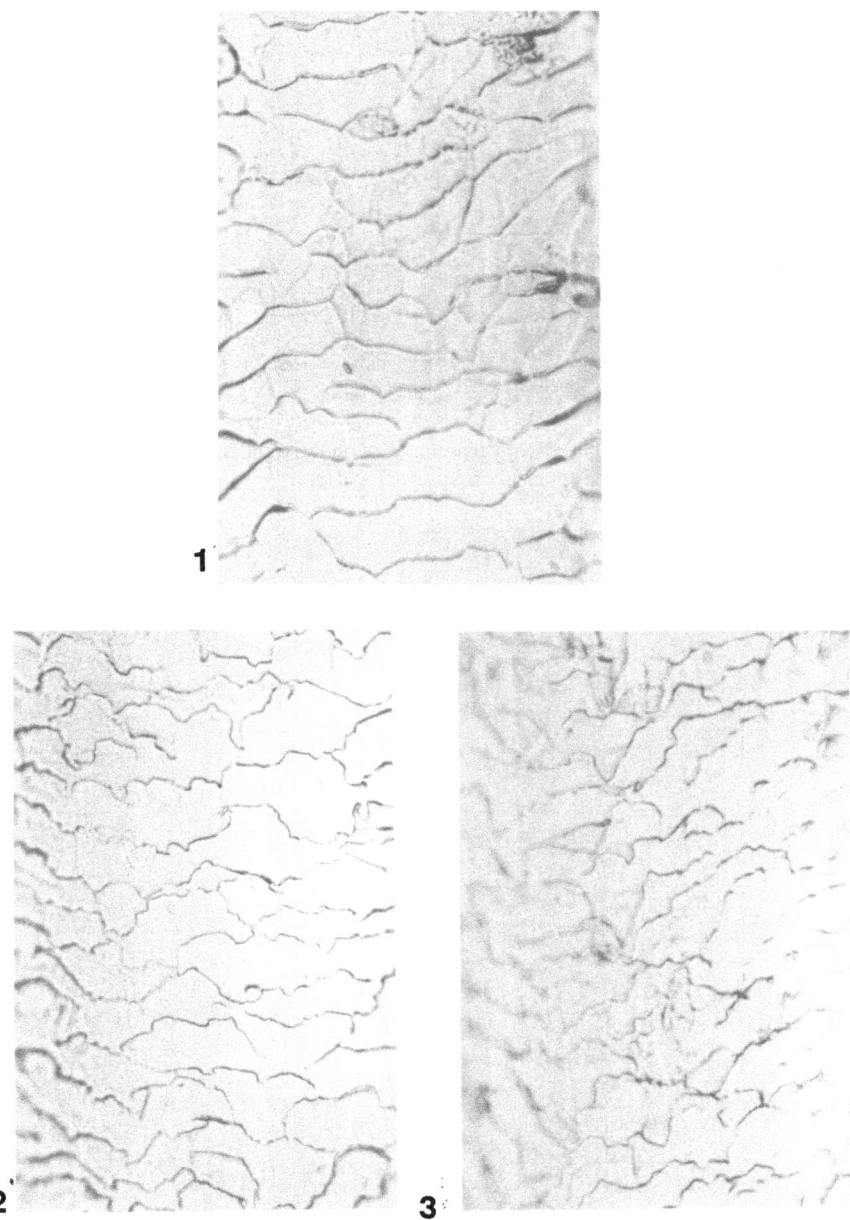

Figure 1   Cast of normal human hair as it merges from the scalp surface
Figure 2   Cast of normal human hair at 2 cm from the scalp surface
Figure 3   Cast of normal human hair at 4 cm from the scalp surface

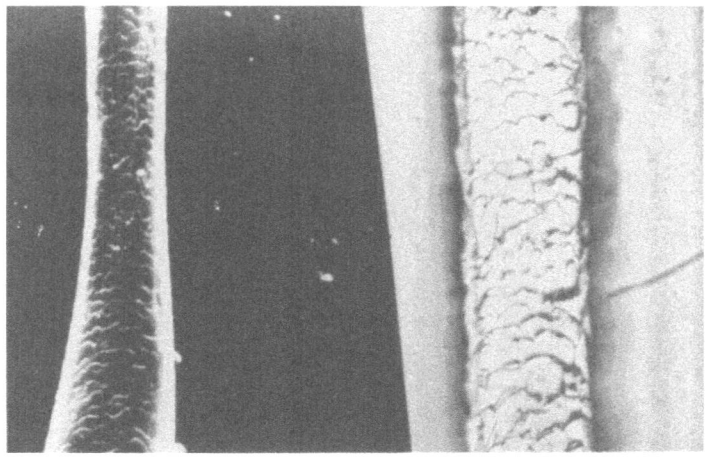

Figure 4 Comparative microscopy pictures (LM on the right, SEM on the left) of segments of monilethrix with roughly normal cuticular cell pattern

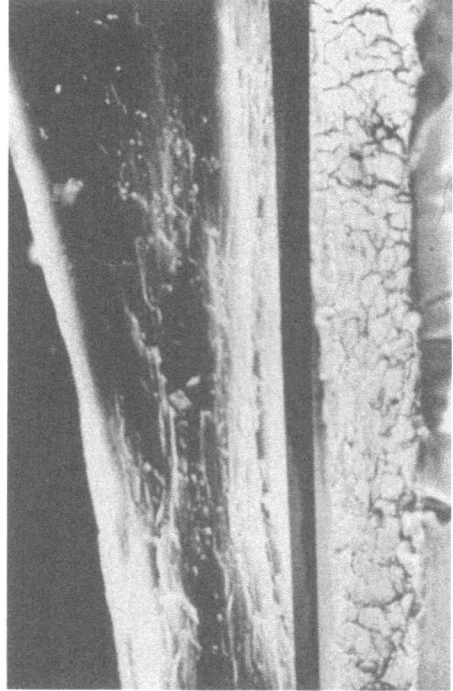

Figure 5 Comparative microscopy pictures (LM on the right, SEM on the left) of premature weathering in monilethrix

176

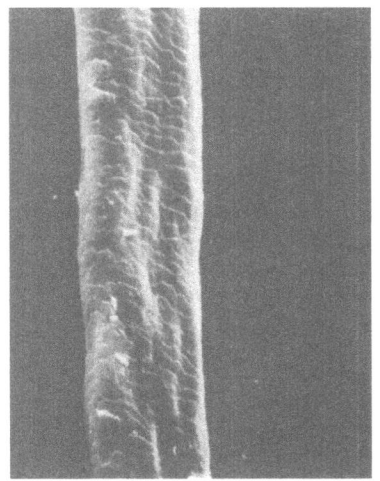
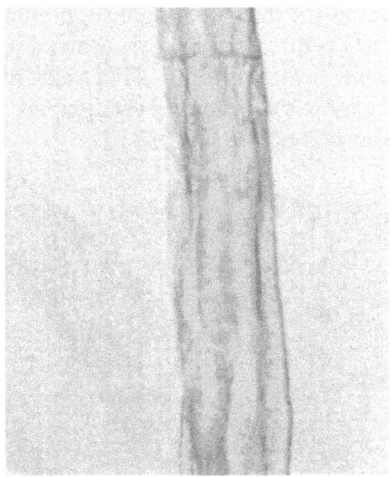

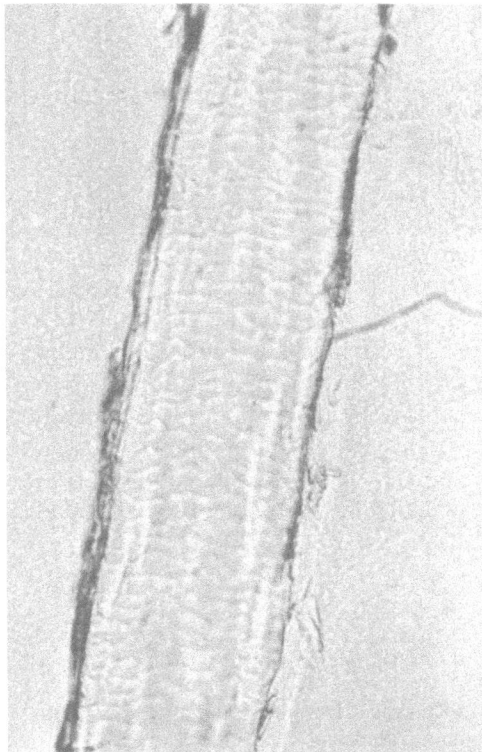

Figure 6 (Top) SEM, LM of the whole shaft and (bottom) cast of the hair surface of TTD hairs

series the most dramatic changes were observed in monilethrix as well on the nodal as on the internodal segments. The nodal segments, with a normal or slightly reduced diameter, showed premature weathering (Figures 4 and 5). The abnormal relief of TTD hairs is also clearly visible: longitudinal fluting and grooves were easily recognized. TRP hairs show a normal pattern of cuticular cell edges (Figure 7).

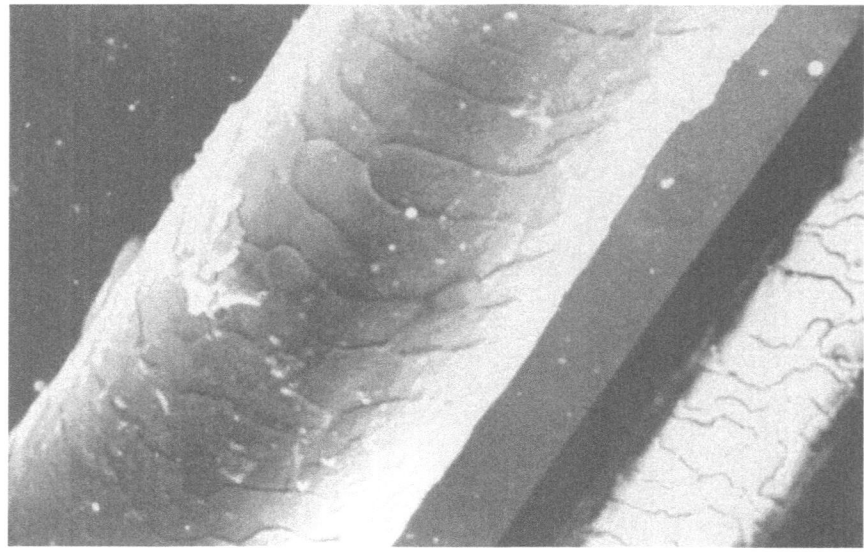

Figure 7   TRP hairs (LM on the right, SEM on the left) show a normal cuticular pattern

The question of whether those cuticular changes represent dynamic changes occurring during their formation along with that of the shaft (cortex and medulla) remains to be determined. It is interesting, in this respect, to mention earlier works showing minor changes along the cuticular cell borders and surface in psoriasis[7] but we have not performed any comparative study with psoriatic hairs and the presently described replica technique.

REFERENCES

1.   Dawber RPR. Weathering of hair in some genetic hair dystrophies. In *Hair, Trace Elements and Human Illness* (Brown A, Crounse RG, eds), pp. 273-280 New York: Praeger, 1980

2.   Van Neste D, Thomas P, Desmons F. Trichoschisis, photosensibilité, retard staturo-pondéral: nouveau syndrome congénital. *Ann Dermatol Syph (Paris)* 107, 718, 1980

3.   Van Neste D, Dumortier M. Tricho-rhino-phalangeal syndrome. Disturbed geometric relationships between hair matrix and dermal papilla in scalp hair bulbs. *Dermatologica*, 165, 16–23, 1982

4. Van Neste D. Une technique simple pour l'étude de la cuticule de la tige pilaire en microscopie optique. *Ann Dermatol Vénéréol*, **112**, 231–233, 1985

5. Van Neste D, Houbion Y. Office diagnosis of changes in hair cuticular cell pattern. *Arch Dermatol*, **122**, 750–752, 1986

6. Schell H, Deinlein E, Haneke E, Schaidt G. Die Darstellung der Haarcuticula durch Abdruck- Eine einfache Method zur Untersuchung der Haaroberfläche in der trichologischen Sprechstunde. *Z Hautkr*, **61**, 1161–1164, 1985

7. Wyatt E, Bottoms E, Comaish S. Abnormal hair shafts in psoriasis on scanning electron microscopy. *Br J Dermatol*, **87**, 368–373, 1972

Part III
Hair and Scalp Diseases and Therapy: Trichothiodystrophy, Pattern Baldness, Alopecia Areata

19

Clinical symptoms associated with trichothiodystrophy: a review of the literature with special emphasis on light sensitivity and the association with xeroderma pigmentosum (complementation group D)

D Van Neste[*], X Miller[**] and E Bohnert[**]

Department of Dermatology [*]Catholic University of Louvain, Brussels, Belgium and [**]University of Heidelberg, Mannheim, Federal Republic of Germany

ABSTRACT

The clinical aspects, and the hair shaft morphology and biochemistry, of trichothiodystrophy are reviewed. A wide spectrum of clinical symptoms has been reported in association with trichothiodystrophy. In this review the authors classify the symptom complexes according to increasing severity, i.e. starting from the isolated hair defect up to the most complex association of defective brain function, growth retardation, ichthyosis and light sensitivity. The authors suggest the existence of an as yet unreported association of hair and nail defect. Recently, the following classification or checklist has been proposed:

A =   **Isolated congenital hair defect**
B =   A   +   **nail dystrophy ?**
C =   B   +   **mental retardation**
D =   C   +   **growth retardation**
D° =   Family studies also showed decreased fertility
E =   D   +   **ichthyosis**
         Lamellar ichthyosis type
                      congenital
                      acquired
F =   E   +   **photosensitivity**
                      defective DNA repair
         in vivo irradiation of the skin
         in vitro irradiation of
                  *peripheral blood lymphocytes
                  *cultured skin fibroblasts
         Complementation with XP ?
         are there other family members with the syndrome?

Hence there is a stepwise increase in the severity of the clinical expression of the disease processes. Even though the presently reported classification of the trichothiodystrophy-associated symptoms offers a schematic way of approaching the trichothiodystrophy patient it has to be specified that it remains unknown if these defects have a common basic abnormality responsible for the hair defect and/or deviations in the other organs.

In recent years a subset of light-sensitive patients has been individualized, and evidence is accumulating that such cases provide a link with the xeroderma pigmentosum syndromes. Finally, there seems to be a biochemical heterogeneity amongst cases with the typical clinical features of Tay's syndrome (IBIDS) without or with light sensitivity (PIBIDS). Two such cases are reported in the next poster.

INTRODUCTION

Fragile, brittle hair has been associated with an ever-increasing number of clinical symptom complexes. In some instances, such as argininosuccinicaciduria, a blockade on a given amino-acid pathway has been discovered, but the specific link between hair abnormalities and the underlying biochemical defect is not always supported by longitudinal studies. Indeed, clinical and physical-chemical improvement of the hair shaft may occur in spite of persistent biochemical deviations[1]. This is but one example of the difficulties encountered when an attempt is made to comprehend the pathophysiology of clinical symptom complexes, involving various systems. Moreover, trichothiodystrophy is no exception to this. It is our purpose to review the published cases where the hair dysplasia is recognizable as such on the basis of morphological or biochemical data even if the term trichothiodystrophy was not specifically included in the title of the report. On the basis of these clinical and investigative reports, further support is given to the concept that this hair dysplasia is a cutaneous marker of a wide range of symptom complexes ranging in severity from isolated hair dysplasia to a constellation of neuroectodermal symptoms. Papers where hair dysplasia is not specifically described or illustrated will not be included in our discussion, but it is tempting to speculate that at least some cases reported in the neuropediatric literature belong to the same neuroectodermal symptom complex associated with this hair shaft abnormality[2,3], hence stressing the importance of accurate examination and identification of the hair shaft changes. The aim of this review is to provide the clinician with a list of symptoms to look for in order to classify his current observation as accurately as possible.

HISTORICAL BACKGROUND

The condition was initially recognized and reported in three complementary papers:

1. In 1968 Pollitt and Stonier[4] described in detail the first biochemical characteristics of this peculiar hair dysplasia;

2. In 1970 it was diagnosed as an isolated abnormality of the differentiating hair follicle in an otherwise perfectly normal girl by Brown et al.[5] and

3. In 1971 it was found to be associated with congenital lamellar ichthyosis, growth retardation and prematurely aged appearance in two siblings reported by Tay[6]. The disease was transmitted as an autosomal recessive character.

Price et al.[7] were the first to coin the term trichothiodystrophy (TTD: from the Greek trichos, hair; thio, sulfur; dys, abnormal; trophe, nutrition) which seems since then to have been widely accepted in the medical literature. However, as will be detailed later on in the biochemistry section, 'sulfur deficiency' does not preclude that there is a specific defective uptake of sulfur or sulfur-containing amino-acids.

Nonetheless, sulfur quantification in hair shafts is a convenient means for probing the more complex protein synthesis and/or breakdown defect of proteins with a high sulfur content and, as a rule, dosage of sulfur-containing amino-acids remains the most convenient and specific way of confirming the clinical diagnosis.

At the present time it is the opinion of several authors to include the patients reported by Tay in 1971 and others within the group of TTD, even though the hair dysplasia was not initially recognized as TTD. Indeed the hair defect has occasionally been confused with other hair dysplasias such as trichorrhexis nodosa, pili torti, bamboo hair, etc. Such cases[8–10] have been reported in a recent review as being 'Tay's syndrome' by Happle et al.[11], who identified TTD by examining published or original micrographs or after personal communication with the authors.

MICROSCOPICAL IDENTIFICATION AND BIOCHEMICAL ASPECTS OF TTD

Microscopic aspects

Hair abnormalities are suspected in almost every case at first glance. The scalp and other hairy areas (eyebrows, lashes,etc.) show weak, short, thin, brittle and rough hair shafts. Hair color is variable from light blonde to darkly pigmented. The length of scalp hairs is usually less than 5 cm in areas subjected to friction (occipital, temporal). If trauma is reduced longer hair shafts can be observed. Almost complete baldness (presence of a limited number of thin hair-like filaments) of the scalp has been reported only exceptionally[12,13]. In such cases the diagnosis of TTD has not yet been confirmed biochemically (M.Gillespie, personal communication concerning observation in ref. 13). Conversely, in two cases reported in this volume as 'TTD variant' the hairs were darker and grew longer than in previously observed cases. Scaliness of the scalp and discrete follicular plugging are usually present, and may be due to acroinfundibular kera-tinization[14] or persistence of the inner hair-root-sheath. In every case the diag-nosis relies upon microscopic examination of cut and/or plucked hair shafts. Hair roots are usually absent after plucking because of hair breakage at the scalp surface; hence, analysis of these hair bulbs can only be performed after scalp biopsy.

Prominent microscopic features of TTD hairs are:

1. Flattened shafts with torsions giving the impression of changing hair diameter[7]. This is analogous to the twisting of ribbon instead of the soft regular twisting of pili torti[15].

2. The contour is irregular with longitudinal grooves and fluting.

3. Short transverse bands of disorganized cortical-cuticular cells where clean transverse fractures happen to occur (trichoschisis 5).

On polarizing microscopy there is a typical diffraction pattern with oblique alternating dark and translucent zones, the angulation of which reverts upon ro-tation either of the hair specimen or of one of the crossed polarizers. Light microscopic study of scalp biopsies[12,16] also showed abnormal polarized light transmission above the keratogenous zone. Furthermore, abnormal persistence of the internal root sheath (IRS) in the acroinfundibulum was demonstrated by the persistence of alkaline-phosphatase activity[12] and rhodamine-toluidine blue staining[14]. The microscopic changes of the hair shaft are seen in greater detail with the scanning electron microscope[12,16–19]). Longitudinal ridging and flut-ing, twisting, premature weathering of the cuticular scale pattern and exposure of cortical cells have been reported. X-ray emission spectra after neutron or electron activation[5,7,17,20] usually reveals relative decreases in sulfur content, giving a first clue as to changes of chemical composition typical of TTD. When plucked hairs are examined under the transmission electron microscope the ker-atogenous zone of the hair cortex displays an abnormal whorled pattern instead of the longitudinal paracrystalline arrangement of fibrillar components em-bedded in the amorphous matrix[21]. There is also malalignment of cuticular cell membranes[17]. Histochemistry with ammoniacal silver nitrate for the detection of sulfur-rich components shows weak staining of normally sulfur-rich cuticular A-layer and exocuticle, and reduced staining of the cortex. This is associated with the presence of cystine-positive inclusions in the endocuticule of cuticular cells and the macrofibrils of the cortex[15,22]. In a more recent ultrastructural-his-tochemical study of a scalp biopsy of TTD hair follicles, severe alterations of protein deposition were found even before the cells of the hair cortex and cu-ticle reached the keratogenous zone[23].

Biochemical aspects of TTD

When clinical and microscopic diagnosis of TTD is suspected the best way to se-cure the diagnosis is to determine the amino-acid composition of the hair shaft.

The most dramatic change is a drop in cystine content which served to forge the name of TTD[7]. A concomitant drop in the amino-acid fractions related to high-sulfur proteins (cys, pro, thre and ser) and an increase in those related to low sulfur proteins (lys, asp, glu, leu, ala and phe) are also acknowledged in the literature. These concurrent changes have been reported in almost every biochemical study of TTD hairs[4,5,7,16,21,24]. Normal peripheral blood levels of cystine and normal *in vitro* incorporation of radiolabeled cystine in scalp biopsies[16] and cultured fibroblasts[24] do not support the earlier hypothesis of a defective cellular transport[7] of this amino-acid. Even though no detailed investigations of the keratin filaments have been performed with the more recently described techniques (see Schweizer, paper 2 in this volume), they do not seem to be specifically altered.

These changes in amino-acid composition reflect the abnormality of the matrix components of the hair cortex[21] and the abnormal distribution and decreased amounts of sulfur as detected histochemically in TTD hairs[22]. These biochemical changes correlate with the abnormal physical properties of TTD hairs[5,21] and could account for the premature weathering in TTD[19].

Moreover, two-dimensional gel electrophoresis of the proteins of normal and TTD hairs show an overall loss of high-sulfur proteins (HSP). This is accompanied by appearance of low molecular weight material and replacement of a fraction of the HSP by components of similar molecular weight but lower cystine content[25,26]. It has been hypothesized on the basis of comparative studies of human hair and sheep wool fibers that the biochemical changes are related to a metabolically induced cystine deficiency and to an altered regulatory gene[25,27]. This fits in well with the recent identification of the 'TTD variant' mentioned above.

Differences between two-dimensional electrophoretic patterns of human TTD hairs from various sources suggest molecular heterogeneity. More in-depth investigation of these patients' hairs and follicles is needed in order to further elucidate the mechanisms regulating the normal protein biosynthesis in human hair. Preliminary data from a family study show no evidence of biochemical changes in hairs taken from obligate heterozygotes[26], and we expect to gain further information by studying hairs from affected siblings.

CLINICAL SYMPTOMS ASSOCIATED WITH TTD

In order to review the complete spectrum of associated defects we collected the observations published after the pioneer biochemical work of Pollitt and Stonier[4] and categorized the patients in subgroups of increasing severity, ranging from those with isolated hair defect to the most complex neuroectodermal symptoms. It is evident that general subheadings cannot account for all the reported clinical variants, but they have the advantage of a schematic clinically relevant ranking system.

(A) Isolated hair defect

There were associated features in all patients reported to date with the notable exception of a single case report by Brown et al.[5] of a girl with no other signs of cutaneous or systemic involvement. Hair changes were, however, similar to those reported in all other patient groups in terms of clinical, microscopic and physical-chemical changes.

(B) Hair–nail dystrophy

Usually nails are involved. In the case of Brown's patient it was stated that 'no defects or dystrophy of the nails were apparent'. But in-depth biochemical studies have not been performed; nor has a long-term follow-up been reported. This may be of importance as clinical expression of nail brittleness, as well as of other characteristics (like ichthyosis, see later), may be delayed. Systematic biochemical investigation of nails[7] should therefore be of prime importance, as nail keratins are actually easy to sample and are helpful in detecting abnormal protein profiles, especially in the cases where alopecia is almost complete[12,13].

(C) TTD with nail changes and mental retardation

Arbisser et al.[18] and Howell et al.[28] reported several family members originating from a small town called Sabinas Hidalgo in northeastern Mexico. This symptom complex comprises congenital hypotrichosis, with brittle hair, typical light and electron microscopical changes of TTD with low sulfur content. Eyebrows and lashes were affected, and there were no visible axillary or pubic hairs in postpuberal subjects. Hair changes were associated with onychodystrophy mild retardation through psychometric examination but normal stature. It was also reported that most patients had accompanying hyperkeratosis of moderate degree on exposed surfaces, but the term 'ichthyosis' was not used. This study of 12 patients originating from five families with decreased fertility also documents the autosomal recessive inheritance of the syndrome. Symptoms occasionally reported were: astigmatism, pale optic discs, and pigmentary retinopathy.

(D) TTD, nail changes with mental and growth retardation

A further series of 25 patients was reported by Watson et al.[17] and Jackson et al.[29] in an Amish population in northern Indiana. Nails which were initially thought to be normal were shown to be affected on closer inspection, and this was confirmed biochemically[21]. In addition, there was mild to severe mental retardation with spastic quadriplegia and frequent seizures in the proband. The other family members were less severely affected but microcephaly and growth retardation were part of the syndrome. Family studies also showed decreased fertility. This symptom complex was finally presented under the acronym

BIDS[21] for Brittle hair–Intellectual impairment–Decreased fertility–Short stature.

(E) TTD, nail changes, mental and growth retardation and ichthyosis

In their early report Pollitt and Stonier[4] reported in detail the brittle hair and nail defects, but patients were also said to have 'dry skin' in association with mental and physical retardation. The patients were noted as being cheerful and of prematurely aged appearance[30]. A peculiar form of congenital ichthyosiform erythroderma was first recognized by Tay[6] and Happle et al.[11] published a new observation and collected several cases from the literature under the heading 'Tay's syndrome'. Lamellar ichthyosis type was reported by Price et al.[7] and Jorrizzo et al.[31]. The latter reported their patients under the acronym IBIDS (Ichthyosis and BIDS). These patients occasionally show tongue plaques, ventricular septal defects and poor teeth. Cataract was not present in Tay's patients but was frequently present in later case reports[7,11].

Another clinical case report appeared in 1986, but no detailed investigations were made[32]. Up to now histological investigations of the ichthyosis reported in this syndrome are few, and show irregular acanthosis with laminated orthokeratosis and focal parakeratosis with a thin but intact horny layer[20,33]. Further examinations of lipid composition, keratin polypeptides and electron microscopy of scales and/or epidermal specimens will provide further means of classifying the ichthyotic changes of the interadnexial epidermis. Emollients such as urea and pyrollidone dicarboxylic acids can occasionally markedly improve the clinical aspect, and the feel of the skin of the affected subjects.

(F) TTD, nail changes, mental and growth retardation, ichthyosis and photosensitivity

The acronym PIBIDS (Photosensitivity and IBIDS) was first used in a short letter by Crovato et al.[34] reporting two light-sensitive patients with the other clinical features of IBIDS. We first noted and emphasized the extreme light sensitivity which was associated with TTD in a young girl of Polish origin[35] and a short clinical report was subsequently published[36]. At this stage however, ichthyosis was not a prominent clinical feature in our patient, and a skin biopsy showed reduced thickness of stratum granulosum and a normal number of cells in S phase[37]; semi-thin sections from a more recent biopsy from an ichthyotic zone showed irregular acanthosis with compact hyperkeratosis and absent granular layer.

Upon closer inspection of published cases it became evident that photosensitivity was documented by Price et al.[7] and in a number of subsequently published cases[15,20,34,38]. The UVB wavelengths[20,36,37] are responsible for a sharply demarcated phototoxic eruption. In a limited number of patients studied there is a normal (M. Carter, personal communication and ref. 39) DNA repair and skin condition is improved by topical application of sunscreens[20]. Defective

DNA repair has been reported after *in vivo* irradiation of the skin (personal unpublished results) or *in vitro* irradiation of peripheral blood lymphocytes[24,37,40] and cultured skin fibroblasts[24,41]. Decreased rates of duplicative DNA synthesis in stimulated lymphocytes, reduced fibroblast survival and low levels of UV-irradiation-induced unscheduled DNA synthesis in G0 (UDS) lymphocytes and in fibroblasts have recently been reported in four subjects, from three apparently unrelated families, with this symptom complex[41]. Further definition of the defect showed that DNA repair was not restored by fusion of TTD cells with xeroderma pigmentosum (XP) group D fibroblasts, while complementation with XP group A cells and normal cells restored the defect[41]. Our observation also shows reduced levels of UDS in cultured fibroblasts (25% of normals) and belongs to XP-D group (unpublished data). Patients without light sensitivity do not show the defect[42]. A further case with light sensitivity, originating from the same area as the previously reported Italian cases, has recently been published[43]. Hence further investigation of PIBIDS patients is expected to uncover coexisting XP, especially in those where low levels of DNA repair have been demonstrated[37]. Early detection of DNA repair defects and prevention of sun-induced skin damage must therefore be the rule in photosensitive TTD patients. In all subjects evaluation of porphyrin metabolism was normal. An isolated abstract reporting abnormal elevated urinary excretion of kynurenin and hydroxykynurenic acid in association with TTD described as flattened hair has not been published in detail after extensive metabolic studies[38].

CONCLUSION

The basic biochemical defect responsible for the hair dysplasia, and most probably also for the wide variety of symptoms occurring in organs derived from the ectoderm and/or neural crest in TTD-associated symptom complexes, has not yet been identified. In typical cases the hair dysplasia is associated with abnormal metabolism of ultra-high and high-sulfur proteins, and it is not known if analogous defects are to be found in other cell systems or if they could account for the clinical aspects of the affected individuals. It is to be hoped that cell cultures from skin (and other tissues) will provide further means of investigating in greater detail the metabolic pathways that could be involved. A step forward has been made in this direction after the recent description of light sensitivity in TTD patients. This opened up new avenues in research, and recent results seem to indicate a possible but not obligatory link between XP and TTD. Once again, clinicians must, however, be cautious about prematurely including new patients in this TTD group if the microscopical observation only is available. Indeed similar morphological changes can occur, especially on very thin hair fibers even in the presence of normal (M. Gillespie, personal communication concerning ref. 13) or low-normal[44] levels of cystine in the hairs.

ACKNOWLEDGEMENTS

The authors thank V.Price and M.Dumortier for their help during the preparation of this manuscript.

REFERENCES

1. Potter JL, Timmons GD, Silvidi AA. Argininosuccinicaciduria: the hair abnormality revisited. *Am J Dis Child*, **134**, 1095–1096, 1980
2. Calderon R, Gonzales-Cantu N. Kinky hair, photosensitivity, broken eyebrows and eyelashes, and non progressive mental retardation. *J Pediatrics*, **95**, 1007–1008, 1979
3. Coulter DL, Beals TF, Allen RJ. Neurotrichosis: hair-shaft abnormalities associated with neurological diseases. *Develop Med Child Neurol*, **24**, 634–644, 1982
4. Pollitt RJ, Jenner FA, Davies M. Sibs with mental and physical retardation and trichorrhexis nodosa with abnormal amino acid composition of the hair. *Arch Dis Childh*, **43**, 211–216, 1968
5. Brown AC, Belser RB, Crounse RG, Wehr RF. A congenital hair defect: trichoschisis with alternating birefringence and low sulfur content. *J Invest Dermatol*, **54**, 496–509, 1970
6. Tay CH. Ichthyosiform erythroderma, hair shaft abnormalities, and mental and growth retardation: a new recessive disorder. *Arch Dermatol*, **104**, 4–13, 1971
7. Price VH, Odom RB, Ward WH, Jones FT. Trichothiodystrophy: sulfur-deficient brittle hair as a marker for a neurectodermal symptom complex. *Arch Dermatol*, **116**, 1375–1384, 1980
8. Salfeld K, Lindley MJ. Zur Frage der Merkmalskombination bei Ichthyosis vulgaris mit Bambushaarbildung und ektodermaler Dysplasie. *Derm Wochenschr*, **147**, 118–128, 1963
9. Leupold D. Ichthyosis congenita, Katarakt, Schwachsinn, Ataxie, Osteosklerose und abwehrdefekt- ein eigenständiges Syndrom? *Monatsschr Kinderheilkd*, **127**, 307–308, 1979
10. Braun-Falco O, Ring J, Butenandt O, Selzle D, Landthaler M. Ichthyosis vulgaris, Minderwuchs, Haardysplasie, Zahnanomalien, Immundefekte, psychomotorische Retardation und Resorptionsstörungen. *Hautarzt*, **32**, 67–74, 1981
11. Happle R, Traupe H, Gröbe H, Bonsmann G. The Tay syndrome (congenital ichthyosis with trichothiodystrophy). *Eur J Pediatr*, **141**, 147–152, 1984
12. Porter PS. The genetics of human hair growth. *Birth Defects*, **12**, 69–85, 1971
13. Stevanovic D, Lalevic B, Vesic S. Kératose pilaire spinulosique décalvante avec kératodermie variante. Syndrome de trichothiodystrophie. *Ann Dermatol Vénéréol (Paris)*, **112**, 478, 1985
14. Van Neste DJJ, Miller X, Bohnert E. Thichothiodystrophie: ein kutanes Merkmal für einen Symptomenkomplex von zunehmendem Schweregrad mit Beziehung zu xeroderma pigmentosum. *Aktuelle dermatologie*, (in press)
15. King MD, Gummer CL, Stephenson JBP. Trichothiodystrophy-neurotrichocutaneous syndrome of Pollitt: a report of two unrelated cases. *J Med Genet*, **21**, 286–289, 1984
16. Van Neste D, Boré P. Trichothiodystrophie: une étude morphologique et biochimique. *Ann Dermatol Vénéréol*, **110**, 409–417, 1983
17. Watson JHL, Weiss L, Jackson CE. Scanning electron microscopy of human hair in a syndrome of trichoschisis with mental retardation. In *The First Human Hair Symposium* (Brown AC, ed), pp. 170–184. New York: Medcom Press, 1974
18. Arbisser AI, Scott CI, Howell RR, Ong PS, Cox HL. A syndrome manifested by brittle hair with morphologic and biochemical abnormalities, developmental delay and normal stature. *Birth Defects*, **12**, 219–228, 1976
19. Venning VA, Dawber RPR, Ferguson DJP, Kanan MW. Weathering of hair in trichothiodystrophy. *Br J Dermatol*, **114**, 591–595, 1986

20. Lucky PA, Kirsch N, Lucky AW, Carter DM. Low-sulfur hair syndrome associated with UVB photosensitivity and testicular failure. *J Am Acad Dermatol*, 11, 340–346, 1984
21. Baden HP, Jackson CE, Weiss L, Jimbow K, Lee L, Kubilus J, Gold RJM. The physicochemical properties of hair in the BIDS syndrome. *Am J Hum Genet*, 28, 514–521, 1976
22. Gummer CL, Dawber RPR, Price VH. Trichothiodystrophy: an electron-histochemical study of the hair shaft. *Br J Dermatol*, 110, 439–449, 1984
23. Gummer CL, Dawber RPR. Trichothiodystrophy: an ultrastructural study of the hair follicle. *Br J Dermatol*, 113, 273–280, 1985
24. Rebora A, Guarrera M, Crovato F. Aminoacid analysis in hair from PIBI(D)S syndrome. *J Am Acad Dermatol*, 15, 109–111, 1986
25. Gillespie JM, Marshall RC. A comparison of the proteins of normal and trichothiodystrophic human hair. *J Invest Dermatol*, 80, 195–202, 1983
26. Van Neste D, Gillespie M, Marshall R. Heterogeneity of trichothiodystrophy: preliminary biochemical results. In *Pediatric Dermatology. Advances in Diagnosis and Treatment* (Happle R, Grosshans E, eds), pp. 170–174. Berlin: Springer, 1986
27. Gillespie JM, Marshall RC. The proteins of normal and aberrant hair keratins. In *Hair Research: Status and Future Aspects* (Orfanos CE, Montagna W, Stuttgen G, eds), pp. 76–83. Berlin: Springer, 1981
28. Howell RR, Collie WR, Cavasos OI, Arbisser AI, Fraustadt U, Marcks SN, Parsons D. The Sabinas brittle hair syndrome. In *Hair Trace Elements and Human Illness* (Brown AC, Crounse RG, eds), pp. 210–219. New York: Praeger, 1980
29. Jackson CE, Weiss L, Watson JHL. 'Brittle' hair with short stature, intellectual impairment and decreased fertility: an autosomal recessive syndrome in an Amish kindred. *Pediatrics*, 54, 201–207, 1974
30. Pollitt RJ, Stonier PD. Proteins of normal hair and of cystine-deficient hair from mentally retarded siblings. *Biochem J*, 122, 433–444, 1971
31. Jorizzo JL, Crounse RG, Wheeler CE. Lamellar ichthyosis, dwarfism, mental retardation, and hair shaft abnormalities. A link between the ichthyosis-associated and BIDS syndromes. *J Am Acad Dermatol*, 2, 309–317, 1980
32. De Prost Y, Lemaistre R, Dupré A. Trichothiodystrophie associée à une ichtyose et à un retard statural et psychomoteur (Syndrome de Tay). *Ann Dermatol Vénéréol (Paris)*, 113, 1016–1017, 1986
33. Jorizzo JL, Atherton DJ, Crounse RG, Wells RS. Ichthyosis, brittle hair, impaired intelligence, decreased fertility and short stature (IBIDS syndrome). *Br J Dermatol*, 106, 705–710, 1982
34. Crovato F, Borrone C, Rebora A. Trichothiodystrophy- BIDS, IBIDS and PIBIDS? *Br J Dermatol*, 108, 247, 1983
35. Van Neste D, Thomas P, Desmons F. Trichoschisis. Photosensibilité. Retard staturopondéral. Nouveau syndrome congénital. *Ann Dermatol Syph (Paris)*, 107, 718, 1980
36. Van Neste D, Boré P, Thomas P, Lachapelle JM. Trichoschisis light sensitivity and growth retardation. *XVI International Congress of Dermatology* (Tokyo), 23-28 May. Tokyo: University of Tokyo Press, p, 79, 1982
37. Van Neste D, Caulier B, Thomas P, Vasseur F. PIBIDS: Tay's syndrome and xeroderma pigmentosum. *J Am Acad Dermatol*, 12, 372–373, 1985
38. Diaz-Perez JL, Vasquez JA. Flattened hair syndrome: a new disease. *Arch Dermatol*, 119, 854–855, 1983
39. Calvieri S, Giustini S, Nini G, Ribuffo D. Trichothiodystrophy: two new cases. In *Clinical Dermatology - The CMD Case Collection* (Wilkinson DS, Mascaro JM, Orfanos CE, eds), pp. 65–66. Stuttgart: Schattauer, 1987
40. Crovato F, Borrone C, Rebora A. The Tay syndrome (congenital ichthyosis with trichothiodystrophy). *Eur J Pediatr*, 142, 233–234, 1984
41. Stefanini M, Lagomarsini P, Arlett CF, Marinoni S, Borrone C, Crovato F, Trevisan G, Cordone G, Nuzzo F. Xeroderma pigmentosum (complementation group D) mutation

is present in patients affected by trichothiodystrophy with photosensitivity. *Hum Genet*, **74**, 107–112, 1986

42. Stefanini M, Lagomarsini P, Giorgi R, Nuzzo F. Complementation studies in cells from patients affected by trichothiodystrophy with normal or enhanced UV-photosensitivity. *Mutation Res*, **191**, 117, 1987

43. Trevisan G, Marinoni S, Stefanini M. PIBIDS syndrome: trichothiodystrophy and photosensitivity with defective UV-repair of DNA. In *Clinical Dermatology - The CMD Case Collection* (Wilkinson DS, Mascaro JM, Orfanos CE, eds), pp. 61–62. Stuttgart: Schattauer, 1987

44. Traupe H, Happle R, Gröbe H, Bertram HP. Polarization microscopy of hair in acrodermatitis enteropathica. *Pediatr Dermatol*, **3**, 300–303, 1986

20

High-sulfur protein deficient human hair: clinical aspects and biochemical study of two unreported cases of a variant type of trichothiodystrophy

D Van Neste[*], H Degreef[†], N Van Haute[†], J Van Hee[†], J Vandermaesen[†], A Taieb[§], A Maleville[‡], D Fontan[¶], N Bakry[¶], JM Gillespie[¶], RC Marshall[¶]

[*]Departments of Dermatology, Catholic University of Louvain, Brussels, Belgium, [†]KU Leuven, Belgium, [‡]Hôpital des Enfants, Bordeaux, France, [§]Department of Pediatrics, Hôpital des Enfants, Bordeaux, France and [¶]CSIRO, Parkville, Australia

ABSTRACT

Two patients with trichothiodystrophy (TTD) are reported. A checklist (ranging from A, isolated hair defect to F, PIBIDS), based on an extensive literature review, has been used for symptom screening and classification of these patients. As compared with the usually associated clinical symptoms, the most striking feature of the hair dysplasia is the presence of slightly longer than usual and darkly pigmented hair. Patient MC, a boy, was seen in Bordeaux for extreme light sensitivity and growth retardation (–1 SD); the presence of all the other symptoms usually recorded under F group allows the patient to be classified as PIBIDS. It is unknown whether the ichthyosis was congenital or acquired. In addition to the symptoms recorded under F, there was a congenital zoniform cataract, low serum concentrations of vitamin B6 and hyper-IgE (6.8 KIU/l). EMG, and cellular immunity *in vitro* were normal. Hypogonadism and fertility, as well as DNA repair, remain to be explored. Patient CC, a girl (3 years), was seen in Leuven for the presence of short, fragile, brittle hair with moderate onychodystrophy and ichthyosiform changes on the trunk, the changes being present since the age of 1 year. There is no consanguinity and the parents originated from Italy. Birth was induced at 42 weeks of gestational age, in the presence of preeclampsia. There was no gross mental deficiency but detailed scoring remains to be made. Clinically, there was no growth retardation (at the age of 3 years and 8 months body weight and size ranged within the 3rd–25th percentiles; CP: 48.3 cm). The thyroid gland was palpated and serum levels of T4 and TBG were increased but there was no clinical or specific biological evidence of hyperthyroidism. In the absence of specific examination for mental retardation, this case is provisionally classified as type E.

In both patients hairs and nails were sampled, and a biochemical study was undertaken. Hair contains intermediate filaments (IF) embedded in a cystine-rich matrix of high-sulfur proteins (about 40%). The decreased cystine content of hairs from patients suffering trichothiodystrophy (TTD) has been found to be due to changes in the high-sulfur group of proteins, comprising the loss of the ultra-high-sulfur (UHS) fraction and the replacement of many normal components by proteins of lower than normal cystine content which have a generally aberrant amino acid composition. Overall, the high-sulfur proteins are reduced to about 25% of normal. We are reporting two cases of TTD in which a different pattern of change is manifested. Both hairs had a lower than normal cystine content, although the decrease was less than that usually found with TTD. The overall amino acid compositions had changed in a direction consistent with decreases in high-sulfur protein content to about 50% of normal with a corresponding increase in proportion of IF. The high-sulfur proteins were isolated from each hair as S-carboxymethyl kerateines and characterized by amino acid analysis and two-dimensional electrophoresis. In amino acid composition both fractions were similar to normal high-sulfur proteins, particularly in containing close to 30 mol% S-carboxymethyl-cysteine, in marked contrast to the usual value of less than 20% for TTD proteins. Electrophoresis of the high-sulfur proteins gave a pattern showing the presence of many normal components, including the UHS fraction, which are absent from he usual TTD pattern. However, the patterns appear somewhat different from the normal control, and whether this is due to a polymorphism or a mutation cannot be determined without the isolation and characterization of individual high-sulfur proteins. On the basis of these studies it is proposed that a subgroup of TTD exists which is characterized by a partial loss of hair high-sulfur proteins without a significant change in their amino acid composition.

INTRODUCTION

Hair contains intermediate filaments (IF) composed of cystine-poor (low-sulfur) proteins embedded in a cystine-rich matrix of IF-associated (high-sulfur) proteins. There are many reports of a clinically and microscopically distinctive dysplasia suggestive of a metabolic defect in man, termed trichothiodystrophy (TTD), which is characterized by the formation of weak, brittle hair and nail of lower than normal cystine content[1-6].

Although only a few individual samples of TTD hair have been examined biochemically, there is general agreement that major changes in the amount and composition of the high-sulfur (HS) proteins are responsible for the altered composition of the hair[2,3,6-9]. The total amount of HS protein is reduced to about 25% of normal, the ultra-high and many normal HS protein components are missing and have been replaced by new components of lower than normal cystine content plus some ill-defined small proteins. The availability of two new samples of TTD hair, in amounts sufficiently large for biochemical study, has provided an opportunity to see whether these biochemical changes are the same for all samples of TTD hair. Particularly from the examination of the electrophoretic patterns of the HS proteins there is evidence that at the very least there is a spectrum of protein changes in TTD and at the most that there is more than one type of syndrome resulting in hair of reduced cystine content.

This paper reports on clinical aspects and biochemical composition of hair and nail samples of two patients with this trichothiodystrophy (TTD) variant syndrome.

As compared with the usually associated clinical symptoms, the only remarkable feature of the hair dysplasia is the presence of slightly longer than usual and darkly pigmented hair. These patients are reported as "TTD variant" because a peculiar biochemical modification has been discovered in their hair and nail samples. Indeed, in both patients, hairs and nails were sampled and analysis of the amino acid composition showed less than normal cystine content which was, however, higher than in other cases of TTD.

MATERIAL AND METHODS

Patients

A checklist (ranging from A, isolated hair defect to F, PIBIDS) based on a an extensive literature review (see Van Neste, Miller and Böhnert, paper 19 in this volume) has been used for symptom screening and classification of these patients.

Patient MC

This boy (Figure 1) was seen in Bordeaux for extreme light-sensitivity and growth retardation (-1 SD); the presence of all the other symptoms usually recorded under F group allows the patient to be classified as PIBIDS.

It is unknown whether the ichthyosis (Figure 2) was congenital or acquired. In addition to the symptoms recorded under F, there was a congenital zoniform cataract, low serum concentrations of vitamin B6 and hyper-IgE (6.8 KIU/l). EMG, and cellular immunity *in vitro* were normal. Hypogonadism and fertility, as well as DNA repair, remain to be explored.

Patient CC

This girl was seen in Leuven for the presence of short, fragile, brittle hair (Figure 3) with moderate onychodystrophy (Figure 4) and ichthyosiform changes on the trunk, these changes being present since the age of 1 year. There was no gross mental deficiency but detailed scoring remains to be made. Clinically there was no growth retardation. The typical changes at scanning microscopic examination of hairs are shown in Figure 5 and 6.

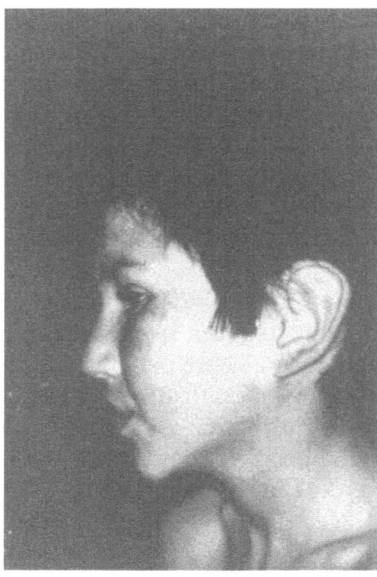

Figure 1 This boy was seen in Bordeaux for extreme light-sensitivity and growth retardation (-1 SD); the presence of long pigmented hairs was considered as an unusual clinical manifestation of TTD; classified as PIBIDS

Figure 2 The ichthyosis presented as small flakes on the trunk. It is not clear whether this was present at birth or not

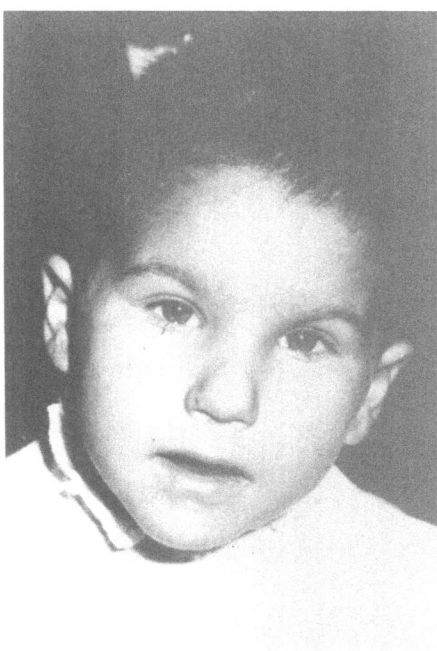

Figure 3 This girl was seen in Leuven for the presence of short, fragile, brittle hair and ichthyosiform changes on the trunk, the changes being present since the age of 1 year

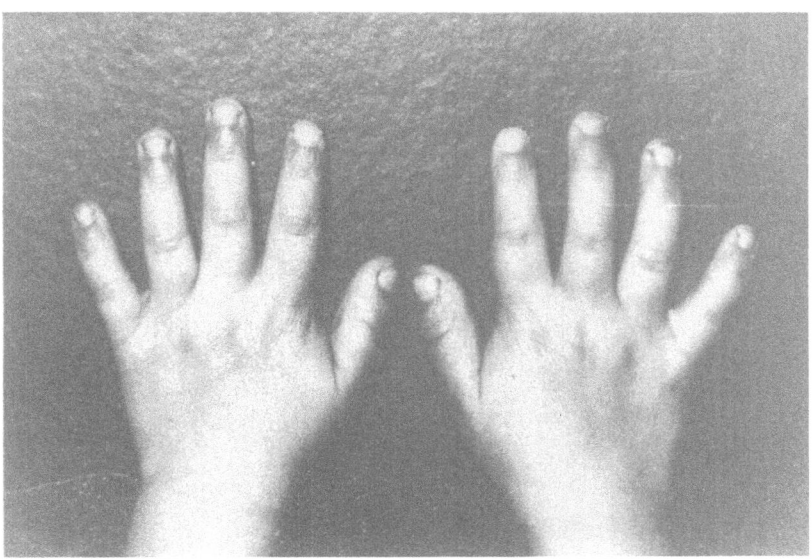

Figure 4 There was also moderate onychodystrophy with thinning of the nail plate

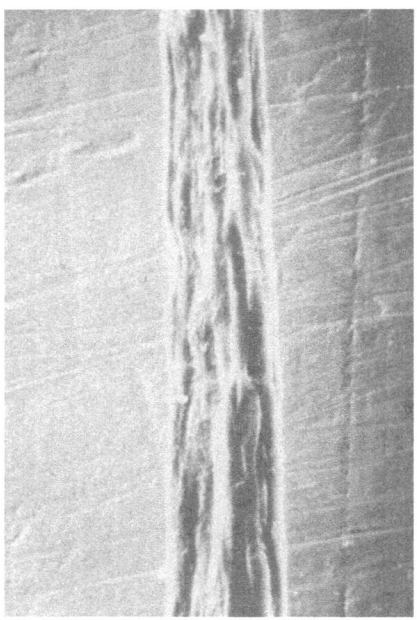

Figure 5 Scanning electron microscopic examination of hairs (patient in Figure 3) shows some of the typical changes such as flattening and longitudinal ridging

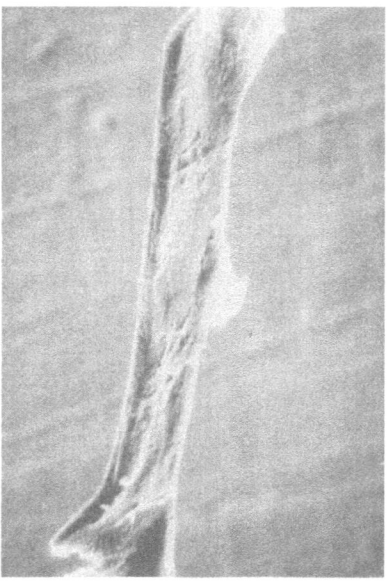

Figure 6 Scanning electron microscopy (hairs of patient in Figure 3) shows extreme flattening. Breakage occurs at zones of fragility (trichoschisis)

200

At the age of 3.75 years body weight and size ranged within the 3rd–25th percentiles; CP, 48.3 cm). The thyroid gland was palpated and serum levels of T4 and TBG were increased, but there was no clinical or specific biological evidence of hyperthyroidism. In the absence of specific examination for mental retardation this case is provisionally classified as type E.

Origin and treatment of hair and nail samples

The TTD hair was the gift of Professor DA Danks, the control was provided by a sample of normal undamaged hair from a 2-year-old boy, the son of one of us (RCM). The two variant TTD hairs are labeled A (CC, originating in Leuven, Belgium) and B (MC, originating in Bordeaux, France). The nails had a similar origin. All were washed with petroleum ether, ethanol and water and then air dried.

Preparation of soluble proteins

The hair samples (100 mg) were solubilised by treatment at 40 °C for 2 h with 10 ml of 0.2 mol/l β-mercaptoethanol in 8 mol/l urea at pH 11, the residue removed by filtration and the cysteinyl residues of the soluble proteins stabilized by alkylation with iodoacetate to convert them to S-carboxymethyl cysteinyl (SCMC) residues. After dialysis the constituent proteins were fractionated by adding zinc acetate to 0.02 mol/l to give a precipitate of IF proteins and a supernatant of HS proteins. Both protein fractions were treated with excess sodium citrate to remove zinc ions, dialyzed and freeze-dried.

Electrophoresis

The HS proteins were compared by electrophoresis in two dimensions. They were first electrophoresed in 10% polyacrylamide (PAA) gel rods (65 x 3 mm) in a buffer system at pH 2.6 containing 4.8 mol/l acetic acid and 2.8 mol/l urea, for 2.5 h at 250 V. In the second dimension the proteins were electrophoresed in continuous-gradient PAA gels (Gradipore: 2.5–27%) in the presence of SDS at pH 7. At the completion of electrophoresis the protein bands were located in the gels by staining with Coomassie brilliant blue G 250.

Amino acid analysis

Hair, nail and protein samples were hydrolyzed in vacuo with 6 mol/l HCl at 108 °C for 22 h and then freeze-dried. Before analysis hair and nail hydrolysates were dissolved in a small volume of water, the pH adjusted to 7–8 and vigorously agitated with air to oxidize cysteine. The amino acids were estimated with a Waters HPLC amino acid analyzer using the ninhydrin detection system.

RESULTS

A comparison of the amino acid and protein composition of normal, TTD and the variant TTD hair

The complete amino acid analyses of normal human hair, a typical sample of TTD hair and two samples (A and B) of variant TTD hair are given in Table 1.

Table 1 Amino acid composition (expressed as residues%) of samples of normal and TTD hair and their constituent high-sulfur proteins (HSP)

	Hair				HSP			
	Control	A	B	TTD	Control	A	B	TTD
Lysine	2.5	3.4	3.2	4.0	0.5	0.7	0.8	1.1
Histidine	0.9	1.0	0.9	1.0	0.8	1.0	1.1	0.7
Arginine	6.4	6.2	6.1	6.8	6.2	5.6	5.6	5.1
Aspartic acid	5.0	6.7	6.4	7.9	2.2	2.6	2.3	4.2
Threonine	7.1	6.0	6.2	5.0	11.2	9.7	9.9	8.8
Serine	11.4	10.8	11.2	9.8	13.1	12.6	12.4	13.3
Glutamic acid	13.0	13.7	14.5	14.0	8.0	8.8	8.4	8.1
Proline	8.0	7.0	7.3	5.9	12.0	12.3	11.9	11.7
Glycine	5.7	6.1	6.2	6.9	5.5	6.2	5.6	7.8
Alanine	4.4	5.7	5.7	6.4	1.9	2.2	2.0	3.9
Half-cystine	17.4	11.8	11.6	8.1	27.2*	26.0*	28.1*	17.6*
Valine	5.4	5.9	5.6	6.0	5.2	4.7	4.5	7.0
Methionine	0.6	0.8	0.4	0.9	0.0	0.0	0.0	0.0
Isoleucine	2.6	3.1	2.9	3.5	1.4	1.8	1.7	2.6
Leucine	6.1	7.8	7.9	8.8	2.2	3.2	2.8	4.6
Tyrosine	2.1	2.4	2.1	2.5	1.5	1.2	1.5	1.5
Phenylalanine	1.6	2.0	1.7	2.6	1.1	1.3	1.3	1.8

* Estimated as S carboxymethyl cysteine

Hair: from this comparison of the amino acid and protein composition of normal, the variant TTD hair (A and B) and TTD hair, it can be seen that hair samples A and B contain more cystine than TTD hair, but very significantly less than normal undamaged hair. The other changes in hairs A and B as compared with normal hair, i.e. less proline but more lysine and leucine, are consistent with the loss of HS proteins and a corresponding gain in IF proteins.

HSP: it can be seen that in most respects the normal HS proteins and those of samples A and B are very close in composition. Their high contents of SCMC and proline serve to distinguish them clearly from the HS proteins isolated from TTD hair (usually less than 20 mol%). There are some differences between the HS proteins of normal hair and samples A and B, notably in arginine, threonine, valine and leucine contents.

It can be seen that hair samples A and B contain more cystine than TTD hair, but very significantly less than normal undamaged hair. The other changes in hairs A and B as compared with normal hair, i.e. less proline but more lysine and leucine, are consistent with the loss of HS proteins and a corresponding gain in IF proteins. The calculated content of HS protein in hair samples A and B is about 20%, a value consistent with the yield on solubilization and a value which is about half that for normal hair.

Table 2 Amino acid compositions (expressed as residues%) of samples of normal and abnormal nails

	Control	A	B	TTD
Lysine	3.1	3.3	3.5	4.1
Histidine	0.9	1.0	0.9	1.0
Arginine	7.0	7.3	6.4	6.8
Aspartic acid	7.0	8.2	7.5	9.1
Threonine	6.0	5.5	5.5	5.0
Serine	10.2	10.2	10.7	8.6
Glutamic acid	13.4	15.2	15.2	16.2
Proline	6.4	4.3	5.6	4.7
Glycine	6.9	6.8	7.6	6.4
Alanine	5.2	6.1	6.1	7.1
Half-cystine	11.4	6.9	8.2	5.2
Valine	5.6	5.5	5.2	5.7
Methionine	0.7	0.8	0.6	1.2
Isoleucine	3.3	3.5	3.2	3.8
Leucine	8.0	9.5	9.3	9.8
Tyrosine	2.9	3.4	2.6	2.6
Phenylalanine	2.2	2.7	2.1	2.5

As compared with normal nail, samples A and B contain less cystine and proline but more aspartic acid, glutamic acid and leucine, differences consistent with a reduction in HS protein content and a corresponding increase in IF proteins. Samples A and B are generally intermediate in composition between normal and TTD nails

The amino acid compositions of HS proteins isolated from control hair, a TTD hair and hair samples A and B are compared in Table 1. It can be seen that in most respects the normal HS proteins and those of samples A and B are very close in composition. Their high contents of SCMC and proline serve to distinguish them clearly from the HS proteins isolated from TTD hair, where in all cases so far examined the latter proteins have been found to have SCMC contents of less than 20 mol%. There are some small but significant differences between the HS proteins of normal hair and samples A and B, notably in arginine, threonine, valine and leucine contents, which may indicate that although these proteins are very similar in composition they are not completely identical.

A comparison of the amino acid compositions of normal and abnormal fingernail

The amino acid compositions of various samples of finger nail are given in Table 2. As compared with normal nail, samples A and B contain less cystine and proline but more aspartic acid, glutamic acid and leucine, differences consistent with a reduction in HS protein content and a corresponding increase in IF proteins. Samples A and B are generally intermediate in composition between normal and TTD nails. Whereas hair samples A and B were almost identical in composition, there are some differences in the composition of their nails. The reason for this is not known, but may be related to sampling variations.

An electrophoretic comparison of high-sulfur proteins isolated from normal and abnormal hair samples.

Figure 7 shows the two-dimensional electrophoretic patterns of HS proteins isolated from normal hair, a typical TTD hair and hair samples A and B. The normal HS proteins (a) show the presence of a large amount of ultra-high sulfur (UHS) proteins in the poorly resolved wedge running from the origin diagonally across the pattern. Most of the other bands are confined to the left-hand quarter of the gel, and represent a typical pattern of human hair HS proteins.

In contrast, the pattern of the TTD HS protein (b) shows the absence of UHS proteins and comparative lack of proteins running in the left-hand quarter of the gel but the presence of abnormal small high-charge proteins evident in the stream to the lower right of the pattern.

In many respects HS proteins from hair samples A and B (c and d) appear to give fairly normal patterns, most of the protein components run in the left-hand quarter of the gel, UHS proteins are present although in reduced amount,

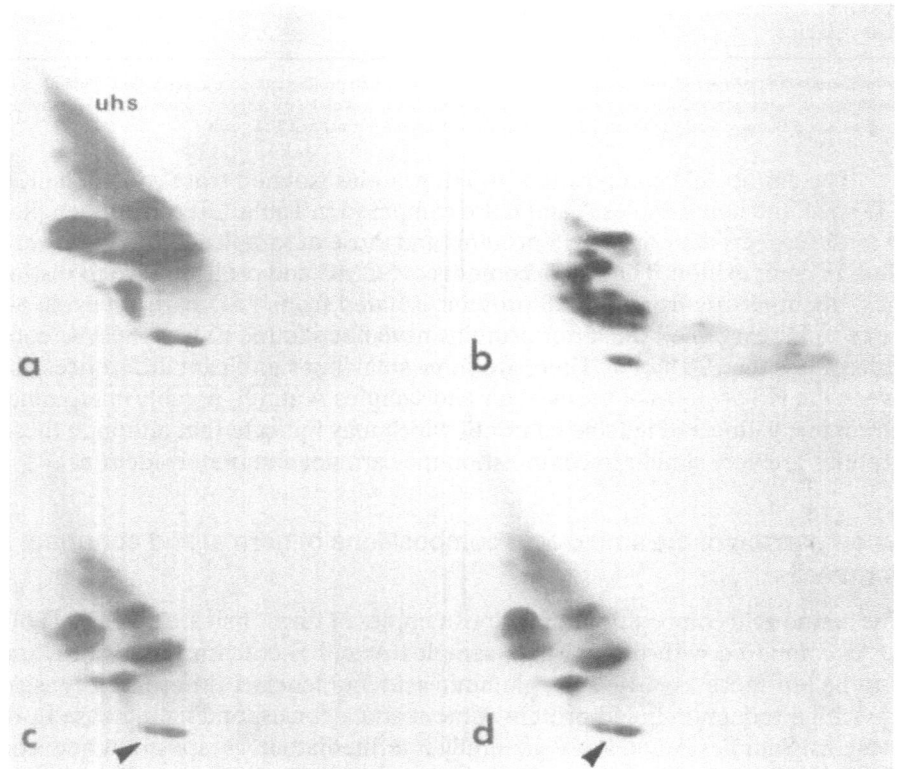

Figure 7 Two-dimensional electrophoresis of human hair HS proteins. Horizontal direction, left to right, at pH 2.6 urea-acetic acid buffer system. Vertical direction, top to bottom, at pH 7 in an SDS buffer: (a) normal hair, (b) TTD hair, (c) variant TTD sample A, (d) variant TTD sample B

and the pattern of bands looks fairly similar to a normal hair pattern. However, a small amount of small high-charge material can be seen on the lower right-hand side of the pattern, and certain components (e.g. the arrowed component), may be abnormal. But without fractionation and characterization of individual components we cannot say whether the proteins from A and B are completely normal and, if not, to what extent they are abnormal.

DISCUSSION

Two samples of human hair (A and B) provisionally classed as trichothiodystrophic, have been found to have cystine contents markedly lower than those found in samples of undamaged normal hair but somewhat higher than the values found previously with other samples of TTD hair. The decreased cystine content of these two samples was found to be primarily due to changes in the HS group of proteins comprising a reduction in their proportions to about 50% of normal without significant changes in their amino acid compositions. There were no significant changes to the IF proteins.

Two-dimensional electrophoretic examination of the HS proteins of samples A and B gave patterns which were similar to those of normal hair, in marked contrast to the very aberrant patterns given by the HS proteins of other samples of TTD hair. Taken at their face value these results suggest that there is a heterogeneity of TTD, and that hair samples A and B represent a variant form characterized by its own mechanism for the depletion of cystine content of hair. It could legitimately be referred to as: high-sulfur protein-deficient human hair. However, the possibility should not be ignored that trichothiodystrophy can manifest itself in a variety of biochemical changes of varying magnitude. It is possible to envisage a continuum of change in hair composition ranging from minor changes where alterations to the proportions of proteins are just detectable, to extreme situations where all the normal HS proteins have been replaced. Samples A and B with relatively minor changes to the proportions of HS proteins may well represent the less severely affected end of the spectrum of TTD hair samples. The hair of patient 1 of Price *et al.* examined by Gillespie and Marshall (1983) may well represent the middle of the spectrum of protein changes. We have recently examined new samples of TTD hair which appear to contain no normal HS proteins, and may well be representative of the most severely affected type. Some correlation between the clinical data and the changes in hair proteins is long overdue.

REFERENCES

1. Brown AC, Belser RB, Crounse RG, Wehr RF. A congenital hair defect: trichoschisis with alternating birefringence and low sulfur content. *J Invest Dermatol*, **54**, 496–509, 1970
2. Pollitt RJ, Stonier PD. Proteins of normal hair and of cystine-deficient hair from mentally retarded siblings. *Biochem J*, **122**, 433–444, 1971

3. Gold RJM, Kachra Z. Molecular defect in hydrotic ectodermal dysplasia. In *Proceedings of the First Human Hair Symposium, Atlanta, 1973* (Brown AC, ed), pp. 260-276. New York: Medcom, 1974
4. Price VH, Odom RB, Ward WH, Jones FT. Trichothiodystrophy: sulfur-deficient brittle hair as a marker for a neuroectodermal symptom complex. *Arch Dermatol*, **116**, 1375–1384, 1980
5. Van Neste D, Boré P. Trichothiodystrophie: une étude morphologique et biochimique. *Ann Dermatol Vénéréol*, **110**, 409–417, 1983
6. Van Neste D, Gillespie M, Marshall R. Heterogeneity of trichothiodystrophy: preliminary biochemical results. In *Pediatric Dermatology. Advances in Diagnosis and Treatment* (Happle R, Grosshans E, eds), pp. 170-174. Berlin: Springer, 1986
7. Baden HP, Jackson CE, Weiss L, Jimbow K, Lee L, Kubilus J, Gold RJM. The physico-chemical properties of hair in the BIDS syndrome. *Am J Hum Genet*, **28**, 514–521, 1976
8. Gillespie JM, Marshall RC. Variability in the proteins of wool and hair. *Proc. 6th Int Wool Text Res Conf Pretoria*, **II**, 67–77, 1980
9. Gillespie JM, Marshall RC. A comparison of the proteins of normal and trichothiodystrophic human hair. *J Invest Dermatol*, **80**, 195–202, 1983
10. Gillespie JM, Marshall RC. The proteins of normal and aberrant hair keratins. In *Hair Research: Status and Future Aspects* (Orfanos CE, Montagna W, Stuttgen G, eds), pp.76-83. Berlin: Springer, 1981
11. Price VH. Strukturanomalien des Haarshaftes. In *Haar und Haarkrankheiten* (Orfanos CE, ed), pp. 387-446. Stuttgart: Fischer, 1979

21

The effect of cyproterone acetate on hair roots and hair shaft diameter in androgenetic alopecia in females

JDR Peereboom-Wynia*[+], AH van der Willigen*, E Stolz* and Th Van Joost*

*Department of Dermatology and Venereology, University Hospital Dijkzigt, Rotterdam, The Netherlands
[+]Bronovo-Nebo Foundation, The Hague, The Netherlands

ABSTRACT

Twenty female patients suffering from androgenetic alopecia were treated for 1 year with 50 μg ethinylestradiol plus 2 mg cyproterone acetate and an additional 20 mg cyproterone acetate on days 5–20 of the menstrual cycle. The control group consisted of eight untreated female patients with androgenetic alopecia. The parameters used to evaluate therapeutic results were trichogram hair shaft diameter of full anagen and number of hairs measuring less than 40 μm. Hair roots were epilated from two locations of the scalp: frontocranial and left temporal (reference point).

After therapy the results of the treated group were compared with the control group. The *trichogram* of the frontocranial scalp region showed an increase of anagens as well as a decrease of telogens. These changes were statistically highly significant. Further, there was a decrease of dysplastic/dystrophic forms. The left temporal scalp region showed no significant differences. The mean hair shaft *diameter* of full anagen ($n = 8$) increased, while the *number of hairs measuring less than 40 μm* ($n = 8$) decreased. The last two findings showed no statistically significant differences. The therapeutic results warrant the conclusion that cyproterone acetate seems to be effective in androgenetic alopecia in women.

INTRODUCTION

Androgenetic alopecia (AA) in females has been generally accepted as belonging to the syndrome known as hyperandrogenism. Hyperandrogenism is an androgen-mediated complex of symptoms such as hirsutism, acne, seborrhea and AA. However, the genetic expression of these symptoms may vary widely. AA results from increased sensitivity of hair follicles to androgen steroids in the frontocranial scalp region in genetically predisposed women[1].

Many female patients complain of hair loss and ask for treatment. Often the diagnosis is given as a diffuse alopecia. Therefore, correct diagnosis is necessary before treatment starts. Diagnosis of AA is mainly based on the clinical picture and the trichogram.

The clinical picture

The characteristic pattern of hair loss in AA starts with a decrease in the density of implantation and diminution of the hair shaft diameter on the cranial region of the scalp. Obviously there is a wide variation in diameter of interindividual hair shafts. Further, there is a progressive decrease in follicular size with each hair growth cycle while the time of each cycle becomes gradually shorter.

Along the frontal hair line a well-preserved fringe of hair is quite characteristic[2].

Trichogram

This is an objective method to confirm diagnosis. On the cranial scalp region there is an increase of telogens and/or dysplastic/dystrophic forms. On the left temporal scalp region (reference point) the trichogram shows normal values.

Therapy studies have shown that the hair shaft diameter is the most sensitive parameter in evaluating results[3]. Cyproterone acetate (CPA) competes with androgens for the cytoplasmatic receptor sites in hair follicles[4]. Since CPA is available in most countries its beneficial effect in the treatment of hirsutism and acne has been proved in clinical studies[5].

An optimal dosage scheme of CPA for women suffering from AA is not yet known. Low CPA dosages are believed to give better results than high dosages[6]. The role of CPA will be considered and studies on the basis of parameters such as trichogram, hair shaft diameter, the number of hairs less than 40 μm in diameter and subjective findings, compared with a non-treated control group.

PATIENTS AND METHODS

On the basis of clinical features and trichogram consistent with AA thirty female patients were selected in retrospect (mean age 33, range 18–40 years). Twenty patients were treated with 50 μg ethinylestradiol (EE) plus 2 mg CPA on days 5–27 and an additional 20 mg CPA on days 5–20 of the menstrual cycle. Ten patients (control group) were left untreated. The patients fulfilled the following criteria: no endocrine disorders, concomitant diseases, pregnancy and/or use of medication. Before the start of the study, and 1 year later, hair roots were removed by a standardized method[7] from two locations: the cranial scalp and left temporal scalp region (reference point).

The trichogram was assessed with the aid of a Euromax microscope type mic. 1025 at 40-fold magnification. The hair shaft diameter was measured at 100-fold magnification, using a measuring eyepiece with screw micrometer type mic. 1179. The hair shaft diameter was measured immediately above the hair root sheath in full anagen, where the shaft is of constant diameter. A single measurement proved to be sufficient[8]. All measurements were performed by the same investigator. The following parameters were used:

1. trichogram
2. hair shaft diameter in full anagen
3. number of hairs less than 40 μm in diameter.

Student's *t*-test was used in statistical analysis.

RESULTS

Trichogram

Tables 1 and 2 show the trichogram of the cranial and left temporal scalp region, respectively, of the treated group (TG) and control group (CG), the standard error of the mean (SEM) of the differences between the initial values and those after 1 year. The TG showed a marked increase in the number of anagens and a decrease in the number of telogens, especially in the cranial scalp region. Highly statistically significant differences between the initial values (B) and those obtained after 1 year (A) were observed in the cranial scalp region in the TG.

In addition there was a marked diminution of the number of dysplastic/dystrophic hair forms in both regions. The CG showed a decrease in the number of anagens and a marked increase in the number of telogens in the cranial scalp region, but not on the left temporal scalp region. The number of dysplastics/dystrophics was diminished slightly in both regions. The differences of the latter findings were not statistically significant.

Table 1 Trichogram (%) before (B) and after (A) 1 year of treatment with Diane™ and additive cyproterone acetate 20 mg dd (days 5–20) ($n = 20$) compared with the control group ($n = 8$) on the *cranial* scalp region

Mean	Treated group B	Treated group A	Control group B	Control group A	Statistical analysis (Student's t-test)
Anagen	49.7	74.4	60.4	48.8	$p < 0.0001$
SEM	±4.8		±5.7		
Catagen/telogen	29.6	16.7	24.9	41.3	$p < 0.0000001$
SEM	±3.6		±4.5		
Dysplastic/dystrophic	20.5	9.0	13.5	10.0	$p = 0.07$
SEM	±2.4		±3.4		

SEM = Standard error of the mean of the differences between the initial values and those obtained after 1 year

Table 2   Trichogram (%) before (B) and after (A) 1 year of treatment with Diane™ and additive cyproterone acetate 20 mg dd (days 5–20) ($n = 20$) compared with the control group ($n = 8$) on the *left temporal* scalp region

Mean	Treated group B	A	Control group B	A	Statistical analysis (Student's t-test)
Anagen	64.7	75.0	65.8	65.8	$p = 0.2$
SEM	± 4.8		± 7.4		
Catagen/telogen	17.5	15.3	14.1	15.1	$p = 0.5$
SEM	± 2.7		± 3.9		
Dysplastic/dystrophic	17.9	9.8	20.1	17.9	$p = 0.3$
SEM	± 3.2		± 4.6		

SEM = Standard error of the mean of the differences between the initial values and those obtained after 1 year

Hair shaft diameter in full anagens

Figures 1 and 2 show the hair shaft diameter (μm) in full anagen before and 1 year after treatment in the cranial and left temporal scalp region respectively. Figure 1 shows an increase in the treated group and a decrease in the control group. Figure 2 shows a decrease in both groups. The differences between the initial values and those obtained after 1 year were not statistically significant either in the TG or in the CG.

The differences between the initial values and those obtained after 1 year were not statistically significant either in the TG or in the CG.

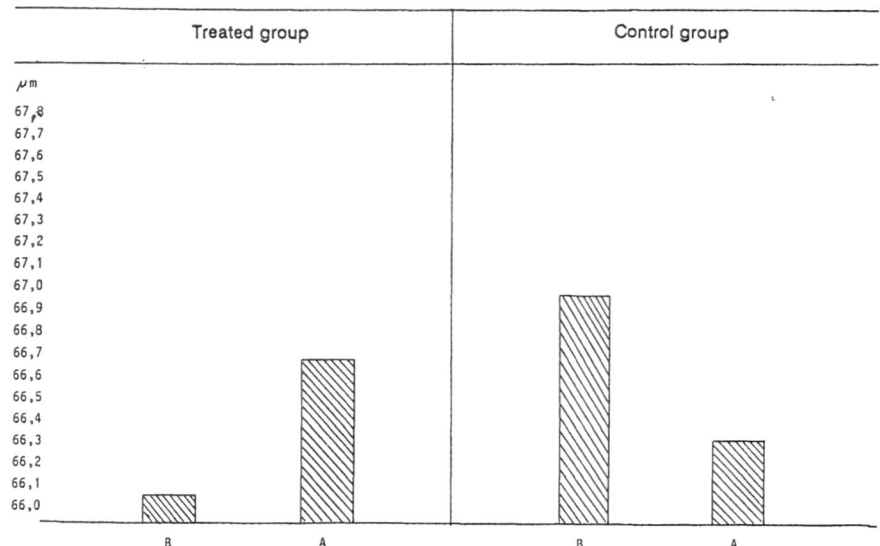

Figure 1   Mean hair shaft diameter in full anagen hair roots before (B) and after (A) 1 year of treatment with Diane™ and additive cyproterone acetate 20 mg dd (days 5–20) ($n = 8$) compared with the control group ($n = 8$) on the *cranial* scalp region

210

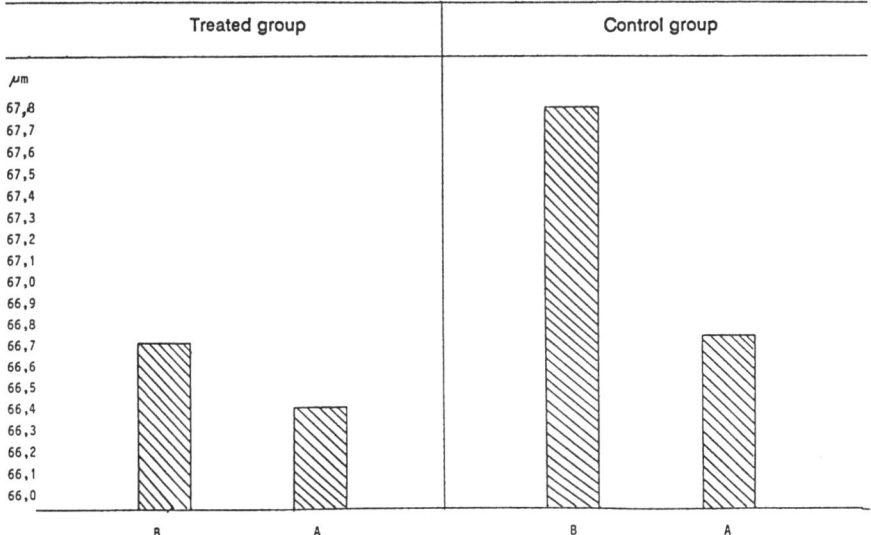

Figure 2   Mean hair shaft diameter in full anagen hair roots before (B) and after (A) 1 year of treatment with Diane™ and additive cyproterone acetate 20 mg dd (days 5–20) ($n = 8$) compared with the control group ($n = 8$) on the *left temporal* scalp region

Number of hairs measuring less than 40 μm in diameter

Hairs measuring less than 40 μm in diameter account for 10% of the total number of hairs in normal persons. Figures 3 and 4 show the number of hairs

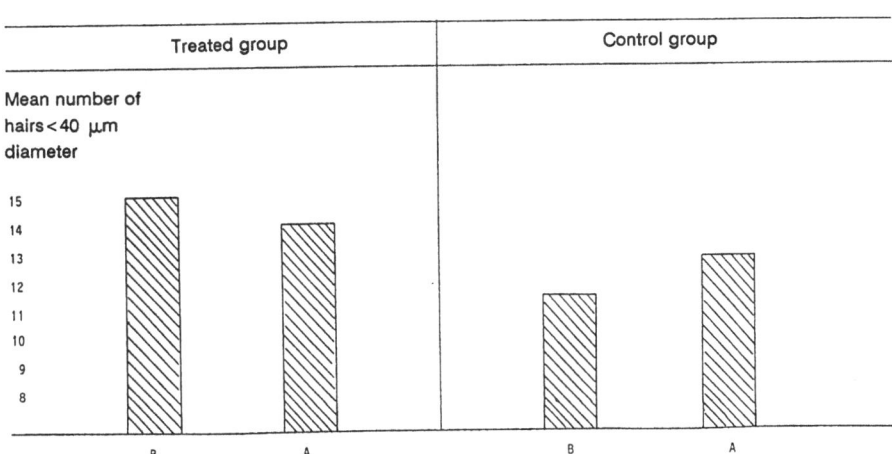

Figure 3   Number of hairs measuring less than 4 μm in diameter before (B) and after (A) 1 year of treatment with Diane™ and additive cyproterone acetate 20 mg dd (days 5–20) ($n = 8$) compared with the control group ($n = 8$) on the *cranial* scalp region

measuring less than 40 μm in diameter before and 1 year after treatment in the cranial and left temporal scalp region respectively. Figures 3 and 4 show a slight decrease in the TG and a slight increase in the CG. In these observations the differences before and 1 year after treatment were not statistically significant.

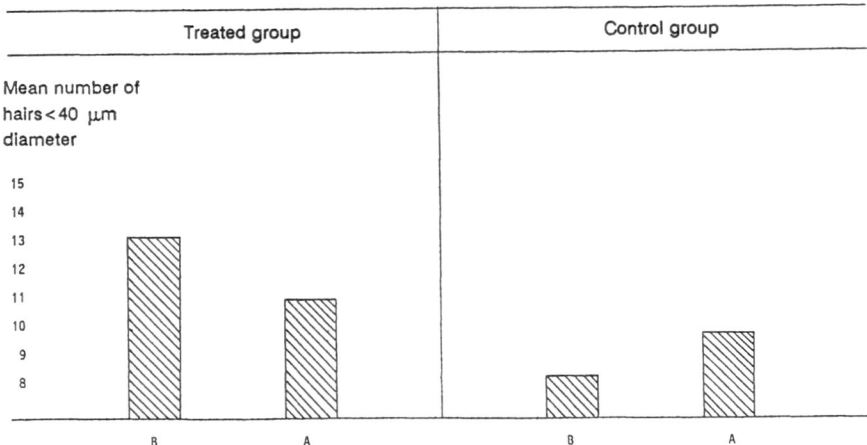

Figure 4 Number of hairs measuring less than 40 μm in diameter before (B) and after (A) 1 year of treatment with Diane™ and additive cyproterone acetate 20 mg dd (days 5–20) (N = 8) compared with the control group (N = 8) on the *left temporal* scalp region

Side-effects in the first 3 and 4 months of treatment were increase of bodyweight (6x), dizziness (1x), nausea (2x) and perspire (1x). These symptoms were transient. It was not necessary to stop treatment.

Subjective findings

In twelve patients of the TG ($n = 20$) improvement of hair growth was marked, in six of them hair loss stopped, while in two patients hair loss did not change. In all patients of the CG ($n = 10$) hair loss continued.

DISCUSSION

The highly significant differences between the initial values and those obtained 1 year later on the cranial scalp region – an increase in anagens and a decrease in telogens – and subjective findings show the beneficial influence of CPA on the hair growth in the cranial scalp region of females with AA. Although these differences of hair shaft diameter in full anagen and the number of hairs measuring less than 40 μm are not significant, these parameters of evaluation indicate a positive trend as regards the effect of the treatment.

A possible explanation for the small differences in hair shaft diameter in full anagen and the number of hairs less than 40 μm might be that AA in women is a slow process. In order to eliminate seasonal influences we chose to evaluate these parameters before treatment and 1 year later. Since there is, until now, no optimal CPA dosage scheme for women suffering from AA, we consider it advisable that various CPA dosages are compared in double-blind placebo-controlled follow-up studies of larger series of patients.

REFERENCES

1. Ludwig E. The role of sexual hormones in pattern alopecia. In *Biopathology of Pattern Alopecia*, (Baccaredda-Boy A, Moretti G, Frey JR eds), vol. I, p. 50, New York: Karger, 1968

2. Ludwig E. Classification of the types of androgenetic alopecia (common baldness) occurring in the female sex. *Br J Dermatol*, **97**, 247, 1977

3. Cottington EM, Kissinger RH, Tolgyesi WS. Observations on female scalp hair population, distribution and diameter. *J Soc Cosmetic Chem*, **28**, 219, 1977

4. Hammerstein J. Anti-androgens – basic concepts for treatment. In *Hair Research*, (Orfanos CE, Montagna W, Stüttgen G, eds), p. 330. Berlin, Heidelberg: Springer, 1981

5. Lebeau M, Vokaer R. Traitement de l'hirsutisme et de l'acné. Leur therapeutique séquentielle inversée anti-androgène/oestrogène. *J Gynecol Obstet Biol Repr*, 1, 715, 1972

6. Moltz L, Meckies J, Hammerstein J. Die kontrazeptive Betreuung androgenisierter Frauen met einem niedrig dosierten cyproteronacetathaltigen Einphasenpräparat. *Deutsche Med Wochenschr*, **104**, 1376, 1979

7. Peereboom-Wynia, JDR. Hair root characteristics of the human scalp hair in health and disease. Thesis, Rotterdam, 1982

8. Peereboom-Wynia JDR. Comparative studies of the diameter of hairshafts in anagen and in telogen phases in male adults without alopecia and in male adults with androgenetic alopecia. In *Hair Research*, (Orfanos CE, Montagna W, Stüttgen G, eds), Vol. I, p. 294. Heidelberg: Springer, 1981

22

Androgenetic alopecia: some thoughts and views about its topical treatment

R Venafra
Med-Import, Como, Italy

In fundamental research the purpose must be, in the first instance, to attempt to understand as much as possible about the microcosm of the hair follicle and the pathway of the different molecular substances involved in hair growth and, of course, hair loss.

Apart from rare exceptions, hair loss has always been a problem for any man or woman affected by this esthetic anomaly.

Independent of its causes, androgenetic alopecia, which is also called common baldness, is the cutaneous aging of a particular zone, the scalp, just as atherosclerosis is the expression of the aging of the arteries.

The fact that these morphological alterations have a variable etiology involving a multiplicity of factors – genetic, metabolic, hormonal, toxic, etc. – does not preclude the fact that any morphological alteration translates itself in practise as a precocious aging of a tissue. Science will never be able to guarantee eternal life, but thanks to continuous research it will become possible to prolong as much as possible the life of an individual, a cell, a tissue or an organ.

This means in the field of androgenetic alopecia, that a baldness of the hypocratic type, once established, cannot be improved substantially by any treatment whatsoever. Spectacular results in terms of regrowth have been seen after the application of certain substances. Unfortunately these results have always been short-lived and reversible. Even then, hair regrowth gives a limited 'cosmetic' result.

Androgenetic alopecia can be summarized as follows:

1. On the one hand atrophy, sclerosis or miniaturization of the hair follicle.

2. On the other hand a progressive shortening of the average duration of the anagen stage, which results in vellus hair before complete disappearance.

With the exception of all other pathological causes which lead to alopecia, the criteria for subjectively and objectively evaluating the tendency to develop androgenetic alopecia before the condition has reached stage II or III (according to Hamilton's classification[1], modified by Ebling, Dawber and Rook (1986) are as follows:

1. The patient complains of having hair loss for a period of several months, whether while washing (shampooing), or while brushing or combing, or on the pillow.

2. A slight regression of the frontal hair line along with bitemporal recession.

3. Generally, if a good trichogram is carried out according to established techniques[2], an anagen:telogen ratio of 4 will be found (80% anagen – 20% telogen)[3].

From a strictly statistical point of view the evaluation of dystrophic and catagen hairs is of little importance except in a morphological analysis which is intended for very precise and sophisticated research.

A phototrichogram according to previously described techniques[4,5] or, preferably a computerized morphometric analysis of the phototrichogram[6,7], can easily be used instead of the more 'invasive' trichogram method.

A biopsy of the hair follicle can also be carried out. It is not certain that this analysis would be easy in clinical practise. As for the treatments which could prolong the life of the hair, three main lines of interest which have emerged from serious research, can be summarized:

1. Certain hypotensive substances exhibiting a vasodilating action have been demonstrated to have a certain effect on the hair follicle; this action, though incontestable, is reversible once the treatment is stopped, resulting in hair loss within 3 months. See the folliculogram before and after treatment with minoxidil on the *Macacca arctoides*, on the one hand, and the increase in the number of terminal or non-vellus hairs before and after treatment of humans, on the other hand (see Chapter 12, Figure 1).

Another interesting fact emerged from a clinical study carried out in the USA[8]; namely a comparable increase of terminal hairs during 4 months treatment with placebo or minoxidil at 2% and 3%. The number of terminal hairs after 4 months treatment was as shown in Table 1.

Table 1   No. of terminal hairs after 4 months treatment with minoxidil

	Before	After 4 months
2% Minoxidil	46.4	54.2
3% Minoxidil	44.1	52.7
Placebo	46.7	53.2

Another study[9] showed that the fairly significant regrowth of hair noted at the end of the first year of treatment receded significantly after 2 years and 9 months of continuous treatment. Nevertheless, because of the very rigorous conditions of these studies it is evident that the substance merits full attention.

2. Trans-retinoic acid shows interesting possibilities, though these still have to be verified and further clinical experience is necessary in order to evaluate the hair-growth stimulating capability and side-effects.

3. Another field of interest involves the combination of natural substances containing well-defined and standardized acid mucopolysaccharides in their formulas, such as high molecular weight hyaluronic acid, chondroitin sulfates and heparan sulfates. The importance of these substances in the hair cycle has been amply cited in earlier reports[10,11].

The problem with these high molecular weight macromolecules was that of their penetration to the level of the hair follicle. A specific vehicle was developed to achieve this goal, and the mucopolysaccharide complex became available on the market under the name Kevis.

Subsequent clinical studies have made it possible to verify the action of this combination on the amount and quality of hair. All these studies, some already published and others in the course of being published, have been checked both before and after treatment with the hair root formula – namely by trichogram, traction test, phototrichogram and computerized trichomorphometry, as well as by subjective parameters. Some were carried out as open trials; others in double-blind versus placebo format.

These studies also discussed androgenetic alopecia of the female type[11].

Since no case of acute, subacute or chronic animal toxicity has been recorded, the studies on humans were performed, and they confirmed absence of toxicity.

Tests of hypersensibility, cutaneous irritation, photosensitivity, phototoxicity, mutagenesis, ocular irritation, etc., as specified in the laws of the Common Market, have made it possible to confirm that this cosmetic mixture is reliable, very easy to handle and without systemic effects.

If this mixture can actually be faulted, it should be for the lack of a longer clinical history, since the treatment lasted for 6 months at the longest.

What is interesting is its statistically highly significant effect on the A:T ratio (and thus not only on the number of hairs on a very short-term basis (2–3 months)). These studies are detailed in other papers in this volume[12,13].

It is useful to emphasize, among other things, three important pharmacological effects of Kevis:

1. highly significant deep hydrating action[14];

2. good effect on cellular oxygenation and on vascular tropism;

3. non-hormonal anti-androgenetic action.

It is clear that, today, use of the mucopolysaccharide complex in the treatment of androgenetic alopecia is a new and promising therapy, combining a proven high significant activity with a very low incidence of side-effects (0.8%).

REFERENCES

1. Hamilton JB. Patterned long hair in man; types and incidences. *Ann NY Acad Sci*, 53, 708–714, 1951
2. Kligman AM. Pathologic dynamics of human hair loss. *Arch Dermatol*, 83, 175–195, 1961
3. Rebora A. The trichogram. In *Capelli e Medecina Estetica – Hair and Aesthetic Medicine*, (Montagna W, Serri F, Bartoletti L, Celleno L, Morganti F, Secchi GF, eds), pp. 39–42, Salus Internazionale, 1984
4. Courtois M, Giland S, Grollier JF. A contribution to the study of the growth and shedding of hair. In *Capelli e Medecina Estetica – Hair and Aesthetic Medicine*, (Montagna W, Serri F, Bartoletti L, Celleno L, Morganti F, Secchi GF, eds), pp. 43–53, Salus Internazionale, 1984
5. Bouhanna P. The phototrichogram: a technique for the objective evaluation of the diagnosis and course of diffuse alopecias. In *Capelli e Medecina Estetica – Hair and Aesthetic Medicine*, (Montagna W, Serri F, Bartoletti L, Celleno L, Morganti F, Secchi GF, eds), pp. 277–280, Salus Internazionale, 1984
6. Pelfini C, Calligaro A. Some notes on the evaluation of hair growth by means of morphometric computerized analysis. *J Appl Cosmetol*, 4, 67–76, 1986
7. Van Neste D, Dumortier M, De Coster W. Phototrichogram analysis. Technical aspects and problems in relation with automated quantitative evaluation of hair growth by computer assisted image analysis. This volume, pp. 151
8. Rietschel RL, Duncan SH. Safety and efficacy of topical minoxidil in the management of androgenetic alopecia. *J Am Acad Dermatol*, 16, 677–685, 1987
9. Olsen E, DeLong ER, Weiner MS. Long-term follow-up of men with male pattern baldness treated with topical minoxidil. *J Am Acad Dermatol*, 16, 688–695, 1987
10. Meyer K, Kaplan D, Steigleder GK. Effect of acid mucopolysaccharides on hair growth in the rabbit. *Proc Soc Exp Biol Med*, 108, 63, 1961
11. Vignini M, Speziali A, Fideli D, Dondini A. Action of a topical product on the scalp. *La Medicina Estetica*, 10, 97–100, 1986
12. Privat Y: A double blind, placebo controlled study with Kevis lotion. This volume, pp. 225
13. Pelfini C. Effects of a topical preparation on some hair growth parameters evaluated utilizing morphometric computerized analysis. This volume, pp. 213
14. Berardesca E, Gabba P, Borroni G, Rabbiosi G. Assessment of the effects of glycosaminoglycans in cutaneous hydration. *Int J Pharm Res*, 8, 69–73, 1988

23
Effects of a topical preparation on some hair growth parameters, evaluated utilizing a morphometric computerized analysis*

C Pelfini, D Fideli, A Speziali and M Vignini
Department of Dermatology
University of Pavia, Italy

ABSTRACT

The action of a topical preparation on some hair growth parameters has been evaluated. The morphometric computerized analysis applied to photographic images of a pre-determined area (with shots after cutting and after 96 h) enabled an estimation of the percentage of elements in active growth phase compared to the total number, the length of all elements and that of the sole elements in active growth phase after 96 h and the growth with respect to the base values; statistically significant differences are observed before and after 60 days treatment.

INTRODUCTION

The problem of hair growth and of the related measurement has been the subject of numerous studies during the last 60 years[1,2], both for anthropological and anatomopathological purposes and for the pharmacological evaluation of products for topical and/or systemic use. Without doubt, the evaluation of such a dynamic phenomenon as hair growth appears to be rather complex; Hamilton et al.[3] evaluated the number and weight of hairs subsequently shaven in standard areas; the most frequently used method, however, proves to be the method of successive linear measurements of shaven hairs[2,4,5,6]. Whereas Saitoh et al.[7] carried out a direct evaluation of hair growth by adopting a millimeter capillary tube which was slipped onto every single shaft, this method is more complicated but also more precise. Orentreich[8] defined hair change by carefully evaluating the number and weight of spontaneously lost hair every week; a similar and more recent

* Reproduced from the *International Journal of Cosmetic Science*, **9**, 1–11 (1987) with permission.

evaluation was conducted by Ciulla and Guarrera[9], in relation to the use of a topical preparation.

Obviously, this problem is made more complex by the need to consider the hair growth cycle which, as is well-known, was identified by Chase in 1954[10], and studied in the dermatological field by Kligman[11]: the evaluation of a hair root pulled out in its anagen–telogen–catagen phase became an essential part of the trichogram, which is extensively used in various normal conditions[5,12,13,15] and pathological conditions[16–20].

Consequently, it was necessary to study not only the growth, but also the duration of each phase of the hair cycle[11]. Decisive progress was made in 1970, with the study effected by Saitoh et al.[21], which consisted of photographs, taken at fixed intervals, of cut hairs in defined and localized areas (temples, upper lip, fingers, arms and legs) of three subjects who were kept under observation for 2 years. It was, therefore, possible to define the length of the single phases of a cycle, both in several follicles and in a single one. This technique was adopted and developed further by others[22–26] under the name of 'phototrichogram', which, by taking a series of repeated photographs in quick succession of a carefully marked area, enables the identification of which hairs are in growth phase and which are not, as well as the determination of their speed of growth and the observation, through time, of the complete evolution cycles up to the elimination of the hair being studied. The morphometric computerized analysis applied to the photographic images taken according to the Saitoh et al. technique (improved by the above-mentioned authors), is a remarkable advancement in this field[27], and enables easier and much more precise linear measurements and evaluations of the ratio between active growth phase hair and rest phase hair.

This technique has been adopted in order to evaluate the action of a topical preparation (supplied by Med-Import International) by taking photographs before and after treatment of a predetermined area of the scalp, both in alopecic patients and in healthy volunteers.

MATERIALS AND METHODS

Eighteen subjects were submitted to investigation, aged between 23 and 32 years (average age: 25.88), divided into two groups (of both sexes) of nine subjects according to clinical data and a preliminary standard trichogram, allocating subjects with not less than 25% telogen phase hair to the pathological group (B). In Group A (subjects with trichogram within normal range), two subgroups were classified, based on the clinical data: subgroup A1, consisting of four healthy subjects and subgroup A2, consisting of five subjects who complained of defluvium (without clinical correspondence) and/or seborrhea.

In Group B, always based on the clinical data, two subgroups were identified, namely B1, consisting of four subjects with alopecia classified as 3rd and 4th degree according to Hamilton[28], and B2, consisting of five subjects with thinning hair and marked defluvium, but lower than the previously mentioned degrees.

No other local or systemic pathology was present in the subjects under investigation.

The topical preparation under study consisted of thioglycoran, HUCP, thurfyl nicotinate, biotin and sodium pantothenate and was applied daily for 60 days. The subjects were allowed to wash their hair weekly with a mild shampoo of the same brand for everyone.

On each subject, the same area between the vertex and occiput was studied (which in alopecic subjects was at least 2 cm distant from the hairless area, also in order to limit the number of dystrophic hairs); for the exact location of these areas during the observation period, long stripsof graduated transparent plastic were used, placed in fixed reference points. Within the space marked by these strips, a 2 cm x 2 cm opening was made. Each subject was provided with individual strips.

The photographs were taken with a reflex camera (Pentax ME Super macro lens and extension tubes) placed on a tripod. After cutting the hair with scissors within the marked area, photographs were taken immediately (base value) and after 96 h. The whole 4 cm^2 area was photographed under standard conditions of mass-produced shots and the negative film was submitted to morphometric analysis using the image analyser Kontron Zeiss Ibas 2.

The analysis consists of the following steps (Pelfini *et al.*, 1985): scale extension of grey levels in the original image on 256 levels (normalization); editing of the image, consisting in the selection and demarcation using an interactive method by means of a graphic table of all elements which can cause erroneous measurements, with elimination of the elements which cannot be evaluated; transformation of the continuous tone image (on 256 grey levels) into binary image (segmentation), suitable for automatic evaluation of the length of the elements located.

Calculation of values

The following values were calculated for each subject before and after treatment:

Average hair length in the area under analysis and its distribution into 25 pre-determined classes after 96 h (Figure 1).

The linear measurement of these elements is carried out (according to the above programme) on a photographic image, and for this reason, in spite of shot standardization, it is affected by the inclination of the single hair shafts and obviously differs from the measurements on hair which is cut or measured *in situ*.

These determinations, however, maintain their validity if evaluated by comparison (e.g. inter-groups or pre- and post-treatment). The elements below 0.2 mm are eliminated from the calculations and graphs; verification has demonstrated that below such a value misleading elements are present: scales, debris, follicle ostia.

Percentage of active growth phase elements

In each subject, 96 h after the haircut the elements appear to be distributed into two different classes (see Figure 1): the first consisting of elements at rest phase (which can also be controlled from the values of the base image) and the second including elements in active growth phase.

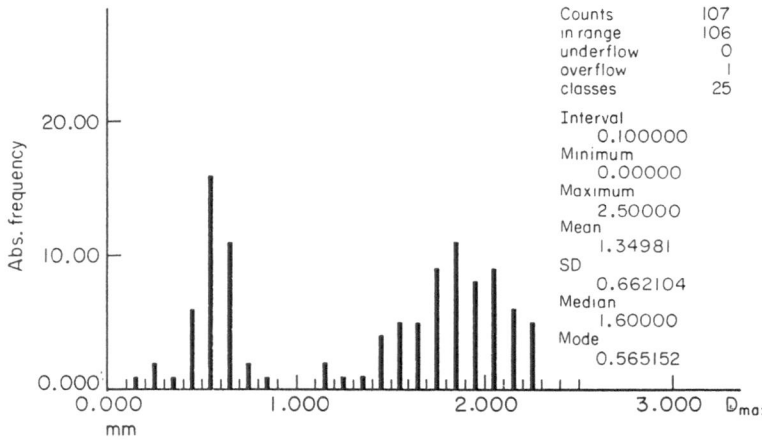

Figure 1 Example of bimodal distribution after 96 h (one of the examined subjects): it is possible to distinguish a class of elements ranging from 0.2 mm to 0.9 mm, corresponding to elements in rest phase, and another class ranging from 1.1 mm to 2.3 mm, corresponding to elements in active growth phase. Gaussian distribution

In both classes, the distribution is of a Gaussian type (normal). By subtracting from the reading taken after 96 h, those elements which are below the mean base value plus two standard deviations (95.4% of the values within a Gaussian curve), i.e. elements which in the same area have not grown, the only remaining elements are those which are in active growth phase and can be referred to the percentage of the total number.

Growth rate after 96 h

The study of only the active growth phase elements gives a precise picture of the degree of growth, expressed in length after 96 h.

Table 1 Evaluation of hair growth parameters

Subjects(n)		Parameters before treatment				Parameters after treatment			
		1	2	3	4	1	2	3	4
Group A	9	84.69	1.6730 ± 0.334	1.471 ± 0.543	1.078	91.62	1.7191 ± 0.341	1.610 ± 0.474	1.24
Sub-group A1	4	81.67	1.7635 ± 0.361	1.518 ± 0.6	1.130	91.47	1.7935 ± 0.341	1.671 ± 0.493	1.335
Sub-group A2	5	87.12	1.5812 ± 0.29	1.425 ± 0.473	1.037	91.74	1.6602 ± 0.33	1.560 ± 0.453	1.164
Group B	9	64.89	1.5335 ± 0.275	1.182 ± 0.54	0.945	80.65	1.6455 ± 0.324	1.425 ± 0.533	1.165
Sub-group B1	4	62.34	1.5524 ± 0.29	1.20 ± 0.584	0.900	82.47	1.6267 ± 0.35	1.459 ± 0.514	1.183
Sub-group B2	5	66.93	1.5186 ± 0.26	1.166 ± 0.53	0.982	79.20	1.6487 ± 0.315	1.405 ± 0.543	1.15

Parameter: 1: % hair in active growth phase in the single groups.
2: after 96 h, length of only the elements in active growth phase.
3: mean length value of all eements, evaluated after 96 h.
4: growth with respect to base
values, after 96 h.

Growth with respect to the base values

This is obtained by subtracting the mean values of the base lengths from the mean values of the lengths of the active growth phase elements after 96 h.

The values obtained before and after application of the topical produce were submitted to statistical analysis: Student's *t*-test for paired data or analysis of varience.

RESULTS

Evaluation of the dynamics of hair growth was carried out before and after treatment in the two groups and four sub-groups under examination, according to the following parameters:

— percentage of elements in active growth phase;

— growth of such elements (length 96 h after cutting);

— length of all elements (both hair in rest phase and that in active growth phase) after 96 h;

— growth (after 96 h) with respect to base values, obviously considering the elements in active growth phase only.

Pre-treatment values

The data gathered from the four parameters considered are reported in Table 1, divided according to the groups and sub-groups of subjects under examination.

Upon statistical analysis with the four sub-groups, significant results were obtained with the comparison of the percentage of the elements in active growth phase with respect to the total number of hairs; the hair length also proved to be statistically significant when all the elements, both in rest phase and in active growth phase, were considered.

The difference between the group of alopecic subjects and the group of apparently healthy subjects is remarkable. Figures 2 and 3 show the distribution into the pre-determined 25 classes of lengths (after 96 h) referred to all the elements evaluated (2), as well as the sole elements in active growth phase (3) in the apparently healthy subjects (Group A). Figures 4 and 5 report the same observations referred to the subjects suffering from alopecia (Group B).

Post-treatment values

Two months after application of the topical product, the same inter-group differences observed before treatment are maintained. The comparison between pre- and post-treatment values related to the four parameters considered proves to be statistically significant (Tables 1 and 2).

Figures 6, 7, 8 and 9 show the distribution of the main lengths and lengths of the sole elements in active growth phase of both Groups A and B.

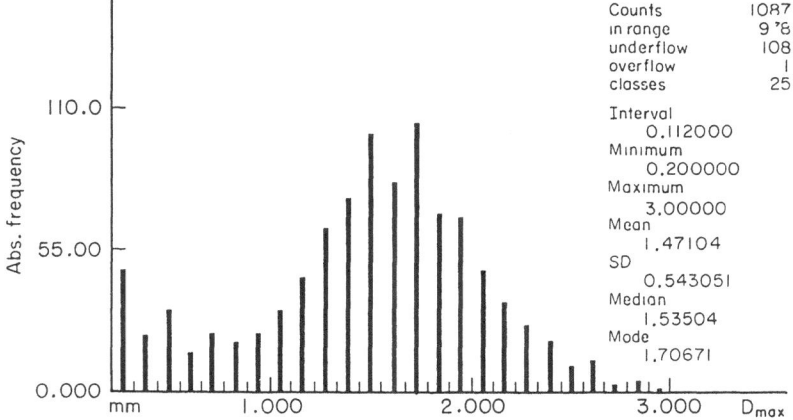

Figure 2 Group A (nine subjects): distribution according to length, in the 25 pre-determined classes, of the elements observed (96 h after cutting) in the 2 < 2 area. Pre-treatment values, mean value ± standard deviation and count of all measured elements

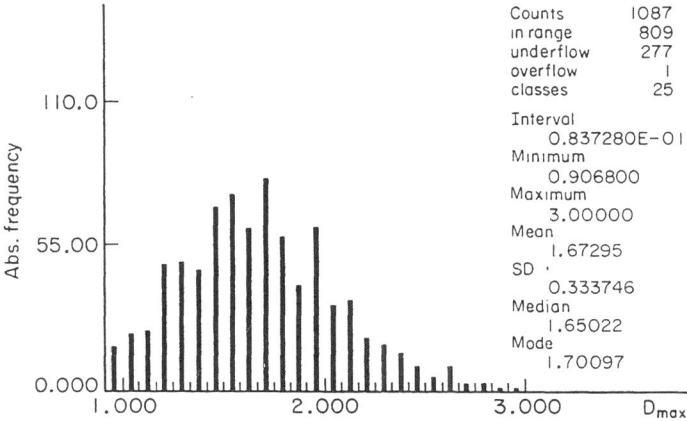

Figure 3 Group A (nine subjects): distribution in the 25 pre-determined classes of elements with growth exceeding base values (+ 2 standard deviation) after 96 h. The mean value, therefore, represents the growth of only the elements in active growth phase after 96 h (before treatment)

CONCLUSION

The morphometric image analysis has demonstrated itself as a valid and accurate method of measurement. The pre-treatment differences, between the groups under examination and particularly between subjects with and without hair pathology, were statistically confirmed by the different percentage of elements in active growth phase as well as by the measurement of mean lengths.

Table 2 Statistical analysis

Comparisons	Result	Probability	Statistical method
Total mean lengths			
pre/post-treatment	$t = 3.5131$	$p < 0.01$	t for paired data
inter-group pre-treatment	$F = 3.3828$	$p < 0.05$	analysis of variance
inter-group post-treatment	$F = 4.7734$	$p < 0.05$	analysis of variance
% active phase growth elements			
pre/post-treatment	$t = 4.89$	$p < 0.001$	t for paired data
inter-group pre-treatment	$F = 11.64$	$p < 0.005$	analysis of variance
group post-treatment	$F = 8.51$	$p < 0.005$	analysis of variance
Lengths of only active growth phase elements			
pre/post-treatment	$t = 3.1552$	$p < 0.01$	t for paired data
inter-group pre-treatment	$F = 1.0326$	ns*	analysis of variance
inter-group post-treatment	$F = 2.0384$	ns*	analysis of variance
Growth with respect to base value			
pre/post-treatment	$t = 5.7718$	$p < 0.001$	t for paired data
inter-group pre-treatment	$F = 1.0772$	ns*	analysis of variance
inter-group post-treatment	$F = 0.01$	ns*	analysis of variance

*ns = not significant

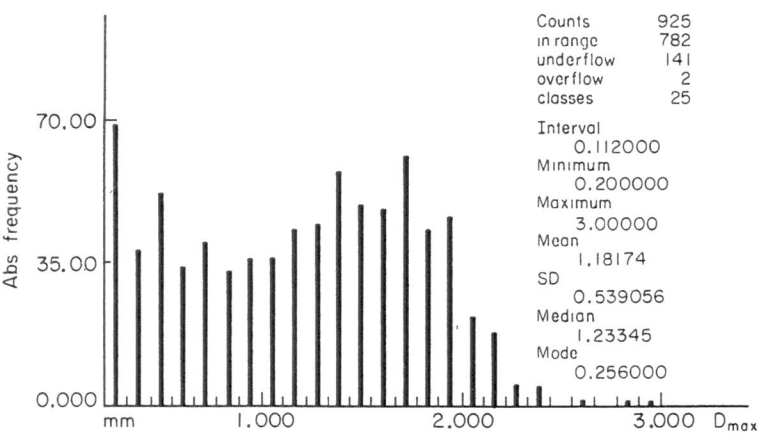

Figure 4 Group B (nine subjects with alopecia): distribution according to the length after 96 h in the 25 pre-determined classes before treatment

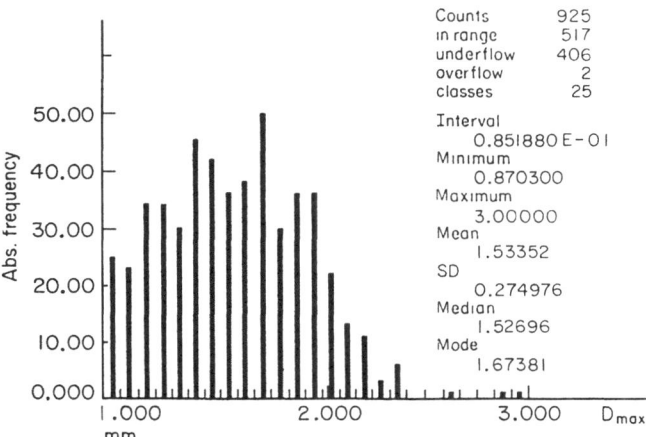

Figure 5 Group B (nine subjects with alopecia): distribution of only the elements in active growth phase in the 25 pre-determined classes before treatment

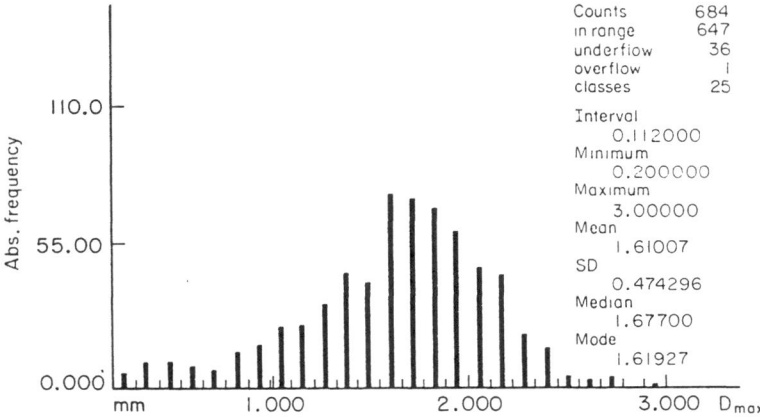

Figure 6 Group A: after treatment (nine subjects): distribution in the 25 pre-determined classes of the elements observed after 96 h, according to the lengths

The differentiation between rest phase hair and active growth phase hair, directly effected measuring the length at various intervals, appears to correspond to the real *in vivo* image of the global hair growth phenomenon. The single measurement of lengths and growth, with respect to the base value of only active growth phase hair, is another parameter which is very useful. The validity and sensitivity of the method appeared to be remarkable, above all in the comparative evaluation of the activity exerted by the treatment.

The topical preparation under test, 96 h after cutting, induced statistically significant differences on the number of elements in active growth phase on the mean hair length on the length of the only elements in the active

227

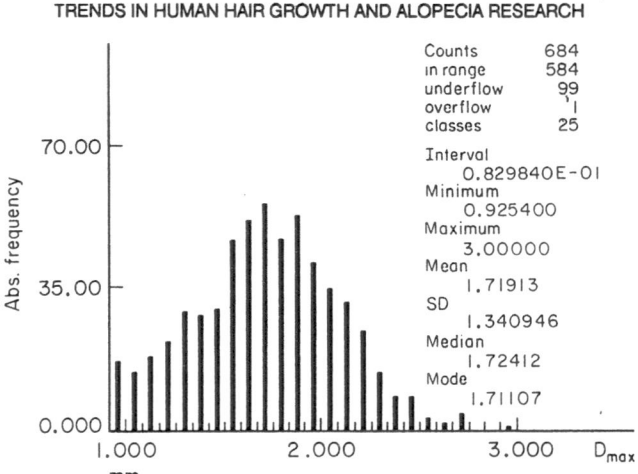

Figure 7 Group A: after treatment (nine subjects): distribution in the 25 pre-determined classes of only the elements in active growth phase according to the lengths

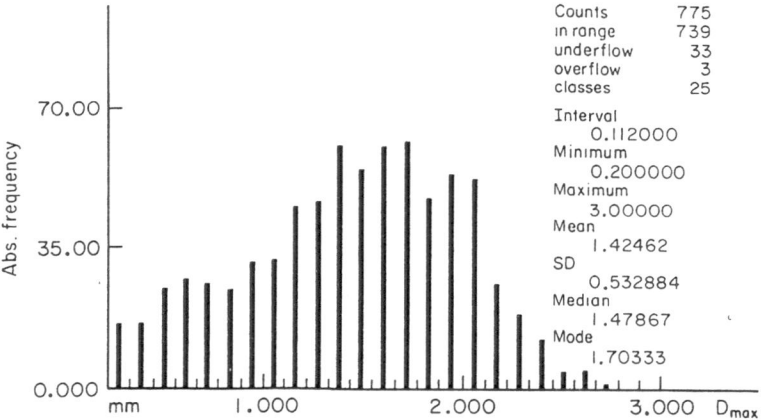

Figure 8 Group B: after treatment (nine patients with alopecia), distribution of lengths referred to 64 h

growth phase, as well as on the growth values with respect to base growth of these elements.

The action of the topical product proved to be positive, but it should be noted that the application time was limited to two months, with immediate control at the end of treatment.

It is not possible to specify how the topical product exerts its action and neither is it the purpose of this report; however, there is a probable stimulation at follicle level, which appears to induce elements to pass from the rest phase to the active growth phase, and the growth of the single element also appears to be strengthened.

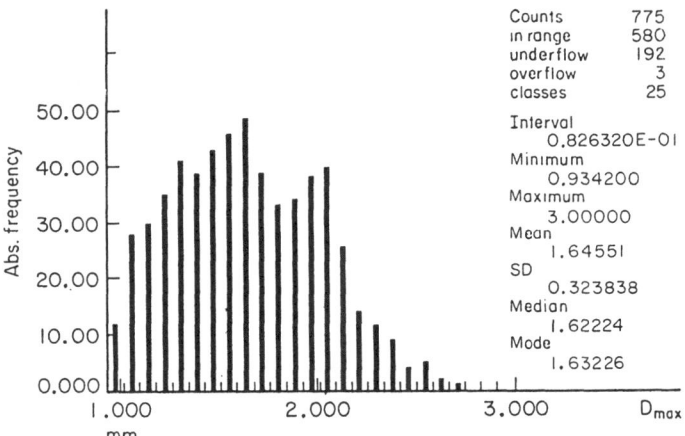

Figure 9 Group B: after treatment (nine subjects with alopecia), distribution of only the elements in active growth phase

Obviously, the objective of this investigation was neither to explain the possible mechanisms by which the above changes are obtained nor to indicate which components of the product could be responsible for such changes.

ACKNOWLEDGEMENT

The equipment was made available by courtesy of the Institute of Histology and General Embryology, University of Pavia, Italy.

REFERENCES

1.   Bulliard H. Influence de la section et du rasage répété sur l'évolution du poil. *Ann Derm Syph* 4, 386–394, 1923
2.   Trotter M. The life cycles of hair in selected regions of the body. *Am J Phys Antrop* 7, 427–437, 1924
3.   Hamilton JB, Terada H, Mestler GE, Tirman W. Hair growth (coarse sternal hairs). In *Advances in Biology of Skin*. (Montagna W & Dobson RB, eds.), Vol. IX, pp. 129–151. Oxford: Pergamon Press, 1969
4.   Myers RJ, Hamilton JB. Regeneration and rate of growth of hair in man *Ann NY Acad Sci* 53 art 3, 562–568 1951
5.   Barman YM, Pecoraro V, Astore I. Method, technique and computations in the study of the trophic state of human scalp hair. *J Invest Derm* 42 421–425, 1964
6.   Pelfini C, Cerimele D, Pisanu G. Hair growth (Aging of the skin and hair growth in man). In: *Advances in Biology of Skin* (Montagna W & Dobson RL, eds.), Vol. IX, 153–160. Oxford: Pergamon Press, 1969
7.   Saitoh M, Uzuka M, Sakamoto H, Kobori T. Hair growth (Rate of hair growth). In: *Advances in Biology of Skin* (Montagna W, Dobson RL, eds.), **Vol. IX**, 183–201. Oxford: Pergamon Press, 1969

8. Orentreich H. Hair growth (Scalp hair replacement in man). In: *Advances in Biology of Skin* (Montagna W, Dobson RL, eds.), Vol. IX, pp. 99–108. Oxford: Pergamon Press, 1969

9. Ciulla MP, Guarrera M. Valutazione dell'efficacia di un trattamento per capelli *La Medicina Estetica*, **2**, 67–74, 1984

10. Chase HB. Growth of the hair *Physiol Rev*, **34**, 113–126, 1954

11. Kligman AM. The human hair cycle *J Invest Derm*, **33**, 307–316, 1959

12. Barman JM, Astore I, Pecoraro V. The normal trichogram of the adult *J Invest Derm*, **44**, 233–236, 1965

13. Barman JM, Astore I, Pecoraro V. Hair growth (the normal trichogram of people over 50 years but apparently not bald). In *Advances in Biology of Skin* (Montagna W, Dobson RL, eds.), Vol. IX, 211–220. Oxford: Pergamon Press, 1969

14. Pecoraro V, Astore I, Barman JM. The pre-natal and post-natal hair cycles in man. In: *Biopathology of Pattern Alopecia* (Baccaredda-Boy, Moretti G, Frey Karger JR, eds), pp. 29–38. Basel, New York, 1968

15. Pelfini C, Vignini M, Zorzi F, Celleno L. Hair and senescence. In: *Hair and Aesthetic Medicine*, pp. 133–139. Roma: Salus Internazionale, 1984

16. van Scott EJ, Reinertson RP, Steinmuller R. The growing hair roots of the human scalp and morphology changes there in following amethopterin therapy. *J Invest Derm*, **29**, 197–204, 1957

17. Witzel M, Braun-Falco O. Uber den Haar-Wurzerl-status am meuschlichen cappilitium unter physiologischenbedingungen. *Arch Klin Exp Derm*, **216**, 221–230, 1963

18. Aron-Brunetiere R, Binet O, Dompmartin-Pernot D. Diagnostic des alopécies diffuses. Une approche objective: le trichogramme. *Rev Médcine*, **18**, 1263–1271, 1977

19. Lambert D, Bordes H, Brenot M, Fontany M, Duserre P. Analytical study on 150 pathologic trichograms. *Hair and Aesthetic Medicine*. pp. 293–295. Roma: Salus Internazionale, 1984

20. Rebora A. The trichogram. *Hair and Aesthetic Medicine* pp. 39–42. Roma: Salus Internazionale, 1984

21. Saitoh M, Uzuka M, Sakamoto M. Human Hair Cycle *J Invest Derm*, **54**, 65–81, 1970

22. Fiquet C, Courtois M. Une technique originale d'appréciation de la croissance et de la chute des cheveux *Cutis*, **3**, 975–984, 1979

23. Cabane J. Etude des variations de la formule pilaire à part d'une nouvelle technique photographique du trichogramme. *Bull Soc Méd*, **8,5**, 150–152, 1980

24. Courtois M, Giland S, Grollier JF. A contribution to the study of the growth and shedding of hair. *Hair and Aesthetic Medicine*, pp.43–53. Roma: Salus Internazionale, 1984

25. Bouhanna P. *The advantage of Phototrichogrm in Hair surgery.* (communication at the International Advanced Hair Replacement Symposium), Birmingham, Alabama, USA, 1982

26. Bouhanna P. The phototrichogram. *Hair and Aesthetic Medicine*, pp. 277–280. Roma: Salus Internazionale, 1984

27. Pelfini C, Calligaro A. Evaluation of hair growth by means of morphometric computerized analysis. *J Appl Cosmet*, **4**, 67–76, 1986

28. Hamilton JB. Patterned loss of hair in man: types and incidence. *Ann NY Acad Sci*, **53** art 3, 708–728, 1951

24
A double-blind, placebo-controlled study with Kevis lotion

Y Privat
Centre Hospitalier Régional, Hôtel Dieu, Place Daviel, 13002 Marseille, France

---

INTRODUCTION

Androgenetic alopecia is characterized by an acceleration of the hair cycle, leading to a decrease in the growth time (anagen period, duration: 2–6 years) without important modifications in the period of involution (duration: 2–3 weeks) and in the period of follicle rest (duration: 2–3 months).

Hair appears which is finer, smaller and more down-like, and which rapidly falls out. All the while, the resources of the hair follicles become exhausted, thus making room for a totally smooth scalp, devoid of hair[1,2].

The hair formula of the normal individual is as follows:
Hair in the growth or anagen stage 84–85%
Hair in the involuted or catagen phase 0–1%
Dead hair, repressed or telogen 15–15%

Various systems of classification have been given for alopecia, all of which include a rate of telogen hairs higher than or equal to 20%.

The aim of this study was to evaluate the effect of a hair care cosmetic lotion on early stages of male pattern baldness.

Kevis lotion is composed of mucopolysaccharides and glycoproteins, associated with substances which favor their bioavailability:

(a) HUCP. Composed of tissue material extracted from the human umbilical cord, characterized by the presence of hyaluronic acid, glycoproteins and amino acids, and endowed with a hydrating and anti-inflammatory action.

(b) Thioglycoran. Natural mucopolysaccaride acids rich in fractions of heparin sulfates and chondroitin sulfates, characterized by the presence of uronic acid, hexosamine and sulfur, and endowed with an anti-inflammatory activity.

(c) Thurfyl nicotinate. Cutaneous vasodilator.

(d)   Sodium pantothenate. Compound which participates in the making of coenzyme A, and is utilized for ailments of the scalp.

(e)   Biotin. Vitamin of the B group, co-factor in numerous carboxylases, employed for skin disorders of the seborrheic type.

Kevis lotion has been submitted to toxicological tests, as well as to primary and ocular cutaneous irritation trials in animals, which have established its innocuousness and good tolerance.

The aim of this clinical study is to determine the effectiveness and the tolerance of Kevis lotion in male patients having androgenetic alopecia, and to establish its trichogenic action against hair loss.

Other parameters which are secondary to androgenetic alopecia, and which can be improved by Kevis lotion, are studied: seborrhea, dandruff and pruritus.

MATERIALS AND METHODS

Selection of patients

Criteria for inclusion

The subjects are male ambulatory patients, aged 18 to 50 years. They manifest an androgenic alcopecia which is in developmental stage I or II according to the Hamilton–Rook classification system (corresponding at the most to degree 5 on a scale from 0 to 10)[1,2]. The percentage of telogen hairs, measured during the first phototrichogram, is 20% in the patients.

Criteria for exclusion

1.   Non-stabilized alopecias dating from less than 3 months.

2.   Alopecias of various origins: congential, iatrogenic, following stress.

3.   Associated treatment with similar therapeutic aims.

4.   Subjects for whom there are reasons to believe that they will not submit themselves to the requirements of the test.

Experiment design

The comparison is done on two parallel groups, with simple randomization and double-blind against placebo. A 'wash-out' period of 15 days previous to the first photograph of the first phototrichogram is established ($D = -20$). A sealed non-self-sealing envelope, containing the randomly established list of treatments, is handed over to the clinical expert. The items involved in the treatment are numbered and handed out in neutral packaging in the numbered order to the patients who have been approved for the test. This is done at the time of the second photograph of the first phototrichogram ($D = 0$).

Treatments compared

1. Kevis: one vial per day for 90 days, applied locally on the alopecic zone. Applying small quantities, rub lightly with the fingertips until the total contents of the vial (6 ml) have been emptied out onto the treatment zone. Then delicately massage the scalp, going from the base to the top of the cranium.

2. Placebo: one vial per day for 90 days, applied locally according to the same principle as for Kevis. The placebo has the following composition:
   1,2-propylene glycol
   ethanol
   perfume (G.I.V. P.L.V. 3531/3)
   distilled water Q.S.P.

The packages carrying the directions for use, etc. are identical and neutral. The vials are packed in three boxes of 30. Two boxes are handed out at the beginning of the study on $D = 0$. The third box is handed out on $D = 60$ during the check-up visit. The treatment lasts for 90 consecutive days. No associated treatment with a similar therapeutic aim is followed, as established in the section 'patient selection'.

Criteria for evaluation

Four criteria are retained for the evaluation of the trichogenic action:

1. the number of hairs pulled out during the traction test at the level of the tonsure;

2. the number of hairs per unit surface area (cm^2) recorded during the phototrichogram;

3. the percentage of telogen hairs recorded during the phototrichogram;

4. the number of hairs counted by the patient during the threecomb-stroke test.

Three criteria are retained for the secondary parameters of androgenic alopecia:

1. seborrhea (presence or absence)

2. dandruff (presence or absence)

3. pruritus (presence or absence)

Gathering of the data

(a) A clinical balance sheet is established before assigning the entrance number in the trial, which is inscribed on the special file provided for the clinician on $D = -20$.

Since the patient has to fill in the criteria of inclusion (with the exception of the telogen percentage, which will be verified during the first phototrichogram), the additional data noted on the sheet are the identity of the subject, his age, the date of consultation, the associated pathologies, the date of appearance of the alopecia and the number of order of inclusion in the trial.

The modalities of the three comb-stroke test are explained to the patient and a record chart is given to him for filling in daily information. This sheet is also used for recording the unforeseen effects noted by the patient.

The patient is required to stop any treatment for alopecia, seborrhea, dandruff, etc., and to wash his hair twice weekly with a mild shampoo (Proteobiol).

(b) Once the patient appears with his hair not having been washed for 3 days, and not having been combed on the day in question, the first photograph of the first phototrichogram is carried out on $D = -4$ (considering the telogen hairs). The record of the data from the three comb-stroke test is verified by the clinician on the chart given to the patient.

(c) The second photograph of the first phototrichogram is taken on $D = 0$. The first treatment kit, carrying the order number attributed to the patient, is given to him for a period of 60 days. The procedure for applying the product is explained to him. The vasodilating effect and the potentially resulting redness are made clear to him (the normal duration of this should not exceed 30 minutes).

The traction test on the tonsure is carried out by the clinician. The number of hairs pulled out is indicated on the clinical chart.

The calculation of the percentage of telogen hairs is performed later. The patient remains included in the trial until the end. The clinical charts of the patients who do not respect these criteria will be withdrawn during the processing of the statistics.

(d) A clinical balance sheet is established during the visit on $D = 60$. The sheet intended for recording the data from the three comb-stroke test and the unforeseen effects is verified.

Eventual unforeseen effects are noted and the recording of this information may be completed during the interview of the patient.

The traction test on the tonsure is carried out by the clinician. The number of hairs pulled out is indicated on the clinical chart. The second treatment kit, carrying the patient order number, is given to him for a period of 30 days.

(e) The first photograph of the second phototrichogram is taken on $D = 86$, the patient's hair not having been washed for 3 days nor having been combed on the day in question (considering the telogen hairs).

(f) The second photograph of the second phototreichogram is taken on $D = 90$. A final clinical balance sheet is established. The clinician's general evaluation of the treatment is given on the individual clinical chart, as well as the decision regarding the end of treatment.

The traction test on the tonsure is carried out by the clinician. The number of hairs pulled out is indicated on the clinical chart.

The chart recording the data from the three comb-stroke test and eventual unforeseen effects is kept by the clinician. Possible comments are noted on the clinical chart by the clinician.

Clinical tolerance

On the chart given to the patient for recording the data relating to the three comb-stroke test, one section is reserved for recording eventual unforeseen effects noted by the patient.

During both the observational consultation and the final consultation, the clinician also notes any eventual side-effects by means of systematic questioning. He also notes whether there is, in his opinion, any cause and effect relationship with the treatment.

Finally, he notes whether the treatment had to be prematurely interrupted and he notes the results at the time of interruption.

Acceptability

During consultations the clinician notes the acceptance of the product by the patient, and whether or not the patient desires to continue the treatment, as well as the reasons which could motivate a negative response.

Test supervision

Each patient taken into account during the study undergoes three consultations:

1. To determine the admissibility of the patient to the trial ($D = -20, -4, 0$), during which the first trichogram and the first traction test on the tonsure are carried out. He receives the treatment kit, covering a period of 60 days, and the record sheet for the data from the three comb-stroke test and eventual unforeseen effects.

235

2. To verify the information gathered by the patient, to carry out the second traction test on the tonsure, to establish an intermediate balance sheet and to give him the remainder of the treatment for 30 days ($D = 60$).

3. In the course of this consultation the final information is gathered: the sheet for the three comb-stroke test, eventual unforeseen effects, patient evaluation, traction test on the tonsure, second phototrichogram and the clinician's conclusion ($D = 86, 90$).

The patients are re-summoned for each consultation.

Phototrichogram

Macrophotographic method derived from the Saitoh technique[3] for the study of the pilar cycles, which makes possible the counting of the number of hairs per unit of surface area (cm^2) and the differentiation of the telogen hairs from the anagen–catagen hairs (the anagen and catagen hairs are regrouped in the enumeration for the ease of counting, only the percentage of telogen hairs being a criterion submitted to statistical processing).

Two photographs are taken, at a 3- and 4-day interval, of a marked zone on the section of the scalp affected by alopecia, on which the hairs have been cut to a length of 1 mm[4–7]. The comparison of the lengths observed for the hairs at the two times allows a detailed account of the hairs at the different phases of their pilar cycle. The different phototrichogram ($D = 0, D = 90$) are carried out on the same marked zone of the section affected by alopecia.

Three comb-stroke test

Daily, before going to bed, the patient makes a 'stroke of the comb', from front to back at the level of the top and the lateral regions respectively of the cranium. The number of hairs retained by the comb after these three strokes of the comb is counted and recorded on the record sheet.

A weekly average is established, which serves for the values used in calculating the variations of the parameter between $D = 0$ (beginning of week 0), $D = 60$ (middle of week 8) and $D = 90$ (end of week 12).

Traction test on the tonsure

For the clinician, this test consists of applying traction on a tuft of hair at the level of the border of the alopecic zone (or tonsure). The traction is carried out in the direction of the implantation of the hair, firmly, though without the purpose of pulling the hair out.

The hairs pulled out are counted and their number recorded on the follow-up chart by the clinician on $D = 0, D = 60$ and $D = 90$.

Analysis of the trial

Population and distribution

The treatment boxes numbered 1 to 100 have been distributed in the random order established by the manufacturer, or producer, or pharmaceutical company, the patients being allocated equally to the two groups.

Included population

Of the 100 subjects originally included, those who finished the study included 40 in the group treated with Kevis lotion and 36 in the group which received the placebo.

Excluded population

Twenty-four observations were not retained. Twenty-two subjects showed a percentage of telogen hairs below 20% in the course of the first phototrichogram. Two subjects did not finish the trial; one quit after the consultation on $D = 60$, and the second did not show up for it. The excluded subjects are divided into 10 exclusions in the group which received Kevis lotion and 14 in the placebo group.

Statistical analysis

The statistical analysis covers:

1. testing of the hypothesis of group identity with respect to the elements recorded at the time of entrance in the trial, by bilateral tests with a risk of alpha = 0.01;

2. the comparison between the two treatments (in view of the rejection of the null hypothesis), with respect to the criteria of effectiveness, by bilateral tests with a risk of alpha = 0.05.

The experimental organization of the test (controlled type) allows a statistical analysis of the results, with a causal interpretation. Seventy-six observations are utilized: 36 in the placebo group, 40 in the Kevis group. The tests utilized are:

1. the Chi-squared test for comparison of the frequencies;

2. after verification of the homogeneity of the variances, the ANOVA (ANalysis Of VAriance) test or the Cochran test for the comparison of the means are employed. To take the matched-pair effect into account, the comparison covers the differences observed for each subject between $D = 60$ and $D = 0$, or between $D = 90$ and $D = 0$.

In the tables are found either frequencies with the corresponding percentages, or the means, their standard deviation (Mean ± SD) and the amount of data.

237

RESULTS

Hypothesis testing of the identity of the groups and description of the patient sample

This concerns the factors recorded at the time of entrance into the trial.

1. Age (cf. Table 1)

2. Duration of the alopecia (cf. Table 2)

3. Significance of the alopecia (cf. Table 3)

4. Presence or absence of seborrhea (cf. Table 4)

5. Presence or absence of dandruff (cf. Table 5)

6. Presence or absence of pruritus (cf. Table 6)

7. Traction test on the tonsure (cf. Table 7)

8. Three comb-strokes test (cf. Table 8)

9. Phototrichogram: (a) number of hairs per unit surface area (cf. Table 9); (b) percentage of telogen hairs (cf. Table 10)

10. Suspensions of treatment. There were no suspensions of treatment.

11. Drop-outs. Two patients dropped out – one in each group.

12. Conclusions. None of the differences observed between the two groups is significant; they can be considered to be comparable. The two patients who dropped out can be excluded from the analysis.

Observance of the treatment

All the patients respected the posology of the treatment. Some subjects, both in the group receiving the Kevis lotion and in the group receiving the placebo, mentioned some omissions which were unrepeated and which could not compromise the results of the test.

Effectiveness of the treatment

The comparison concerns the criteria of effectiveness.

Trichogenic action

Phototrichogram

1. Number of hairs per unit of surface area (cf. Table 9). This increases more in 90 days in the Kevis group than in the placebo group, but the difference is not statistically significant.

238

2.   Percentage of telogen hairs (cf. Table 10). This diminishes more in 90 days in the Kevis group than in the placebo group, and this in a statistically significant way.

Three comb-stroke test (cf. Table 8)
The number of hairs lost decreases more (both after 60 and 90 days) in the Kevis group than in the placebo group, and this in a statistically significant way.

Traction test (cf. Table 7)
The number of hairs pulled out decreases more (both after 60 and 90 days) in the Kevis group than in the placebo group, and this in a statistically significant way.

Secondary effects

1.   Presence or absence of seborrhea (cf. Table 4). This is not modified in a statistically significant way.

2.   Presence or absence of dandruff (cf. Table 5). This is not modified in a statistically significant way.

3.   Presence or absence of pruritis (cf. Table 6). The pruritis diminishes slighly more – in 90 days – in the Kevis group than in the placebo group, but not in a statistically significant way.

Tolerance

1.   Tolerance of the product (cf. Table 11). The ratio of the average tolerance of the products does not differ significantly between the two groups, either at $D = 60$ or at $D = 90$.

2.   Side-effects (cf. Table 11). The number of patients showing side-effects does not differ significantly between the two groups, either at $D = 60$ or at $D = 90$.

Conclusion of the statistical study

In this experiment, which allows a causal interpretation for comparable groups, the effectiveness of Kevis in comparison with a placebo is revealed in a statistically significant manner:

1.   On the percentage of telogen hairs: in 90 days it decreases by 16% in the Kevis group, and only by 6% in the placebo group;

2.   On the number of hairs counted in the three comb-stroke test:
     (a)   in the Kevis group it decreases by 56% in 60 days and by 59% in 90 days;

(b)   in the placebo group it only decreases by 18% in 60 days and by 16% in 90 days.

3.   On the number of hairs pulled out in the traction test:

(a)   in the Kevis group it decreases by 29% in 60 days and by 47% in 90 days,

(b)   in the placebo group it only decreases by 5% in 60 days and by 7% in 90 days.

The number of hairs per unit surface area is not altered in a statistically significant way.

There is no apparent statistically significant action of Kevis on seborrhea, dandruff or pruritus. Concerning this last criterion, it tends to decrease more in the Kevis group than in the placebo group.

There is a good tolerance and it is the same for both groups.

Table 1 Subject: age Mean ± SD

Treatment	Time $D = 0$
Placebo $(n = 36)$	42.28 ± 0.846
Kevis $(n = 40)$	39.97 ± 0.922
Comparison between the two treatments	$F^1_{74} = 3.34$ N.S.
Total number of patients $(n = 76)$	41.07 ± 0.639

Table 2 Subject: duration of the alopecia (months), Mean ± SD

Treatment	Time $D = 0$
Placebo $(n = 36)$	37.58 ± 2.717
Kevis $(n = 40)$	30.67 ± 2.267
Comparison between the two treatments	$F^1_{74} = 3.86$ N.S.
Total number of patients $(n = 76)$	33.95 ± 1.788

Table 3 Subject: significance of the alopecia (from 0 to 10), Mean ± SD

Treatment	Time $D = 0$
Placebo ($n = 36$)	2.36 ± 0.165
Kevis ($n = 40$)	2.05 ± 0.172
Comparison between the two treatments	$F^1_{74} = 1.69$ N.S.
Total number of patients ($n = 76$)	2.20 ± 0.120

Table 4 Subject: seborrhea

	Time					
	$D = 0$		$D = 60$		$D = 90$	
Treatment	Presence	Absence	Presence	Absence	Presence	Absence
Placebo ($n = 36$)	13 (36.1%)	23 (63.9%)	8 (22.2%)	28 (77.8%)	8 (22.2%)	28 (77.8%)
Kevis ($n = 40$)	8 (20.0%)	32 (80.0%)	5 (12.5%)	35 (87.5%)	5 (12.5%)	35 (87.5%)
Comparison between the two treatments	$\chi^2 = 2.45$ N.S.		$\chi^2 = 1.26$ N.S.		$\chi^2 = 1.26$ N.S.	
Total number of patients ($n = 76$)	21 (27.6%)	55 (72.4%)				

Table 5 Subject: dandruff

	Time					
	$D = 0$		$D = 60$		$D = 90$	
Treatment	Presence	Absence	Presence	Absence	Presence	Absence
Placebo ($n = 36$)	16 (44.4%)	20 (55.6%)	12 (33.3%)	24 (66.7%)	12 (33.3%)	24 (66.7%)
Kevis ($n = 40$)	9 (22.5%)	31 (77.5%)	9 (22.5%)	31 (77.5%)	6 (15.0%)	34 (85.0%)
Comparison between the two treatments	$\chi^2 = 4.13$ N.S.		$\chi^2 = 1.11$ N.S.		$\chi^2 = 3.52$ N.S.	
Total number of patients ($n = 76$)	25 (32.9%)	51 (67.1%)				

241

Table 6 Subject: pruritus

	Time					
	$D = 0$		$D = 60$		$D = 90$	
Treatment	Presence	Absence	Presence	Absence	Presence	Absence
Placebo ($n = 36$)	10	26	6	30	7	29
	(27.8%)	(72.2%)	(16.7%)	(83.3%)	(19.4%)	(80.6%)
Kevis ($n = 40$)	10	30	6	34	2	38
	(25.0%)	(75.0%)	(15.0%)	(85.0%)	(5.0%)	(95.0%)
Comparison between	$\chi^2 = 0.07$		$\chi^2 = 0.039$		$\chi^2 = 3.78$	
the two treatments	N.S.		N.S.		N.S.	
Total number of	20	56				
patients ($n = 76$)	(26.3%)	(73.7%)				

Table 7 Subject: traction test on the tonsure, Mean ± SD

	Time		
Treatment	$D = 0$	$D = 60 - D = 0$	$D = 90 - D = 0$
Placebo ($n = 36$)	4.11 ± 0.248	-0.20 ± 0.266	-0.30 ± 0.287
Kevis ($n = 40$)	3.80 ± 0.224	-1.12 ± 0.193	-1.80 ± 0.261
Comparison between	$F^1_{74} = 0.87$	$F^1_{74} = 8.10$	$F^1_{74} = 14.91$
the two treatments	N.S.	$p < 0.001$	$p < 0.001$
Total number of	3.95 ± 0.166		
patients ($n = 76$)			

Table 8 Subject: three comb-strokes test, Mean ± SD

	Time		
Treatment	$D = 0$	$D = 60 - D = 0$	$D = 90 - D = 0$
Placebo ($n = 36$)	16.48 ± 1.719	-2.96 ± 0.604	-2.60 ± 0.784
Kevis ($n = 40$)	13.85 ± 1.060	-7.70 ± 0.510	-8.24 ± 0.534
Comparison between	$F^1_{74} = 1.89$	$F^1_{74} = 35.76$	$F^1_{74} = 37.86$
the two treatments	N.S.	$p < 0.001$	$p < 0.001$
Total number of	14.93 ± 0.949		
patients ($n = 76$)			

Table 9 Subject: number of hairs per unit surface area, Mean ± SD

	Time	
Treatment	$D = 0$	$D = 90 - D = 0$
Placebo ($n = 36$)	132.5 ± 2.37	2.83 ± 2.468
Kevis ($n = 40$)	123.8 ± 2.16	10.45 ± 3.151
Comparison between	$F^1{}_{74} = 0.70$	$F^1{}_{74} = 3.51$
the two treatments	N.S.	N.S.
Total number of	131.1 ± 1.59	
patients ($n = 76$)		

Table 10 Subject: percentage of telogen hairs, Mean ± SD

	Time	
Treatment	$D = 0$	$D = 90 - D = 0$
Placebo ($n = 36$)	22.97 ± 0.407	-1.44 ± 0.514
Kevis ($n = 40$)	24.45 ± 0.722	-3.77 ± 0.642
Comparison between	$F^1{}_{74} = 3.18$	$F^1{}_{74} = 7.80$
the two treatments	N.S.	$p < 0.01$
Total number of	23.75 ± 0.432	
patients ($n = 76$)		

Table 11 Subject: tolerance and side-effects of the product

	Time			
	$D = 60$		$D = 90$	
Treatment	Medium	Good	Medium	Good
Placebo ($n = 36$)	2	34	0	36
	(5.6%)	(94.4%)	(0%)	(100%)
Kevis ($n = 40$)	6	34	2	38
	(15.0%)	(85.0%)	(5.0%)	(95.0%)
Comparison between	$\chi^2 = 0.514$		$\chi^2 = 1.84$	
the two treatments	N.S.		N.S.	
Total number of	8	68		
patients ($n = 76$)	(10.5%)	(89.5%)		

DISCUSSION

This double-blind trial of Kevis lotion versus placebo was carried out on a sample of 100 male patients, 76 of whom completed the test (Kevis $n = 40$, placebo $n = 36$) and were statistically processed. The effectiveness of Kevis lotion was evaluated by reference techniques such as the phototrichogram, the three comb-stroke test, and the traction test on the tonsure.

The effectiveness of Kevis lotion in the treatment of androgenic alopecia is assessed by:

1. the decrease in the percentage of telogen hairs after 90 days of treatment ($p < 0.01$);

2. the decrease in the number of hairs pulled out during the traction test performed on the tonsure after 60 and 90 days of treatment ($p < 0.01$);

3. the decrease in the number of hairs counted during the three comb-stroke test after 60 and 90 days of treatment ($p < 0.001$).

The tolerance was judged to be good. The side-effects were judged to be minor.

Kevis lotion did not demonstrate its effectiveness as to certain criteria secondary to androgenic alopecia: seborrhea, pruritus and dandruff. The effectiveness of Kevis lotion on androgenic alopecia translates into an anti-falling-out effect, which was objectified by the decrease in the percentage of telogen hairs. This decrease is noted, even when the number of hairs per unit surface area does not show a significant difference. It can thus be directly correlated with an increase in the number of anagen hairs; this correlation can be associated with the regrowth effect exercised by the Kevis lotion.

This regrowth effect can equally be linked to the decrease in the number of hairs pulled out during the traction test on the tonsure, which translates into a better tonicity of the hair follicle.

In summary, Kevis lotion can be considered to have demonstrated an 'anti-falling-out and in certain cases regrowth' action in the course of its use with subjects showing an androgenic alopecia. It has also demonstrated a satisfactory tolerance. Attention should be paid to the painful erythema which can occur during the application of the product.

REFERENCES

1. Hamilton JB. Patterned long hair in man; types and incidence. *Ann NY Acad Sci*, **53**, 708–714, 1951

2. Hamilton JB. Age, sex, and genetic factors in the regulation of hair growth in man: a comparison of caucasian and japanese populations. In *The Biology of Hair Growth* (Montagna W, Ellis RA, eds), pp. 399–433, New York: Academic Press, 1958

3. Saitoh M, Uzuka M, Sakamoto M. Human hair cycle. *J Invest Dermatol*, **54**, 65–81, 1970

4. Courtois M, Giland S, Grollier JF. A contribution to the study of the growth and shedding of hair. In *Capelli e Medecina Estetica – Hair and Aesthetic Medicine* (Montagna W, Serri F, Bartoletti L, Celleno L, Morganti F, Secchi GF, eds), pp. 43–53, Salus Internazionale, 1984

5. Bouhanna P. The phototrichogram: a technique for the objective evaluation of the diagnosis and course of diffuse alopecias. In *Capelli e Medecina Estetica – Hair and*

Aesthetic Medicine (Montagna W, Serri F, Bartoletti L, Celleno L, Morganti F, Secchi GF, eds), pp. 277–280, Salus Internazionale, 1984

6.   Guarrera M, Ciulla MP. A quantitative evaluation of hair loss: the phototrichogram. *J Appl Cosmetol*, **4**, 61–66, 1986

7.   Pelfini C, Calligaro A. Some notes on the evaluation of hair growth by means of morphometric computerized analysis. *J Appl Cosmetol*, **4**, 67–76, 1986

25
Topical minoxidil used before and after hair transplantation surgery

P Bouhanna
Hair Department
Hôpital Saint-Louis
Paris, France

ABSTRACT

A 2% topical minoxidil solution was applied on the recipient bald scalp of sixteen patients aged 25 to 52 years with Hamilton classification of androgenetic alopecia from III to IV. Therapy began 4 weeks before surgery, then stopped during 3 weeks and started again for 3 months. 4 mm grafts were inserted into 3.5 mm recipient holes. A macrophotographic follow-up was done for 3 months on four grafts near a tattooed located area. On about 71% of the 64 grafts, partial or total hair is still growing without the shedding that usually occurs 2–4 weeks after transplantation. Topical minoxidil seems to be an adjunct for a better evolution of grafts after hair transplant surgery.

INTRODUCTION

Since 1974 in our own practice we have used the punch graft technique[1,2] for the treatment of androgenetic alopecia[3,4]. Until 1981 we used a macrophotographic study and the phototrichogram technique for the follow-up of grafts and flaps[5]. We have carried out 64 of 4 mm punch grafts on 16 individuals. Patients were treated with a 2% solution of topical minoxidil. Therapy began 1 month before hair transplantation and started again 3 weeks after transplantation for 3 months. A macrophotographic follow-up of located grafts was done for 3 months. Several patients demonstrated hair growth in the grafts without the shedding that usually occurs 2 to 4 weeks after surgery (Figure 1). Hairs are still growing, whereas regrowth begins 3–5 months after surgery in untreated patients. Contrary to the opinion of many authors[6] we have found that the postoperative shedding phase which occurs in the grafts about 3 weeks after transplantation is an anagen defluvium and not a telogen effluvium (Figure 2).

MATERIAL AND METHODS

Sixteen healthy male patients aged 25–52 years with Hamilton classification of androgenetic alopecia from III to IV, who were undergoing a hair transplant procedure, participated in this open controlled study. Each patient was given a complete physical and biological examination. Beginning 1 month before surgery, each subject applied minoxidil 2%, 1 ml twice daily on the recipient area. This local treatment was stopped for 3 weeks and started again for 3 months. Sixty-four 4 mm punch grafts were harvested with a 4 mm power punch. The occipital area was infiltrated with a solution of 1% lidocaine and epinephrine. Saline solution was administered to increase tissue turgor. Twenty to 30 min elapsed between the harvesting and cleaning of the grafts and their insertion into the recipient area. During this period the grafts were placed in a saline solution at room temperature. All 4 mm grafts were transplanted into a 3.5 mm hole at an angle of about 60°.

A macrophotographic follow-up was done for 3 months on four grafts near a tattooed located area for each of the 16 individuals (Figure 3).

The macrophotographic equipment is an Olympus OM2 with a 50 mm macro-objective, a telescopic tube, a lateral flash Olympus T32 (Figure 4) and a grid of our own fabrication screwed on the objective which outlines 0.25 cm^2 areas[7,8]. The grid is applied on each located graft to be studied and the central 0.25 cm^2 area is photographed. Three successive macrophotographs are taken on the grafted area and on each located graft on Day 0 and Day 90 (Figure 5). This macrophotographic technique enables objective assessment of hair loss and hair regrowth of each graft.

Results

We carried out 64 punch grafts of 4 mm on 16 healthy male individuals aged 25–52 years with a 2% minoxidil topical treatment. Hairs on grafts were counted at Day 0, Day 30 and Day 90.

DISCUSSION

A 2% topical minoxidil solution used in preoperative and postoperative transplantation sessions seems to be effective on postoperative shedding and regrowth of hair on transplants. Contrary to many authors the postoperative shedding phase is not a telogen effluvium but an anagen defluvium. It is an explanation of the shedding hair which occurs 2–4 weeks after hair transplantation and the regrowth which begins 3–5 months after surgery in untreated patients. We have not found any report of immediate hair growth after hair transplantation without a prior shedding of hair.

It is of considerable interest that, 30 days after a hair transplant session, hairs are still growing on about 71% of grafts but hair loss was less than 50% in about 31% of grafts (Table 1). Three months after transplantation hair loss

248

was less than 50% on about 84% of grafts (Table 2). On the grafts some thick hairs 2–4 cm in length form the primarily growing hair, and some fine and short hairs form the new growing hair. Topical minoxidil seems to allow an unceasing anagen stage and therefore to be an important adjunct for better evolution of grafts after hair transplantation (Figure 6).

Table 1   Evaluation of the hair loss on grafts at Day 30

Rate of hair loss (%)	Number of grafts	Rate of grafts (%)
100	18	28.12
75–99	13	20.34
50–75	13	20.34
25–50	11	17.18
0–25	9	14.09

Table 2   Evaluation of the hair loss on grafts at Day 90

Rate of hair loss (%)	Number of grafts	Rate of grafts (%)
100	2	3.12
75–99	4	6.25
50–75	4	6.25
25–50	18	28.12
0–25	36	56.25

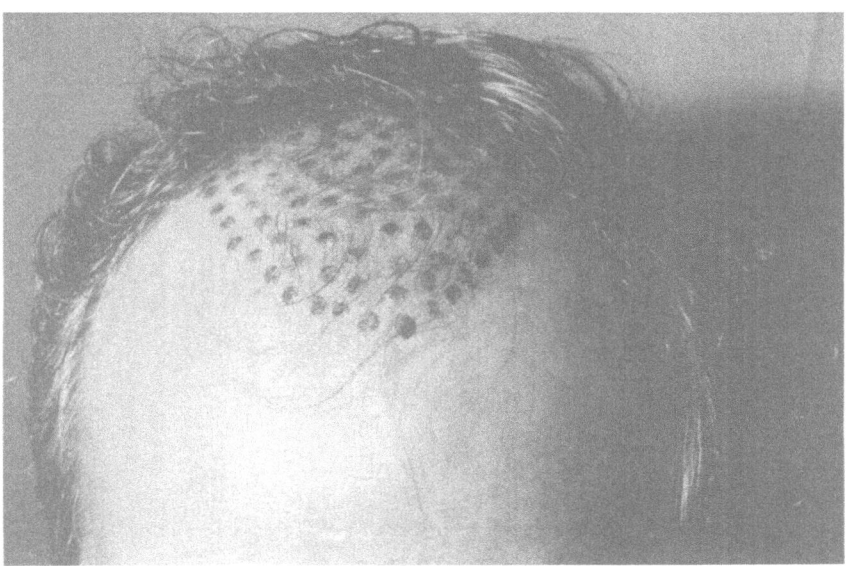

Figure 1A

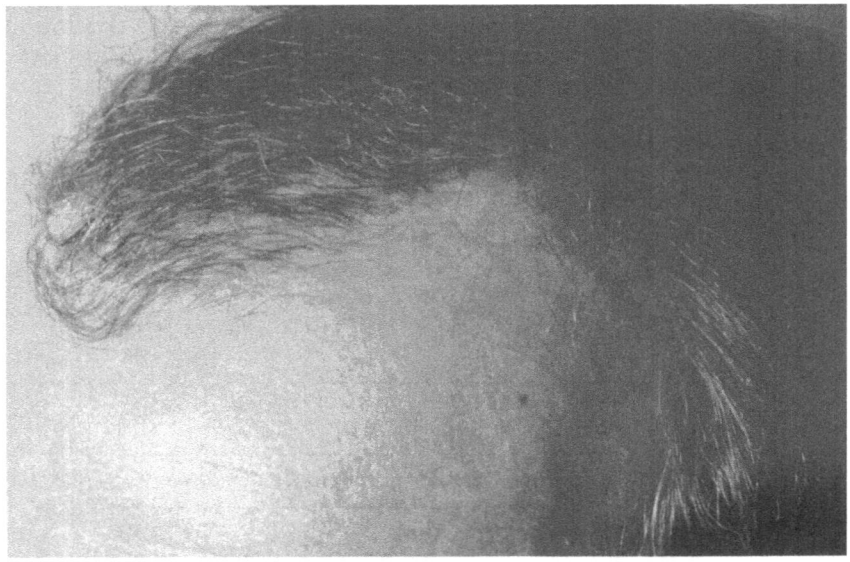

Figure 1B

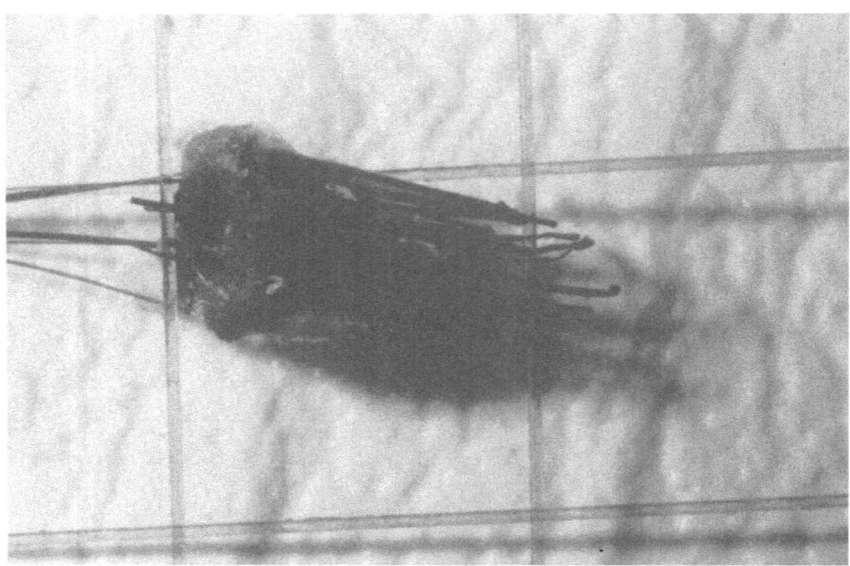

Figure 2

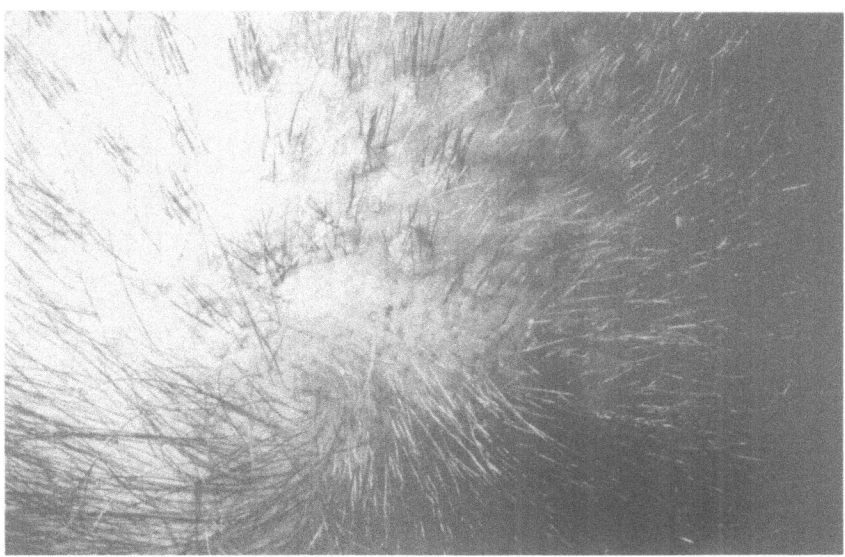

Figure 3A

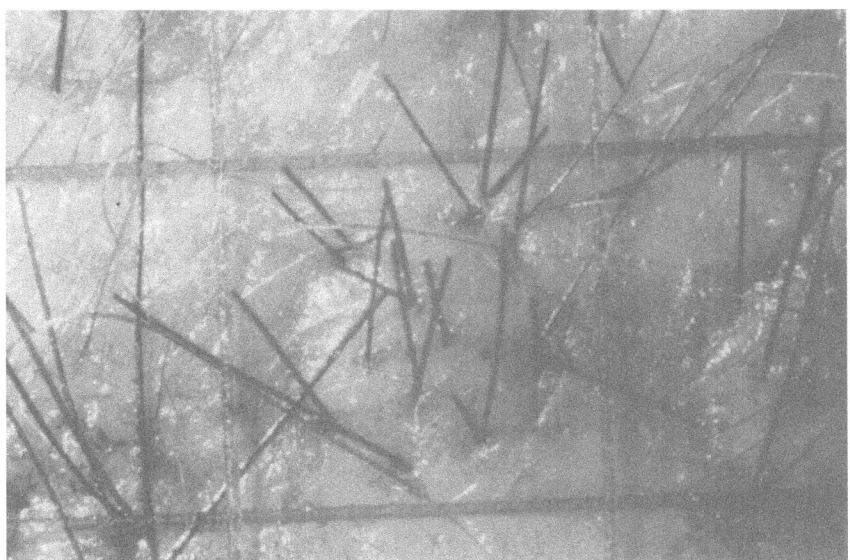

Figure 3B

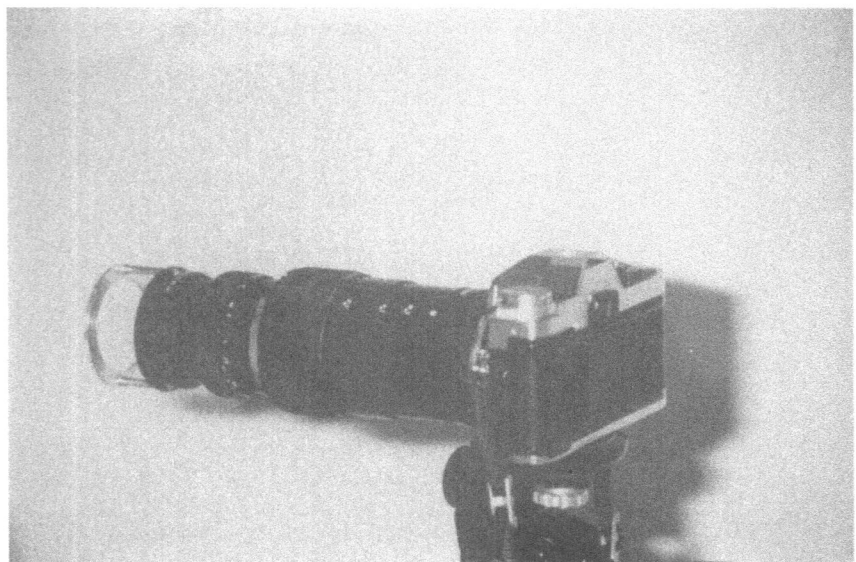

Figure 4

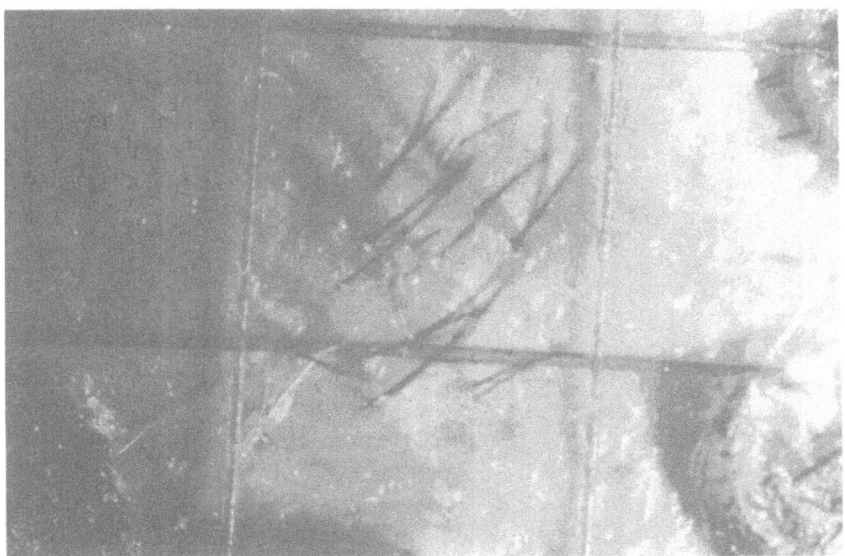

Figure 5A

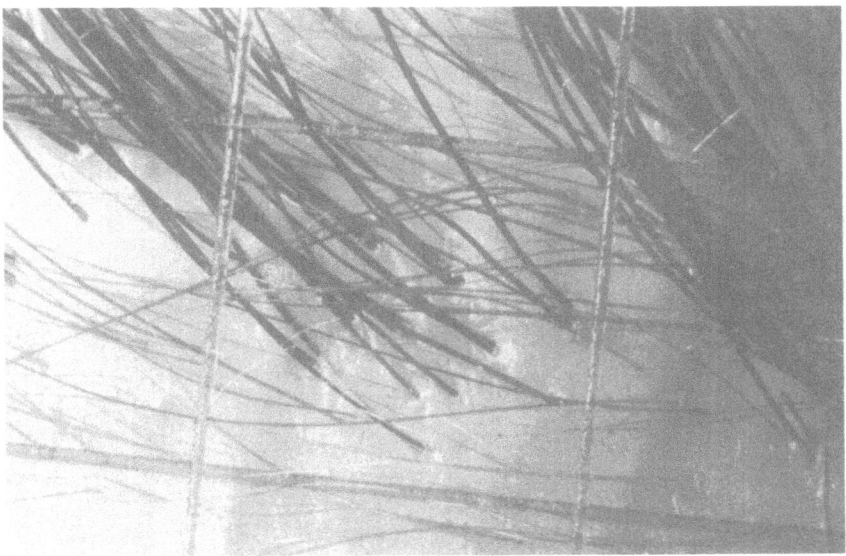

Figure 5B

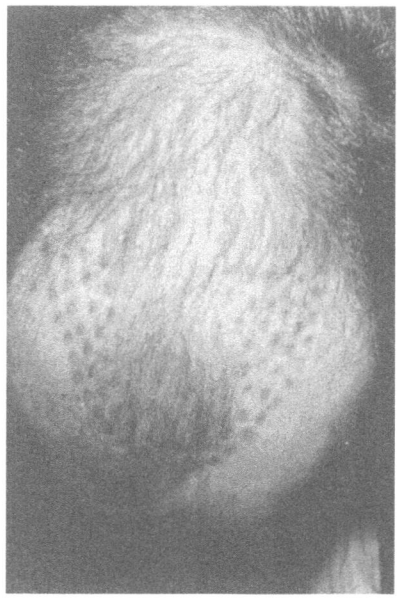

Figure 6A

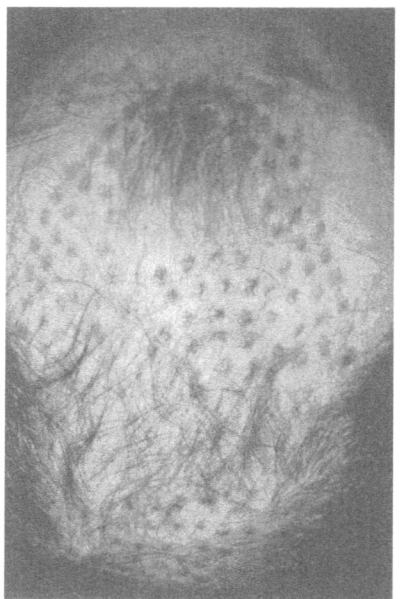

Figure 6B

REFERENCES

1. Okuda S. The study of clinical experiments and hair transplantation. *Jpn J Dermatol Urol*, October: 537, 1939
2. Orentreich N. Autografts in alopecias and other related dermatologic conditions. *Ann NY Acad Sci*, **83**, 403, 1959
3. Bouhanna P. Le cuir chevelu. Les alopécies définitives et leurs traitements. Thesis, Paris, 1976
4. Bouhanna P, Nataf J. A propos des transplantations du cuir chevelu. Critiques et propositions. *Rev Chir Esth*, **7**, 17–23, 1976
5. Bouhanna P. The advantage of phototrichogram in hair surgery. The international advanced hair replacement symposium. Birmingham, Alabama, 3–4 February, 1982
6. Kassimir JJ. Use of topical minoxidil as a possible adjunct to hair transplant surgery. *J Am Acad Derm*, **16**, 685–687, 1987
7. Bouhanna P. The phototrichogram. A technique for the objective evaluation of the diagnosis and course of diffuse alopecias. In *Hair and Esthetic Medicine* (Montagna W, ed.), Rome: Salus ed, 1983
8. Bouhanna P. The phototrichogram: an objective technique used in hair replacement surgery evaluation. In *Hair Transplantation*, 2nd edn (Unger PW, Nordström RE, eds). New York: Marcel Dekker, 1987
9. Bouhanna P. Topical minoxidil used in hair surgery. The international congress for hair replacement surgery. Los Angeles, California, 21–24 May, 1987

26
Clinical and macrophotographic study of the percutaneous implantation of synthetic hair (Nido SHI)

P. Bouhanna
Hair Department,
Hôpital Saint Louis,
Paris, France

ABSTRACT

A clinical study was made on scalp at 3 days, 1 month, 3 months and 6 months following implantation of synthetic fibers developed as artificial hair in Japan. Sixteen male and female patients with cicatricial or androgenetic alopecia were implanted. The clinical follow-up was completed by macro-photography of the same located areas. We have evaluated the density, durability and complications after synthetic hair implantation of small located bald areas (0.25 cm^2).

INTRODUCTION

There have been some clinical studies of the evolution of the implanted synthetic hair on scalp. We examined 16 individuals from a total of 20 patients. Four were excluded. Sixteen patients were implanted with Nido synthetic hair on located bald areas. A macrophotographic follow-up of these areas was carried out for 6 months.

MATERIAL AND METHODS

The polyester fibers and implantation needles used were all developed by the Nido company. The fiber, made from polyethylene terephthalate about 0.09 mm diameter, has an alpha-shaped loop root portion[1]. The fiber was implanted on the galea through the epidermis, dermis and hypodermis with a 0.23 mm special needle[2]. Sixteen healthy male and female patients aged 20–45 years, with Hamilton classification of 13 androgenetic alopecia from grade III to VI or 3 with non-evolutive cicatricial alopecia undergoing a test with Nido synthetic hair implant, participated in this controlled study. Each patient was given a complete physical and clinical examination and a complete scalp evaluation from 0 to 3 of seborrhea, pruritus, dandruff, thickness and

Table 1 Implantation of Nido synthetic hair

			Sex	Age	Type of alopecia	Seborrhea	Pruritus	Dandruff	Thickness	Laxity
1	BEL	Fatima	F	20	Cicatricial alopecia	+	0	0	+	0
2	BER	Philippe	M	37	A A M IV	+ +	0	0	+ + +	+ + +
3	DUP	Henry Paul	M	42	A A M III	0	0	0	+	+ + +
4	FLA	Jean François	M	30	A A M V	+ +	+ +	+ +	+	+ +
5	FOU	Monique	F	36	A A F II	+ +	+	0	0	+ +
6	GRI	Jean Yves	M	37	A A M III	+ +	0	0	+	+
7	HOU	Jean Claude	M	38	A A M V	+ + +	0	0	+	+ +
8	LAB	Patrick	M	34	A A M IV	+ + +	0	0	+	+ +
9	LEB	Marc	M	29	A A M V	0	0	0	+ + +	+ +
10	MEK	Lounes	M	37	A A M V	+	0	0	+ + +	+ +
11	PAU	Alain	M	32	Cicatricial alopecia	0	+	+	+	0
12	QUE	Franck	M	22	A A M IV	+ +	0	0	+	+ +
13	RAM	Mohamed	M	31	A A M V	+ +	+	0	+	+ +
14	TIL	Ali	M	45	A A M VI	+ + +	+	+ +	+	+ + +
15	GES	Pascal	M	24	Cicatricial alopecia	+	0	0	0	+ + +
16	BAL	Christian	M	29	A A M V	+	+	+	+	+ + +

laxity (Table 1). Macrophotographic equipment comprising an Olympus OM2, a 50 mm macro-objective, a telescopic tube, and a lateral flash Olympus T32 was used[3] (Figure 1). A grid of our own fabrication[4] was screwed on the macro-objective and permitted outlines of 0.25 cm[2]. Synthetic hairs were implanted on four tattooed areas for each of the 16 individuals (Figure 2).

The grid was applied on each located implanted area and the central 0.25 cm[2] area was photographed (Figure 3). Synthetic hairs were counted on the three successive macrophotographs at Day 0, Day 90 and Day 180 (Figures 4–6). Tolerance was evaluated from bad to fair, good or very good. Complications such as folliculitis, seborrheic dermatitis (Figures 7 and 8) seborrheic follicular deposits and pits were noted (Figure 9).

RESULTS

The results after implantation (Table 2) were as follows:

Table 2   Results after implantation of Nido synthetic hair (SHI)

			Complications	Tolerance	Day 0	Day 90	Day 180
1	BEL	Fatima	SFD	+ + +	35	29	29
2	BER	Philippe		+ + +	41	40	39
3	DUP	Henry Paul	SFD, folliculitis	+	33	27	25
4	FLA	Jean François		+ +	16	9	—
5	FOU	Monique		+ + +	43	39	—
6	GRI	Jean Yves	Pits, SFD	+	40	—	19
7	HOU	Jean Claude	Folliculitis	+ +	41	—	30
8	LAB	Patrick	Seborrheic dermatitis	+	27	20	13
9	LEB	Marc	Folliculitis	+ +	45	44	32
10	MEK	Lounes	SFD	+ + +	41	36	—
11	PAU	Alain	SFD	+ + +	36	32	30
12	QUE	Franck	SFD, folliculitis pruritus	+	38	28	23
13	RAM	Mohamed		+	24	—	0
14	TIL	Ali	Folliculitis	+ + +	37	35	33
15	GES	Pascal	SFD	+	33	—	26
16	BAL	Christian		+ +	20	11	—

SFD: seborrheic, follicular, deposits

1. the average density of hair implant per cm[2] was 137.48 at Day 0, 116.64 at Day 90 and 99.64 at Day 180 (Table 3)

2. the average fixation rate was 84.4% at Day 90 and 72.47% at Day 180;

3. the average rate of complications was 31.25% with folliculitis, 6.25% with seborrheic dermatitis, 6.25% with pits, 43.7% (seven patients) revealed seborrheic follicular deposit in relation with the few care by unrepeated shampoo (Table 4);

4.   the average rate of tolerance is 31.25% very good, 25% good, 43.75% fair and bad none (Table 5)

We have not found any foreign body granuloma[1,5,6] reaction during the 6-month follow-up of this study.

Table 3   Results after implantation of Nido synthetic hair (SHI)

	Day 0	Day 90	Day 180
Average density SHI/cm^2	137.48	116.64	99.64
Average shedding rate	0%	15.16%	27.53%
Average fixation rate	100%	84.84%	72.47%

Table 4   Complications after Nido – SHI

	No. of patients	Average rate (%)
Seborrheic follicular deposits	7	43.70
Folliculitis	5	31.25
Seborrheic dermatitis	1	6.25
Pits	1	6.25

Table   5   Tolerance after Nido – SHI

	No. of patients	Average rate (%)
Very good	5	31.25
Good	4	25
Fair	7	43.75
Bad	0	0

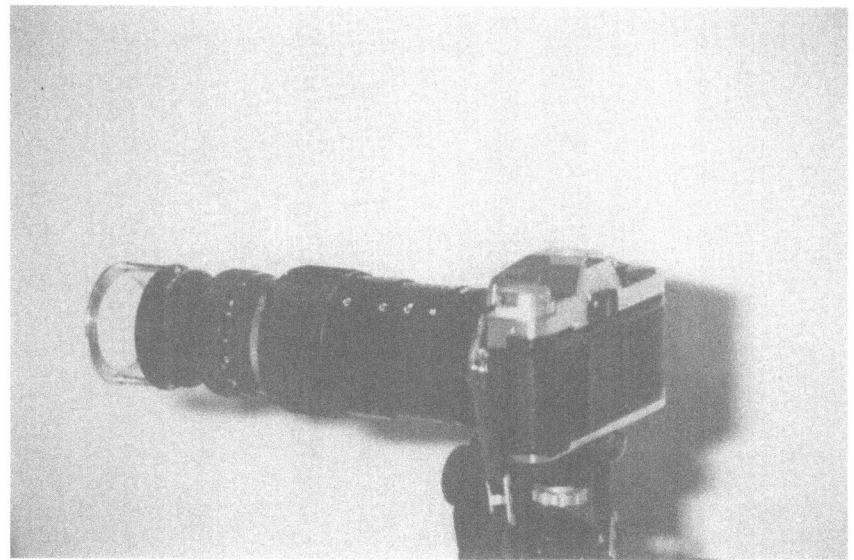

Figure 1 Macrophotographic equipment

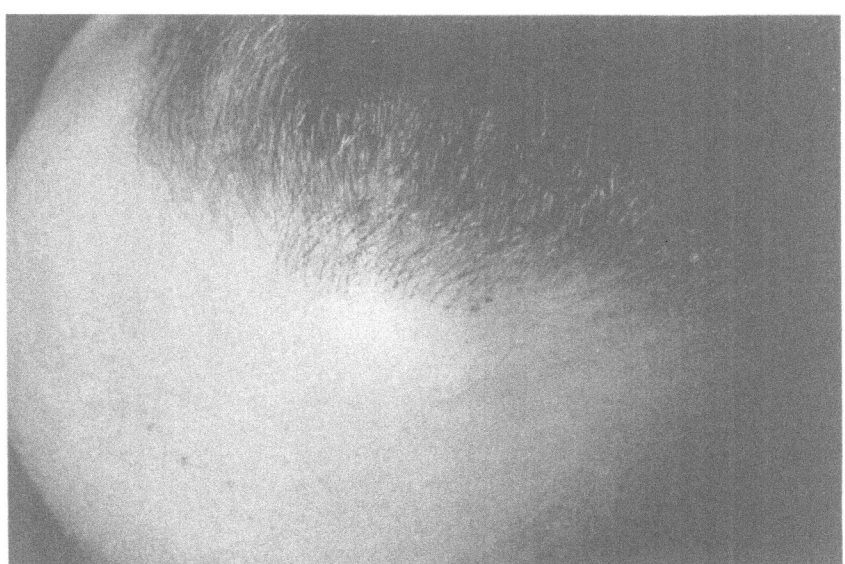

Figure 2 Scalp with implants on four tattoed areas

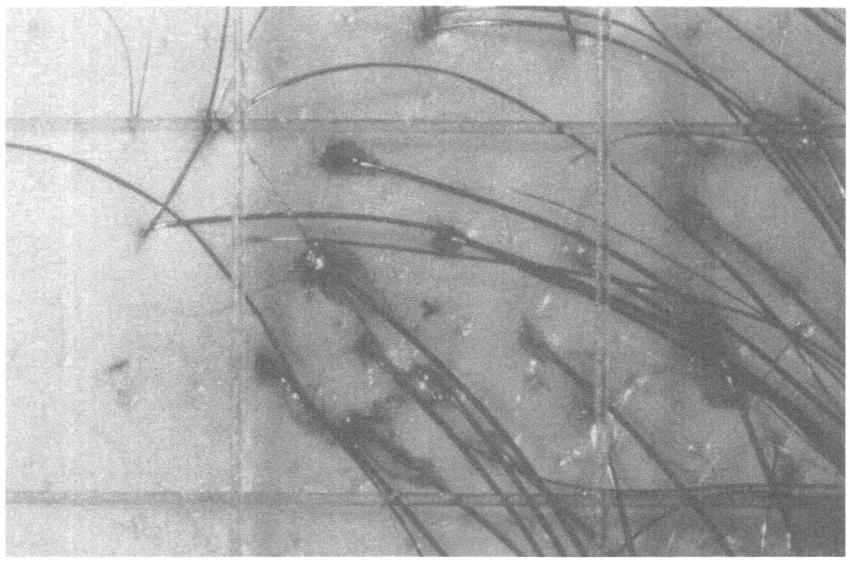

Figure 3   Macrophotograph of an 0.25 cm^2 located area immediately after implantation

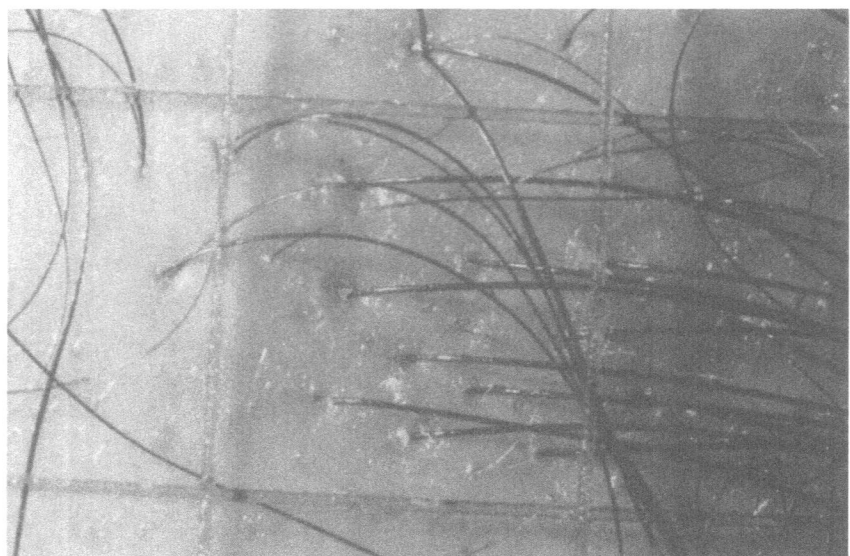

Figure 4   Same patient, same area, 3 months later

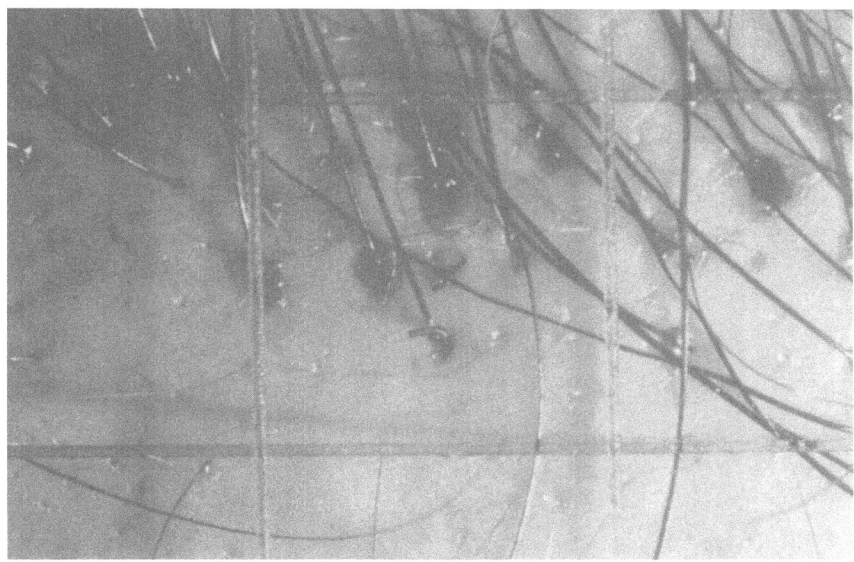

Figure 5   Spontaneous shedding of a hair implant immediately after implantation

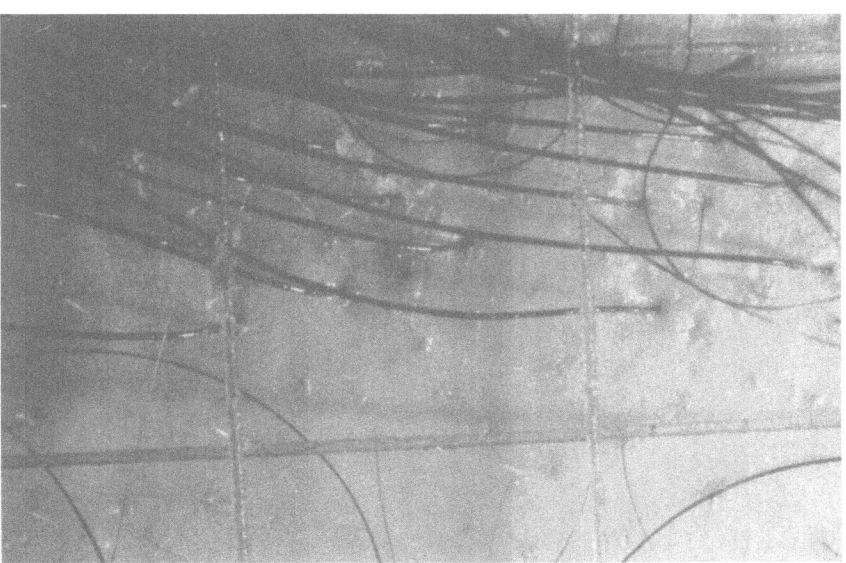

Figure 6   Same area – without residual sequellae

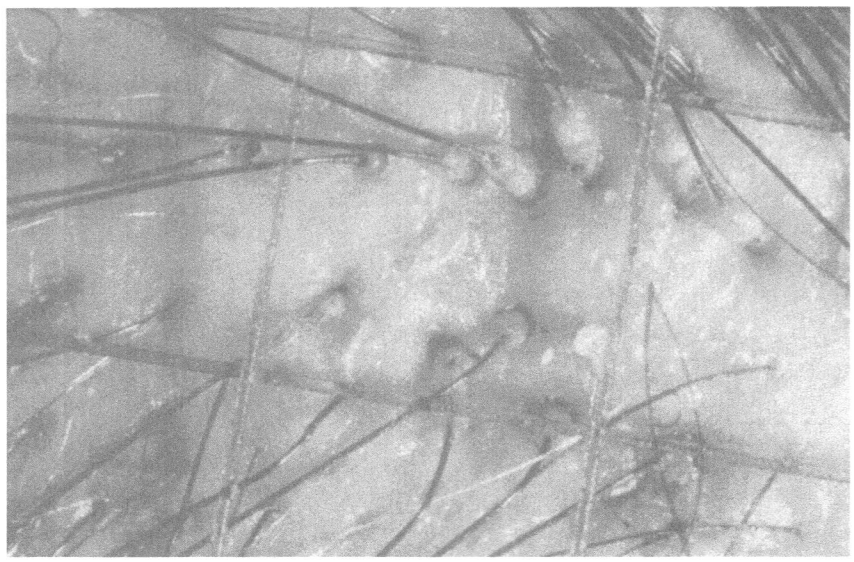

Figure 7 Day 180 – seborrheic follicular deposits

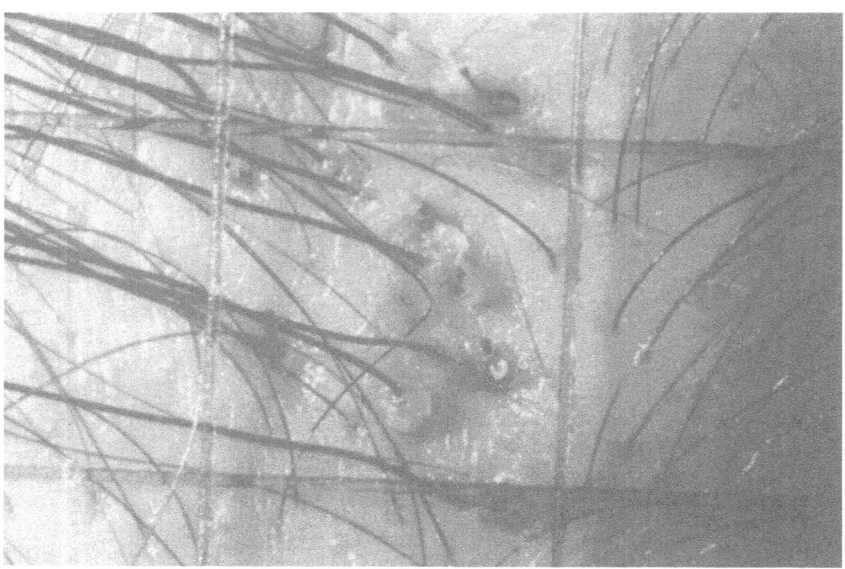

Figure 8   Day 180 – shedding hair implant

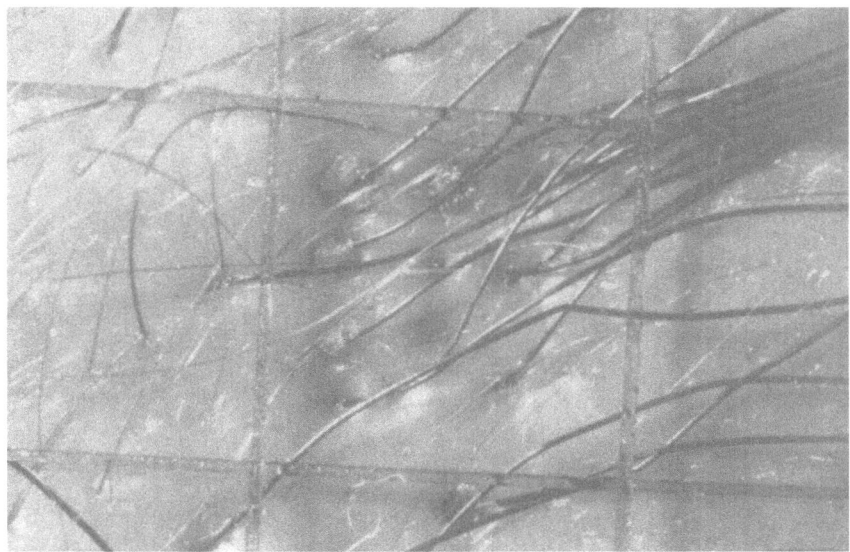

Figure 9   Day 180 – pits

REFERENCES

1.   Kobayashi T, Kamiyama G, Akagawa T, Akamatsu T. Research and investigation of artificial hair implantation. JSAPS, **3**, 12–40, 1981
2.   Taniguchi . Histopathological study of the percutaneous implantation of polyester fibers. *Aesth Plast Surg*, **8**, 67–74, 1984
3.   Bouhanna P. The advantage of phototrichogram in hair surgery. T*he International Advanced Hair Replacement Symposium*. Birmingham, Alabama, 3–4 February, 1982
4.   Bouhanna P. The phototrichogram: an objective technique used in hair replacement surgery evaluation. In *Hair Transplantation* (Unger WP, Nordström RE, eds), pp. 837–883, New York: Dekker, 1987
5.   Hanke CW, Bergfeld WF. Hair implant complications. *J Am Med Assoc*, **245**, 1344–1345, 1981
6.   Lepaw MI. Therapy and histopathology of complications from synthetic fiber implants for hair replacement. *J Am Acad Dermatol*, 195–204, **3**, 1980

27
Patch testing procedures in patients suffering from suspected allergic contact dermatitis to minoxidil

JM Lachapelle, D Tennstedt, B Leroy, V Van den Haute and F Naert

Unit and Laboratory of Occupational and Environmental Dermatology
Catholic University of Louvain, 30, Clos Chapelle-aux-Champs
B-1200 Brussels, Belgium

ABSTRACT

Two patients presenting androgenetic alopecia were treated with Regaine® solution. Both of them developed during the second week of application, allergic contact dermatitis of the scalp, extending to the ears, the neck and the face. When lesions were healed, the patients were patch tested. Patch test results were as follows: Regaine® solution as is: + +; Minoxidil *pro analysi* 2% in petrolatum: –; 2% in ethanol: –; 2% in a mixture propylene glycol 20%/water 80%: + +. The control test with propylene glycol was negative. A repeated open application test[1] (Roat Test: Ref *Contact Dermatitis*, **14**, 221–227, 1986) with minoxidil in propylene glycol gave a positive response after five applications in the first case, and after seven applications in the second case, but was negative when minoxidil was dissolved in ethanol. In conclusion, when a patient is suspected to be allergic to minoxidil, it is necessary to test minoxidil dissolved in propylene glycol. This indicates that the choice of vehicle is essential at the patch test clinic.

INTRODUCTION

In recent years minoxidil, or 2,4-diamino-6-piperidino pyrimidine-3-oxide, was found to be topically active for treating some cases of androgenetic alopecia and/or alopecia areata. Since its widespread use in many countries, a few cases of allergic contact dermatitis to the molecule itself and/or to some components of the vehicle were reported in a number of dermatological clinics[2-8]. The authors reporting those observations used closely related patch testing procedures.

In Belgium, minoxidil is marketed under the trade name Regaine®, the chemical formulation of which is as follows: minoxidil 2%, propylene glycol 10%, ethanol 70% and distilled water *ad* 100 g.

We planned to summarize the various procedures that can be used to investigate patients suspected to be allergic to minoxidil itself or other components of the vehicle. This is of prime importance for giving advice to patients as regards continuation or discontinuance of the treatment.

CASE REPORTS

Patient 1

A male patient (GLB), aged 23, suffered from androgenetic alopecia (type II pattern, after Hamilton) and started topical application of minoxidil (Regaine® solution) in May 1987. About 12 days later he experienced itching in the neck and on both ears. An erythematovesicular rash appeared in the next few hours (Figure 1) and allergic contact dermatitis was readily suspected.

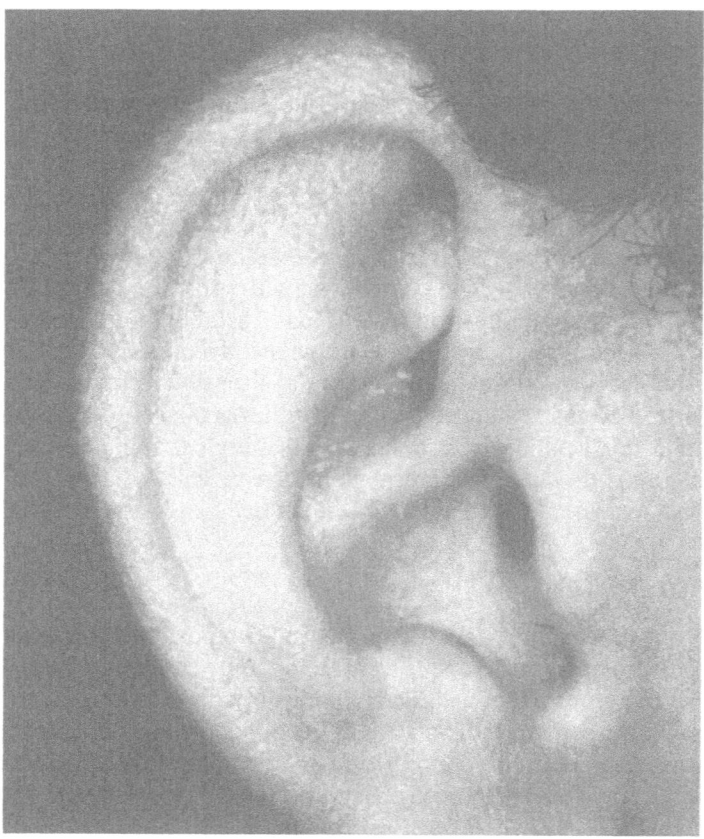

Figure 1 Allergic contact dermatitis to Regaine® solution, 12 days after starting the treatment

Treatment was discontinued and the lesions disappeared progressively in the next few days. Patch tests were made 2 weeks later. The following tests were made: Regaine® Upjohn solution, as is; minoxidil (*pro analysi* grade) 2% in petrolatum, 2% in ethanol and 2% in a mixture containing 20% propylene glycol and 80% distilled water. A 20% aqueous solution of propylene glycol was used as control. The tests were read at 72 h (Figure 2).

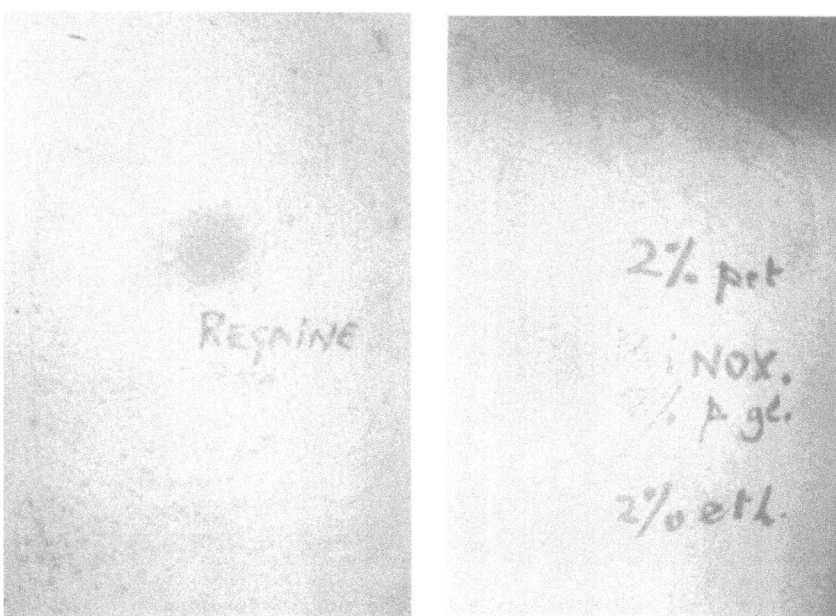

Figure 2   Positive patch test reactions to Regaine® solution and to minoxidil 2% in a 20% aqueous solution of propylene glycol at 72 hours

Table 1   Patch test results at 72 hours

	Patient 1	Patient 2
Regaine® as is	+ +	+ +
Minoxidil 2% in petrolatum	–	–
Minoxidil 2% in ethanol	–	–
Minoxidil 2% in an 20% aqueous solution of propylene glycol	+ +	+ +
Propylene glycol 20% in water	–	–

The patch tests results are presented in Table 1. A repeated open application test (ROAT), following the method of Hannuksela and Salo[1], was performed on the volar aspect of the forearms near the cubital fossa (on the left side with Regaine® solution as is, and on the right side with minoxidil 2% in a 20% aqueous solution of propylene glycol). The solutions were applied twice daily (without washing); a positive reaction was observed on both sides after the fifth application (Figure 3).

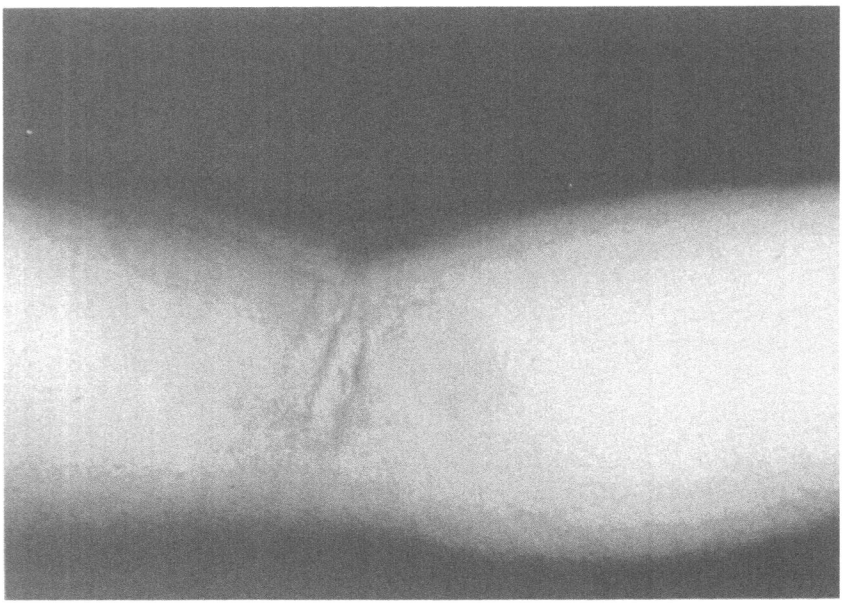

Figure 3   Positive ROAT test to Regaine® solution after five applications

The patient was advised to discontinue treatment, taking into account his problem of intolerance, severe enough to discomfort him despite the good results obtained so far.

Patient 2

A male patient (ADM), aged 27, suffered from male pattern alopecia (type II pattern, after Hamilton). He started topical application of minoxidil (Regaine® solution) in July 1987. About 20 days later he developed a severe allergic contact dermatitis on the scalp. Treatment was discontinued and the lesions subsided progressively, but not completely. Itching and an erythematosquamous rash of the scalp were still present after a few weeks. Patch tests were performed as in patient 1. Results are presented in Table 1. The ROAT test provided useful information: an erythematous, edematous, faintly vesicular eruption appeared simultaneously on both cubital fossae after seven applications of either Regaine® solution as is, or minoxidil 2% in a 20% aqueous solution of propylene glycol.

270

Here again, the patient was discouraged to continue the treatment, due to the severity of allergic side-effects.

DISCUSSION

Allergic contact dermatitis to minoxidil seems to be rare, taking into account its widespread use in dermatological practice. According to Benezra (personal communication) the chemical structure of the molecule is such that it appears to be a moderately active hapten. The uncommonness of allergic reactions is emphasized by the study of Weiss et al.[8]; one out of 48 patients under treatment developed allergic contact dermatitis to minoxidil itself.

Complaints of irritation occur in some patients, whose scalp becomes itchy, erythematous and scaly. Sometimes it is clinically difficult to differentiate irritation from contact allergy: patch testing and applying ROAT tests are therefore two useful tools of differential diagnosis between both types of reactions.

It must be stressed that some patients could also develop immediate or delayed reactions to propylene glycol. Such reactions are important to detect since they would not lead to an automatic discontinuation of minoxidil therapy; indeed, in such cases minoxidil could be applied using another vehicle.

REFERENCES

1. Hannuksela M, Salo H. The repeated open application test (ROAT). Contact Derm, 14, 221–227, 1986
2. Alomar A, Smandia JA. Allergic contact dermatitis from minoxidil. Contact Derm, 18, 51–52, 1988
3. Degreef H, Hendrickx I, Dooms-Goossens A. Allergic contact dermatitis to minoxidil. Contact Derm, 13, 194–195, 1985
4. Tosti A, Bardazzi F, De Padova MP, Caponeri GM, Melino M, Veronesi M. Contact dermatitis to minoxidil. Contact Derm, 13, 275–276, 1985
5. Valsecchi R, Cainelli T. Allergic contact dermatitis from minoxidil. Contact Derm, 17, 58–59, 1987
6. Van der Willigen AH, Dutree-Meulenberg ROGM, Stolz E, Guersen-Reitsma AM, Van Joost Th. Topical minoxidil sensitization in androgenetic alopecia. Contact Derm, 17, 44–45, 1987
7. Weiss VC, West DP. Topical minoxidil therapy and hair regrowth. Arch Dermatol, 121, 191–192, 1985
8. Weiss VC, West DP, Fu TS, Robinson LA, Cook B, Cohen RL, Chambers DA. Alopecia areata treated with topical minoxidil. Arch Dermatol, 120, 457–463, 1984

28

Histopathology of alopecia areata: the relation with clinical parameters and response to a topical sensitizer

H. Uno* and G. Orecchia**

*Wisconsin Regional Primate Research Center and Department of
Pathology and Laboratory Medicine,
School of Medicine, University of Wisconsin,
Madison, Wisconsin, USA
**Clinica Dermatologica
Università di Pavia
Italy

ABSTRACT

Correlation between the clinical features of alopecia areata including therapeutic response to squaric acid dibutylester and histopathological changes was
studied using the biopsied scalp skins from 23 patients. Thirteen cases which
showed no therapeutic response exhibited a reduced size of anagen follicles
(microfollicles) showing dystrophic changes in the suprabulbar portion of the
follicles accompanied by dense infiltration of lymphocytes in the perifollicular
dermis. Moreover, these patients had a long duration, over 5 years, of symptoms.
Eight cases which showed either good or moderate response had medium to
normal sized anagen follicles and most of them showed mild pathological
changes in the follicular milieu. Longstanding refractory lesions cause regressive
changes of the hair follicles concomitant with latent inflammatory changes in
the dermis.

INTRODUCTION

The focal or diffuse hair loss of alopecia areata is primarily caused by disruptive
epilation of hair from degenerated anagen follicles. In early progressive and recurrent stages, the anagen follicles are involved with a varying degree of
degeneration in the lower follicular sheath concomitant with disintegration of
the suprabulbar hair matrix. These changes are often associated with dense perifollicular infiltration of lymphocytes and occasionally with perivascular infiltration in the dermis of involved scalp skin[1–11]. These degenerative anagen follicles
appear to undergo premature entry to the telogen phase through a short
catagenic course[3,9]. Remission of alopecia areata may occur when anagen fol-

273

licles regrown in the new cycle involve no recurrent lesions. The lesion, however, often recurs and some cases extend over the total scalp (alopecia totalis) or to the follicles in other body regions (alopecia universalis). The hair follicles in these refractory lesions exhibit persistent changes of degeneration and inflammation and marked reduction of follicular size[1,3,8].

In cases showing successful therapeutic approaches by prednisone[1] or minoxidil[7], the dermal and perifollicular inflammation subside and the follicles grow back to normal size and structure.

In the present study, we attempted to correlate the histopathological types of lesions based on severity of follicular degeneration, reduction of the follicular size, and associated inflammatory changes and therapeutic successful grade of 23 alopecia areata patients during the treatment with squaric acid dibutylester.

MATERIAL AND METHODS

Twenty-three patients, 9 males and 14 females, ranging in age from 16 to 54 years, suffered from alopecia areata (9), alopecia totalis (10), and universalis (11). The extent of hair loss in alopecia areata patients varied from 5 to 80% but the majority of them had more than a 50% loss. The duration of the disease in patients extended from less than a year (10), 1–5 years (12), to over 5 years (13). The onset of disease in these patients, divided into different age groups, was juvenile (14), adolescent and adult (11), and over 30 years (15). Topical application of squaric acid was carried out using four dilutions (0.1, 0.2, 0.5 and 0.8%), depending on the result of a sensitivity test in each patient[13,14]. The duration of treatment varied in each patient from 3 months to 3 years. However, the majority of them had received the treatment for approximately 6 to 12 months at the time of biopsy.

Skin biopsy (4 mm punch) was taken from the scalps of patients at varying times after treatment (5 months to 2 years). The skin specimens were fixed with 10% formalin solution and cut vertically to the skin surface. Serial paraffin sections (10 μm thick) were stained with hematoxylin–eosin.

Folliculogram[8,12]: all hair follicles appearing in each section were serially traced by the use of a microvideo computer-image apparatus with McVision program. Approximately 50 to 60 follicles traced in all sections from one biopsied skin were recorded through their cyclic growth phases (telogen, early to mid anagen, late anagen and catagen) and size (depth of an individual follicle from the epidermal surface to the base of the hair follicle). Using these parameters, the bargraphs representing the proportional population (percentages) of each cyclic phase and the size of follicles were made by using a computer program.

RESULTS

1. Histopathological types

Overall histopathological changes in each case were recorded in the following categories: the size of hair follicles (micro, medium and large), degree of disruption (dystrophy) of the hair matrix, particularly at the suprabulbar level of the anagen follicle, degeneration of the lower follicular and bulbar structures, and density of perifollicular and dermal perivascular lymphocytic infiltration or of lamellar proliferation of perifollicular fibrous tissue. The size of follicles including the early, mid, and late anagen and telogen follicles was a rather representative feature of each individual case in the present series. The analysis of the folliculogram further confirmed the overall size of the follicles in four random cases (see below). The microfollicles were defined so that the bottom or the bulb of the follicle laid in the dermal collagenous layer at the level either above or slightly below the sebaceous glandular level (Figure 1(a)). The bulb portion of the medium and large follicles belonging to the late anagen phase reached into the adipose tissue layer; the former laid in the upper and the lat-

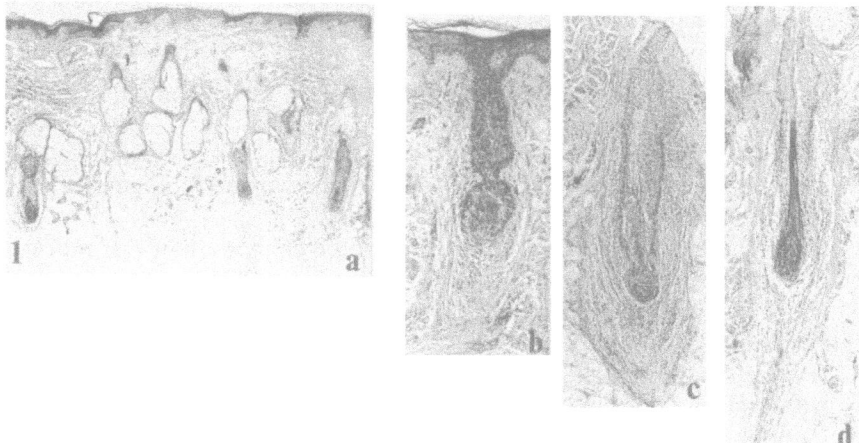

Figure 1(a)   Microfollicle; 3 small anagen follicles associated with perifollicular proliferation of fibrous tissue and some lymphocytic infiltration. The bulbar portion lies in the level slightly below the sebaceous glands. x12

Figure 1(b)   A small early anagen follicle is surrounded with lamellar fibrous tissue with lymphocytic infiltration and shows a disproportional shape of the primordial bulb and epithelial stalk. x50

Figure 1(c)   A small mid anagen follicle is surrounded with dense fibrous tissues and lymphocytic infiltration and shows shrinkage of the lower follicular sheath and disruption of the hair matrix. x31

Figure 1(d)   A small late anagen follicle is surrounded with fibrous tissues and lymphocytic infiltration and shows an irregularity of the outer root sheath and splitting of the hair matrix in the pilar canal. The presence of the fibrous sheath below the follicle suggests suppression of the follicular growth. x31

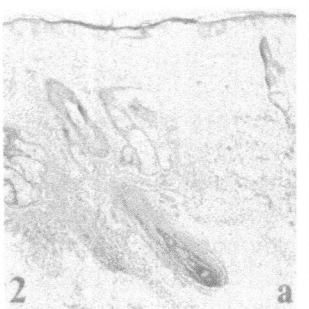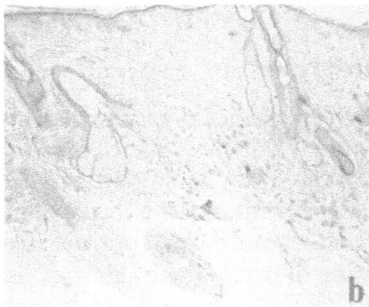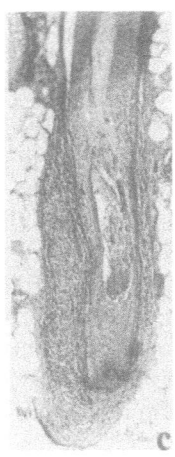

Figures 2(a) and (b) Medium follicles showing dense infiltration of lymphocytic cells and proliferation of perifollicular fibrous tissue. The bulb portion lies in the upper layer of adipose tissue and one microfollicle (arrow) in the dermal collagenous layer. x14

Figure 2(c) A medium-sized anagen follicle is associated with dense infiltration of lymphocytes and disruption of the hair matrix. x34

ter in the lower level, respectively (Figures 2(a), (b) and Figure 3(a) and Figure 4).

The cases were then classified into the following four types combined with the size of follicles and the nature and degree of associated follicular and perifollicular lesions.

Type 1; microfollicles with severe associated changes (hair disruption, follicular degeneration and perifollicular inflammation): Figures 1(b), (c), (d).

Type 2; microfollicles and medium follicles with severe associated changes: Figures 2(a), (b), (c).

Type 3; medium sized follicles with moderate associated changes (including proliferation of perifollicular fibrous tissue): Figures 3(a) and (b).

Type 4; large follicles with mild or no associated changes: Figure 4.

2. Histological types and clinical features

The cases classified into the four histological types were retrogradely examined according to their clinical features such as the type of lesions (alopecia areata, totalis and universalis), duration of the disease, age of onset of symptoms, and the degree of hair regrowth after the treatment with squaric acid (good, moderate, poor and none). Table 1 shows numerical representation of histological types and clinical features of the 23 cases studied.

The Type 1 lesion (microfollicles with severe associated changes) appeared to have a long duration of disease and the poorest response to treatment. The Type 2 lesion (a mixture of microfollicles and medium follicles with severe associated changes) showed largely poor response. The Type 3 lesion (medium follicles with moderate associated changes) showed much better response than the former types. The Type 4 lesion (large follicles with mild or no changes) appeared to show good response in most cases though some had a long duration of disease. Although the total number of Type 2 and 3 lesions was so low, there were no significant differences in the onset age group and the clinical type of alopecia which correlated with the histological lesions in all types.

Table 1   Histological type

Clinical features		(1) Microfollicle follicle with sev. changes	(2) Micro & med follicle with sev. changes	(3) Medium follicle with mod. changes	(4) Large follicle mild changes or normal
Total cases		11	4	2	6
A. areata (13)		6 (54)	1 (25)	2 (100)	4 (66)
A. totalis (2)		1 (09)	1 (25)	–	–
A. universalis (8)		4 (36)	2 (50)	–	2 (33)
Disease duration	< 1y (1)	–	–	–	1 (16)
	1–5y (5)	1 (09)	2 (50)	1 (50)	1 (16)
	> 5y (17)	10 (90)	2 (50)	1 (50)	4 (66)
Age of onset	< 12y (9)	4 (36)	1 (25)	–	4 (66)
	13–30y (8)	5 (45)	2 (50)	1 (50)	–
	> 30y (6)	2 (18)	1 (25)	1 (50)	2 (33)
Response to treatment (after 4 mo)	Good (3)	–	1 (25)	2 (100)	–
	Moderate (5)	–	–	–	5 (83)
	Poor (1)	1 (09)	–	–	–
	None (14)	10(90)	3(75)	–	1 (16)

( )Percentage in each type

3.   Folliculogram analysis

The folliculogram represents the proportional population (percentage) of different phases of the follicular cycle and the length of follicles obtained in a biopsied scalp skin of an individual patient.

In a patient who had about 5% hair loss at several months after the onset of symptoms, the folliculogram showed that more than half of the follicles were late anagen follicles and the rest telogen, early to mid anagen, and catagen follicles (Figure 5(a)). This pattern suggests that the follicles undergo active cyclic growth. Late anagen follicles were largely of medium size (approximately 2.5 mm length) and some vellus size (below 1.5 mm). Histologically, most anagen follicles showed a moderate degree of follicular degeneration and perifollicular

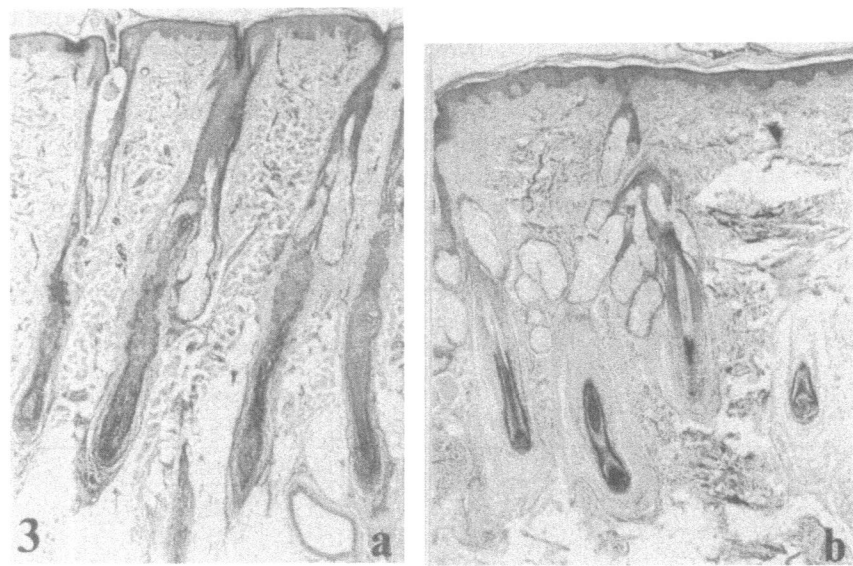

Figures 3(a) and (b) Four medium sized anagen follicles show perifollicular proliferation of fibrous tissue and lymphocytic cell infiltration (a) and multi-layered lamellar fibrous tissues (b) x16

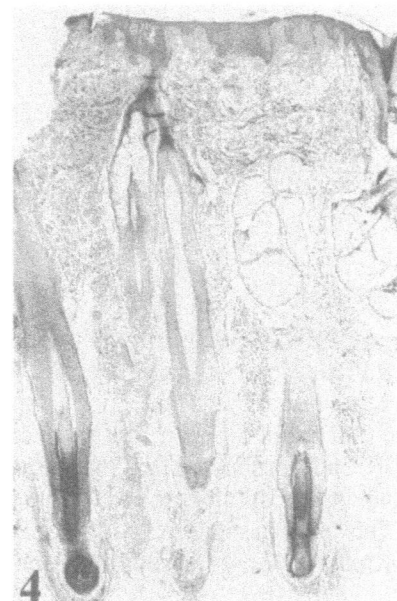

Figure 4 Three large anagen follicles show normal follicular structure and hairs and some degree of retained fibrous tissues around the lower follicles x18

cell infiltration; the size and pathological changes correspond to those seen in Figure 2(a) and (b) and histological feature Type 2.

The folliculogram obtained from a patient who had alopecia areata, 70% hair loss, for about 15 years, showed that the size of most telogen and anagen

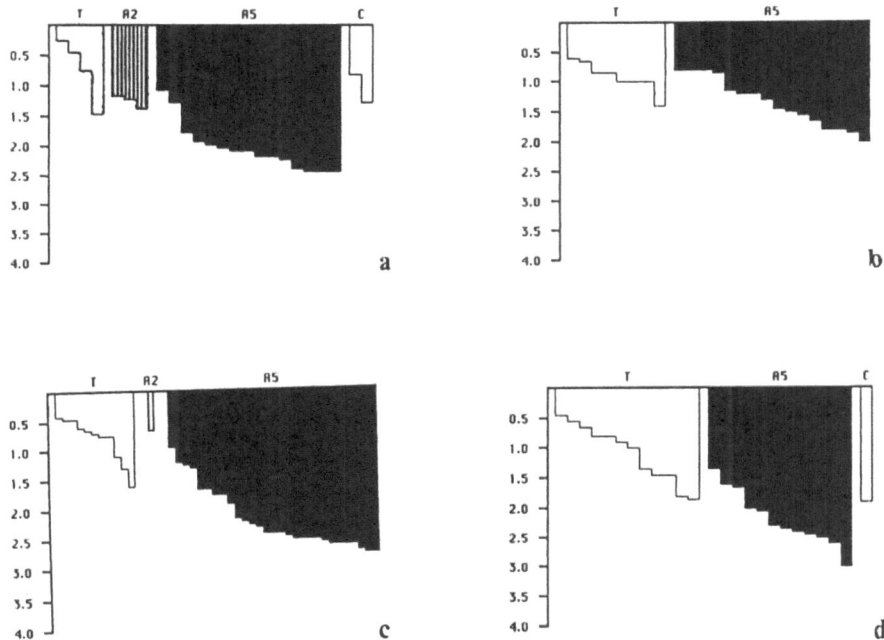

Figure 5 Folliculograms represent the proportional population (abscissa, percentage) of different cyclic phases of the hair follicles (T = telogen; A₂ = early to mid anagen; A₅ = late anagen; C = catagen) and the length of follicles (ordinate, millimeter). a) alopecia areata (31 years, female), 5% hair loss with 2 months duration; b) alopecia areata (18 years, female), 70% hair loss with 8 years duration; c) alopecia areata (22 years, male), 50% hair loss with 17 years duration; and d) alopecia areata (29 years, male), 70% hair loss with 18 years duration.

follicles was very small and they consisted of microfollicles (less than 1 mm in telogen, 1.5 mm in anagen) (Figure 5(b)). Histologically, the majority of anagen follicles showed severe degeneration and inflammatory change. This case possessed the typical histological features of Type 1.

The folliculograms (Figure 5(c) and (d)) obtained from the patients having 50 to 70% hair loss over 15 years showed a mixed population of microfollicles and medium sized follicles for both telogen and anagen follicles. Histologically, most anagen follicles exhibited severe dystrophic and inflammatory changes and the cases were classified as Type 2.

DISCUSSION

The histopathological classifications of 23 patients with alopecia areata, totalis and universalis were made at various times after the treatment of squaric acid dibutylester. The classifications were based on the size of anagen follicles, from normal to medium and micro size, and the severity of degeneration of follicular structures and inflammation of the perifollicular region. Type 1 represents all hair follicles showing markedly reduced size (microfollicles), and severe degeneration of the lower follicular sheath and accompanied inflammation was found in the scalp skin of patients with a long duration of disease who showed no sign of therapeutic response. The extent of hair loss and age of disease onset were not significantly correlated.

Type 2 representing a mixture of microfollicles and medium sized follicles associated with severe inflammation and degeneration of the follicular milieu had no response to the treatment in 3 of 4 patients. The scalp skins containing medium and normal (large) follicles and moderate to mild associated lesions were found in the patients who had good or moderate response to treatment.

Although the numbers in each type were not large enough and sequential study (before and after treatment) was not attempted, the lesions consisted of mainly microfollicles with severe associated changes showing no response to the treatment compared to the other types (medium to large follicles). Furthermore, scalp skin containing large numbers of microfollicles had a long duration of disease. Folliculogram analysis and histological study revealed that the reduction in size of anagen follicles and latent inflammatory degeneration of the follicles were characteristic features of long standing refractory lesions.

As described in the previous studies, the hair follicles in the scalp undergo a years-long anagen phase; thus the normal adult scalp contains nearly 90% of hair follicles belonging to anagen follicles[15]. A rather rapid episode of hair loss in alopecia areata is initially caused by disruptive epilation of hair from degenerative anagen follicles. Degeneration of the lower follicular sheath and bulbar structures of affected anagen follicles appears to induce premature catagenic involution. The resultant telogen follicles enter a new cycle, but usually latent inflammatory changes in the dermis appear to interfere with follicular growth. Occasionally, new anagen follicles involve abnormal melanocytic migration; white hairs grow in dark hairs and vice versa. Dermal interference to follicular remodeling causes not only abnormal and dystrophic anagen follicles, but also causes a miniaturization of the anagen follicles. Recent immunological studies suggest that a triggering mechanism of alopecia areata is considered to be an autoimmune process occurring in the hair follicular structure, particularly in the suprabulbar region of the anagen follicle[6]. Subsequent local or systemic immunologic change may cause the spread of the lesion. The histological changes were also related to the presence of organ and non-organ specific autoantibodies (anti-nuclear, anti-DNA, anti-reticulin, anti-parietal cells, anti-microsomes, anti-thymoglobulin, anti-duodenum, anti-smooth muscle, anti-mitochondria), determined with the direct immunofluorescence method (all autoantibodies) or with a haemoglutination test (anti-microsomes and anti-thyreoglobulin). Moreover, a relationship was researched with the helper/suppressor ratio of peripheral blood lymphocytes, measured with a cell sorter. Finally, 9 out of 23 patients were HLA typed (loci A, B, C, Dr)[16].

Remission often occurs in alopecia areata, but is usually rare in alopecia totalis and universalis patients. However, the present study revealed that the cases having a prolonged duration of symptoms, over 5 years, showed a marked reduction of follicular size with latent severe inflammatory lesions and had no therapeutic response to a topical sensitizer in all 3 types of alopecia patients.

ACKNOWLEDGEMENTS

Research supported by NIH RR00167 to the W.R.P.R.C. The author wishes acknowledge Adrienne Cappas for her technical assistance.

REFERENCES

1. Van Scott EJ. Morphologic changes in pilosebaceous units and anagen hairs in alopecia areata. *J Invest Dermatol*, **31**, 35–43, 1958
2. Van Scott EJ. Evaluation of disturbed hair growth in alopecia areata and other alopecia. *Ann NY Acad Sci*, **83**, 480–490, 1959
3. Braun-Falco O, Zaun H. Uber die beteiligung des gesamten capillitiums bei alopecia areata. *Haut Argt*, **13**, 342–348, 1962
4. Thies W. Vergleichende histologische untersuchungen bei alopecia areata und narbig-atrophisierenden alopecien. *Arch Klin Exp Dermatol*, **277**, 541–549, 1966
5. Messenger AG, Bleehen SS. Alopecia areata: light and electron microscopic pathology of the regrowing white hair. *Br J Dermatol*, **110**, 155–162, 1984
6. Messenger AG, Bleehen SS. Expression of HLA-DR by anagen hair follicles in alopecia areata. *J Invest Dermatol*, **85**, 569–572, 1985
7. Uno H, Mori O, Cappas A, *et al*. The effect of topical minoxidil on sequential histological changes in alopecia totalis and universalis, abstracted. *J Invest Dermatol*, **86**, 512, 1986
8. Uno H. The histopathology of hair loss. *Current Concepts*, 1–47, Upjohn, 1988
9. Messenger, AG, Slater, DN, Bleehen, SS. Alopecia areata: alterations in the hair growth cycle and correlation with the follicular pathology. *Br J Dermatol*, **114**, 337–347, 1986
10. Ioannides G. Alopecia: a pathologist's view. *Int J Dermatol*, **21**, 316–328, 1952
11. Van Scott EJ, Ekel TM. Geometric relationships between the matrix of the hair bulb and its dermal papilla in normal and alopecic scalp. *J Invest Dermatol*, **31**, 281–287, 1958
12. Uno H. Biology of hair growth. *Semin Reprod Endocrinol*, **4**, 131–141, 1986
13. Giannetti A, Orecchia G. Clinical experience on the treatment of alopecia areata with squaric acid dibutylester. *Dermatologica*, **167**, 280–282, 1983
14. Orecchia G, Giacomo R. Squaric acid dibutylester in alopecia areata: is discomfort really necessary? *J Am Acad Dermatol*, **17**, 876, 1987
15. Kligman AM. The human hair cycle. *J Invest Dermatol*, **33**, 307–316, 1959
16. Orecchia G, Cuccia Belvedere M, Martinetti M, Capelli E, Rabbiosi G. Human leukocyte antigen region involvement in the genetic predisposition to alopecia areata. *Dermatologica*, **175**, 10–14, 1987

29
In situ immunophenotyping of follicular keratinocytes in alopecia areata

HW Niedecken, G Lutz, R Bauer and HW Kreysel
Department of Dermatology,
Rheinische Friedrich-Wilhelms-Universität Bonn,
Federal Republic of Germany

ABSTRACT

Histological and immunological findings indicate that alopecia areata (AA) is an immunologically mediated disease. Previous investigations could demonstrate the expression of the MHC class II antigen HLA-DR on follicular keratinocytes in the progressive stage of AA. The expression of MHC class II antigens by epithelial cells represents a reaction of unknown function, and it is not clear whether the expression of HLA-DR by follicular keratinocytes is a primary or a secondary event in the pathogenesis of AA. Nevertheless this was considered as an indication for the involvement of the follicle in immunological reactions, and as a confirmation of the immunological nature of this disease. Meanwhile we know that keratinocytes in diseased or healthy skin can react with different monoclonal antibodies against MHC class II antigens. For this reason we investigated the reactivity of follicular keratinocytes with a series of monoclonal antibodies against MHC class II antigens HLA-DR, -DQ, -DP *in situ*. Scalp biopsies from 40 patients with AA were compared with biopsies from normal individuals using the avidin–biotin–immunoperoxidase method.

INTRODUCTION

Alopecia areata, a disease of unknown etiology[1], is characterized by peribulbar, perifollicular and perivascular infiltrates of activated T cells and by degenerative changes of the suprapapillary matrix and the presumptive cortex of the anagen follicle[2,3]. We do not know if the follicular changes are a primary event in the pathogenesis of alopecia areata, leading to the activation of a T cell response, or if the lesional lymphocytic activity induces the follicular changes. In this context expression of MHC class II antigens by follicular keratinocytes may be of special interest.

The expression of these antigens by epithelial cells is a widely distributed and not very well understood epithelial reaction. The induction of these antigens on keratinocytes depends on interferon gamma[4] – a gamma interferon receptor on keratinocytes is documented[5] – and results from the interaction of epidermal and activated lymphocytic cells[6,7].

HLA-DR is the best examined of this group of antigens. While the expression of HLA-DR in normal skin is restricted to Langerhans cells and the acrosyringia[8], in diseased skin it was proved on keratinocytes in many dermatoses[9–11]. As a rule HLA-DR was found in dermatoses characterized by lymphocytic infiltrates[12], although occurrence of this antigen on keratinocytes in dermatoses without predominant lymphocytic infiltrates such as the oral hairy leukoplakia is reported[13].

During the past year other MHC class II antigens like HLA-DQ and HLA-DP were seen in, e.g. contact reactions, cutaneous T cell lymphomas and lichen planus[14–16]. We examined the expression of MHC class II antigens HLA-DR, HLA-DQ and HLA-DP in biopsies of alopecia areata *in situ*.

MATERIAL AND METHODS

The investigations were carried out on biopsies of 40 patients with AA. Biopsies were taken from peripheral regions of typical AA lesions. The age of the lesions studied varied from 4 weeks to 2 years. Seventeen biopsies of normal skin, including seven biopsies of scalp skin, served as controls.

The specimens were snap-frozen in liquid nitrogen immediately after biopsy and stored at –70 °C. Cryostat sections (4 μm thick) were air-dried, fixed in acetone, and labeled by means of the avidin–biotin–peroxidase complex (ABC) method described earlier[17]. After incubation with normal horse serum the preparations were coated with the monoclonal antibodies anti-HLA-DR, anti-HLA-DQ (anti-Leu 10), anti-HLA-DP (Becton-Dickinson) in appropriate dilutions. Biotinylated horse–antimouse IgG was used as secondary antibody. Afterwards, incubation was carried out with the avidin–biotin–peroxidase complex. The chromogenic reaction was performed with 0.05% diaminobenzidine solution and 0.01% hydrogen peroxide. Counterstaining was carried out with methylene blue. The preparations were rinsed several times with phosphate buffered saline between the incubations. All incubations with antisera were performed in a moist chamber at room temperature.

Negative controls comprised leaving out the primary antibody, coating the preparations with non-immune mouse serum as a first layer as well as substitution of the primary antibody by irrelevant antibodies.

RESULTS

Interfollicular epidermis

Expression of HLA-DR was found in eight of 40 biopsy sections. In three of these specimens HLA-DQ was found as a second class II antigen, while HLA-

DP was not found in 18 biopsies. HLA-DQ was seen only in specimens containing HLA-DR positive keratinocytes in the same regions. The expression of these antigens in interfollicular epidermis was restricted to later lesions of AA and was lacking in early progressive stages (Figure 1).

Expression of class II antigens by keratinocytes was not found in normal epidermis.

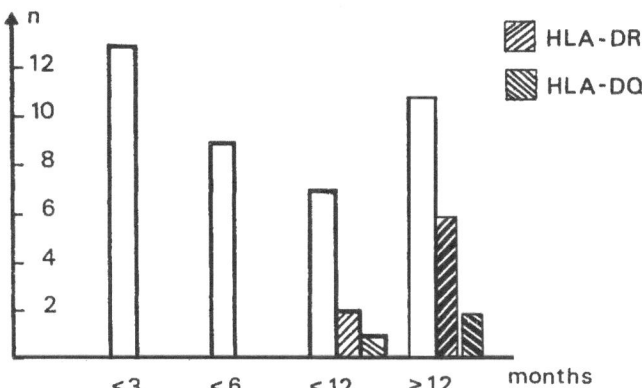

Figure 1   Distribution of specimens with keratinocytes expressing MHC class II antigens in interfollicular epidermis. Forty cases of AA with different-age lesions were examined. HLA-DR and HLA-DQ expressing keratinocytes were seen only in later lesions. HLA-DP was not found in interfollicular epidermis

Follicular epidermis

HLA-DR expressing keratinocytes in the cortical matrix and the presumptive cortex were found in 13 of 116 follicles (8/40 cases) (Figure 2). In 12 of 114 follicles (6/40 cases) this antigen was seen in the infundibular part (Table 1).

Table 1   Specimens with keratinocytes expressing different MHC class II antigens (number of follicles in parentheses)

	AA		
Antigen	*Infundibulum*	*Inferior segment*	*Normal skin*
HLA-DR	6/40 (12/114)	8/40 (13/116)	0/17
HLA-DQ	2/39 (3/105)	0/39	0/17
HLA-DP	0/18	0/18	0/12

Expression of HLA-DQ was restricted in three of 105 follicles (2/39 cases) to the infundibulum; in the inferior segment of the follicle HLA-DQ and HLA-DP were not seen.

285

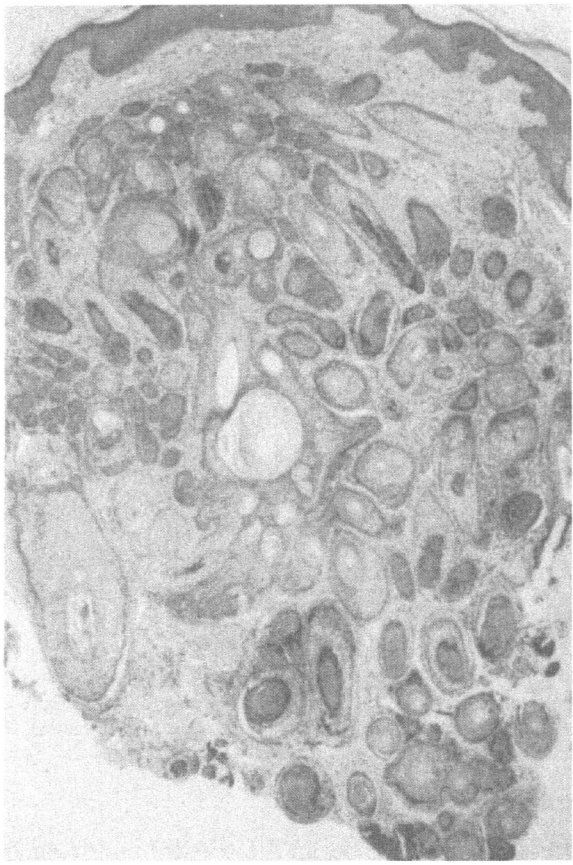

Figure 2   HLA-DR expression by cortical keratinocytes (alopecia areata, x200)

In the follicles of normal skin these antigens were expressed only by Langerhans cells.

Demonstration of HLA-DR in parts of the inferior segment of the follicle was seldom in early lesions, frequent in lesions older than 6 months and lacking in cases older than 12 months (Figure 3), while HLA-DR and HLA-DQ in the infundibular part occurred in long-standing cases of AA and corresponded to the findings in interfollicular epidermis.

DISCUSSION

The functional importance of the expression of MHC class II antigens by follicular keratinocytes in alopecia areata is not clear. Inferior segments of the follicles are of special interest, because this is where the primary degenerative changes and the lymphocytic infiltrates are located.

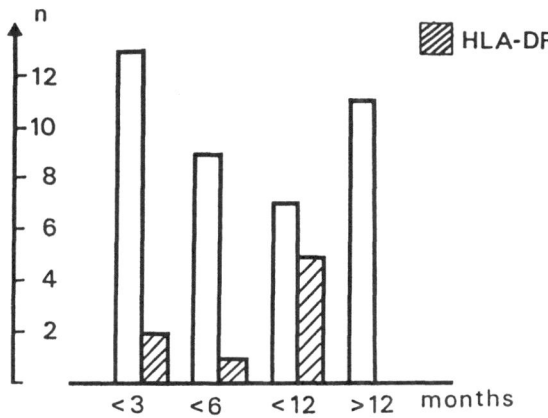

Figure 3 Distribution of specimens with keratinocytes expressing HLA-DR in the inferior part of the follicle (precortical matrix, cortex). In 40 cases of different age HLA-DR expressing keratinocytes were found infrequently in early lesions and were lacking in later lesions. HLA-DQ and HLA-DP were not found

The results of our study show that expression of HLA-DR in these regions of the follicle was very infrequent in early stages of AA. Therefore expression of HLA-DR may be rather a secondary than a primary event in the pathogenesis of AA.

Table 2 Specimens with keratinocytes expressing HLA-DR (number of follicles in parentheses): results of previous studies

Cases	Localization/stage	Reference
9/9 (25/37)	precortical matrix, presumptive cortex	19
3/9 (6/37)	lower hair bulb, inner, outer root sheath	
2/5	matrix (progressive AA)	20
1/5	matrix (stable AA)	
0/8	first attack of progressive AA	18
5/10	longstanding AA	21

Our findings correspond to previous divergent results (Table 2) Peereboom-Wynia et al.[18] could not detect HLA-DR expressing keratinocytes in very early stages of progressive AA, while Messenger and Bleehen[19] found HLA-DR in precortical matrix and presumptive cortex in 24 of 37 AA follicles, and in the deep matrix and the inner or outer root sheath in six of 37 follicles. Happle et al.[20] found HLA-DR in the matrix in two of five cases of progressive, and in one of five cases of inactive, AA. Kietzmann and Sterry[21] have seen HLA-DR and HLA-DQ in follicular localization in 50% of their 10 cases.

In the inferior part of the follicles in AA we could not detect other class II antigens like HLA-DQ and HLA-DP. This finding is in contrast to that of the small series cited above[21].

It is well known from studies with other cell types that HLA-DR and HLA-DQ, -DP are the results of different regulating mechanisms[22,23]. In keratinocytes HLA-DR is well induced, and HLA-DQ is much less induced by interferon gamma *in vitro*[24]. Furthermore we know from sequential *in situ* studies of epidermal contact reactions that keratinocytes express HLA-DQ and HLA-DP later than HLA-DR[14].

Obviously the expression of HLA-DQ and HLA-DP by keratinocytes is the result of a qualitative alteration of the keratinocyte–lymphocyte interaction, which is occurring in, e.g. cutaneous T cell lymphomas or contact reactions[14–16], but not in alopecia areata.

In conclusion we have shown that the expression of MHC class II antigens by keratinocytes in the suprabulbar area of the follicle in AA is restricted by the age of the lesion and by the type of the antigen. HLA-DR was seen frequently in cases of medium duration, but was scarce in early lesions, what may be an advice for the secondary nature of this phenomenon. On the other hand we could not find expression of HLA-DQ and HLA-DP in this region of the follicles in AA. This may be due by the special, but as yet unknown, quality of the interaction between keratinocytes and lymphocytes in alopecia areata, which is capable of inducing the expression of HLA-DR, but not the expression of HLA-DQ and HLA-DP.

REFERENCES

1. Runne U. Alopecia areata. In *Haar und Haarkrankheiten* (Orfanos CE, ed.), pp. 505–544. Stuttgart, New York: Fischer Verlag, 1979

2. Thies W. Vergleichende histologische Untersuchungen bei Alopecia areata und narbig-atrophisierenden Alopecien. *Arch Klin Exp Dermatol*, **227**, 541–549, 1968

3. Perret C, Wiesner-Menzel L, Happle R. Immunohistochemical analysis of T cell subsets in the peribulbar and intrabulbar infiltrates of alopecia areata. *Acta Derm Venereol (Stockh)*, **64**, 26–30, 1984

4. Basham TY, Nickoloff BJ, Merigan TC, Morhenn VB. Recombinant gamma interferon induces HLA-DR expression on cultured human keratinocytes. *J Invest Dermatol*, **83**, 88–92, 1984

5. Nickoloff BJ. Binding of 125 I-Gamma interferon to cultured human keratinocytes. *J Invest Dermatol*, **89**, 132–135, 1987

6. Czernielewski JM, Bagot M. Class II antigen expression by human keratinocytes results from lympho-epidermal interactions and γ-interferon production. *Clin Exp Immunol*, **66**, 295–302, 1986

7. Nickoloff BJ, Basham TY, Merigan TC, Torseth JW, Morhenn VB. Human keratinocyte–lymphocyte reactions in vitro. *J Invest Dermatol*, **87**, 11–18, 1986

8. Carr MM, McVittie E, Guy K, Gawkrodger DJ, Hunter JAA. MHC class II antigen expression in normal human epidermis. *Immunology*, **59**, 223–227, 1986

9. Lampert IA. Expression of HLA-DR (Ia like) antigen on epidermal keratinocytes in human dermatoses. *Clin Exp Immunol*, **57**, 93–100, 1984

10. Smolle J. HLA-DR-antigen bearing keratinocytes in various dermatologic disorders. *Acta Derm Venereol (Stockh)*, **65**, 9–13, 1985

11. Auböck J, Romani N, Grubauer G, Fritsch P. HLA-DR expression on keratinocytes is a common feature of diseased skin. *Br J Dermatol*, **114**, 465–472, 1986
12. Aiba S, Tagami H. HLA-DR antigen expression on the keratinocyte surface in dermatoses characterized by lymphocytic exocytosis (e.g. pityriasis rosea). *Br J Dermatol*, **111**, 285–294, 1984
13. Daniels TE, Greenspan D, Greenspan JS, Lennette E, Schiodt M, Odont D, Peterson V, de Souza Y. Absence of Langerhans cells in oral hairy leukoplakia, an AIDS-associated lesion. *J Invest Dermatol*, **89**, 178–182, 1987
14. Gawkrodger DJ, Carr MM, McVittie E, Guy K, Hunter JAA. Keratinocyte expression of MHC class II antigens in allergic sensitization and challenge reactions and in irritant contact dermatitis. *J Invest Dermatol*, **88**, 11–16, 1987
15. Volc-Platzer B, Groh V, Wolff K. Differential expression of class II alloantigens by keratinocytes in disease. *J Invest Dermatol*, **19**, 64–68, 1987
16. Niedecken HW, Lutz G, Bauer R, Kreysel HW. Differential expression of MHC class II antigens on human keratinocytes. *J Am Acad Dermatol* (in press).
17. Hsu SM, Raine L, Fanger H. The use of avidin–biotin–peroxidase complex (ABC) in immunoperoxidase techniques. A. A comparison between ABC and unlabeled antibody PAP procedure. *J Histochem Cytochem*, **29**, 577–580, 1981
18. Peereboom-Wynia JDR, van Joost T, Stolz E, Prins MEF. Markers of immunologic injury in progressive alopecia areata. *J Cutan Pathol*, **13**, 363–369, 1986
19. Messenger AG, Bleehen SS. Expression of HLA-DR by anagen hair follicles in alopecia areata. *J Invest Dermatol*, **85**, 569–572, 1985
20. Happle R, Klein HM, Macher E. Topical immunotherapy changes the composition of the peribulbar infiltrate in alopecia areata. *Arch Dermatol Res*, **278**, 214–218, 1986
21. Kietzmann H, Sterry W. Activation of lymphocytes and keratinocytes in alopecia areata. *J Invest Dermatol*, **89**, 316, 1987
22. Wang CY, Al-Katib A, Lane CL, Kozinei B, Fu SM. Induction of HLA-DC/DS (Leu 10) antigen expression by human precursor B cell lines. *J Exp Med*, **158**, 1757–1762, 1983
23. Capobianchi MR, Ameglio F, Tosi R, Dolei A. Differences in the expression and release of DR, BR and DQ molecules in human cells treated with recombinant interferon gamma: comparison to other interferons. *Hum Immunol*, **13**, 1–11, 1985
24. Basham TY, Nickoloff BJ, Merigan TC, Morhenn VB. Recombinant gamma interferon differentially regulates class II antigen expression and biosynthesis on cultured normal human keratinocytes. *J Interferon Res*, **5**, 23–27, 1985

30
Expression of Langerhans cell antigens in the hair follicles in alopecia areata

HW Niedecken, G Lutz, R Bauer and HW Kreysel
Department of Dermatology
Rheinische Friedrich-Wilhelms-Universität Bonn
Federal Republic of Germany

ABSTRACT

In the normal hair follicle Langerhans cells (LC) are located predominantly in the outer root sheath. The majority of LC was found in the supraseboglandular part of the follicle, while in the infraseboglandular parts only single LC could be demonstrated. Progressive stages of alopecia areata (AA) are characterized by an increase of CD1-positive cells in the hair bulb, and this was considered as an indication for the involvement of dendritic follicular cells in the pathogenesis of AA. While CD1 is suggested as the best immunomorphological marker for LC, besides electron microscopic characterization, monoclonal antibodies against MHC class II antigens and the CD4 antigen characterize different subsets of functional active LC populations. Therefore the expression of LC antigens CD1, CD4, HLA-DR, -DQ, -DP was examined using the avidin–biotin–peroxidase method *in situ* in interfollicular and follicular epidermis of 40 patients with untreated AA. The results were compared with those of scalp biopsies from normal controls.

INTRODUCTION

Since alopecia areata is characterized by peribulbar and perifollicular infiltrates and progressive degeneration of the keratinizing matrices[1,2] the main aim of dermatological research is directed to the composition of the infiltrates and the involvement of keratinocytes in the pathogenesis of AA[3-6]. On the contrary, activity, distribution of LC and differential expression of LC antigens in AA are not well studied to date.

In the normal hair follicle LC are mainly located in the outer root sheath. The majority of these cells is found in the infundibular region of the follicle[7,8] while in the inferior segment only single cells can be demonstrated[9].

Progressive stages of AA are characterized by large numbers of LC in the infundibulum and small numbers in the deeper parts of the follicle[9]. An increase of cells expressing the LC antigen CD1 was found in the hair bulbs of AA and in the peribulbar infiltrates[10,11].

We have now studied the expression of different LC antigens in follicular and interfollicular epidermis in patients with AA *in situ*.

MATERIAL AND METHODS

The investigations were carried out on biopsies of the peripheral region of typical lesions in 40 patients with AA. Seventeen biopsies of normal skin and scalp skin ($n = 7$) served as controls.

The specimens were snap-frozen in liquid nitrogen immediately after biopsy and stored at –70 °C. Cryostat sections (4 μm thick) were air-dried, fixed in acetone, and labeled by means of the avidin–biotin–peroxidase complex (ABC) method[12]. The preparations were coated with the monoclonal antibodies anti-Leu 6, anti-HLA-DR, anti-HLA-DQ (anti-Leu 10), anti-HLA-DP, anti-Leu 3a, anti-Leu 4 (Becton-Dickinson) in suitable dilutions (Table 1).

Table 1   Antibodies with predominant reactivities

Antibody	Antigen	Predominant reactivity
Anti-Leu 6	CD1	thymocytes, Langerhans cells
Anti-HLA-DR	HLA-DR	B cells, monocytes, macrophages, activated T cells
Anti-HLA-DQ (anti-Leu 10)	HLA-DQ	B cells, monocytes
Anti-HLA-DP	HLA-DP	B cells, monocytes
Anti-Leu 3a	CD4	T helper/inducer cells
Anti-Leu 4	CD3	T cells

Biotinylated horse–anti-mouse-IgG was used as secondary antibody. Afterwards, incubation was carried out with the avidin–biotin–peroxidase complex. The chromogenic reaction was performed with 0.05% diaminobenzidine solution and 0.01% hydrogen peroxide. Counterstaining was carried out with methylene blue. All incubations with antisera were performed in a moist chamber at room temperature.

Negative controls comprised omission of the primary antibody, coating the preparations with non-immune mouse serum as a first step as well as substitution of the primary antibodies by irrelevant antibodies. Statistical analysis was carried out using Tukey's studentized range test and the Bonferroni *t*-test.

RESULTS

Interfollicular epidermis

In interfollicular epidermis numbers of LC expressing CD1 antigen were found in the same range as in normal skin. Cells expressing MHC class II antigens HLA-DR, HLA-DQ, HLA-DP showed a slight but not significant increase in number, while comparison of LC expressing CD4 antigen showed a statistically significant difference between AA and normal skin (Figure 1). Langerhans cells expressing this antigen were rarely found in normal epidermis but were present in the majority of AA specimens.

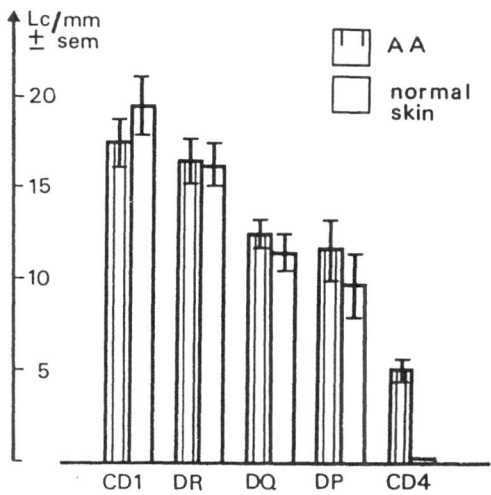

Figure 1 Comparison of Langerhans cell numbers in AA and normal skin. Langerhans cells expressing different antigens are counted in serial sections per mm interfollicular epidermis (medium values ± standard error of mean).

Follicular epidermis

In hair follicles of AA the number of LC expressing CD1 and MHC class II antigens seemed not significantly increased (Table 2).

A quantification as done in interfollicular epidermis was not possible, because of the anatomical situation of the hair follicle, the peripheral localization of LC in the outer root sheath of the follicle and the problem of finding corresponding serial sections. In the inferior segment of the follicle only single cells expressing these antigens were seen in AA and in normal skin.

On the other hand follicles of AA showed CD4 positive dendritic cells (Figure 2). These cells were rarely seen in normal hair follicles (Table 2).

293

Table 2 Semiquantitative comparison of Langerhans cells expressing different antigens in serial sections of hair follicles in AA and normal skin (NS)

Antigen	Follicles		Infundibulum		Inferior segment	
	AA	*NS*	*AA*	*NS*	*AA*	*NS*
CD1	110	32	+/++	+/++	−/+	−/+
HLA-DR	112	30	+/++	+/++	−/+	−/+
HLA-DQ	104	28	+/++	+/++	−/+	−/+
HLA-DP	43	21	+/++	+/++	−/+	−/(+)
CD4	108	31	−/++	−	−/+	−

In early lesions we found more cells expressing this antigen than in later ones. These cells were mainly located in the infundibular part of the follicle but single cells were found in the inferior part. Control stainings performed with anti-Leu 4 demonstrating T cells (CD3) showed that these CD4 positive cells were not T cells.

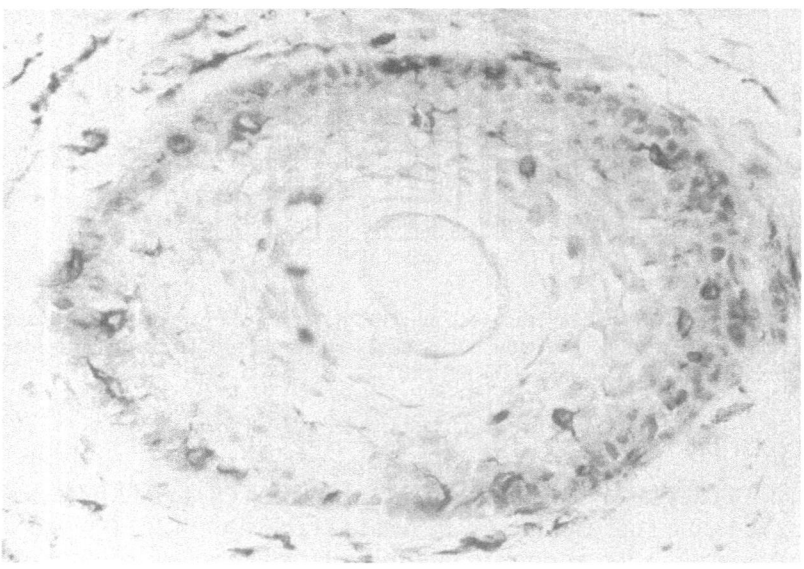

Figure 2 Cross-section of a hair follicle with Langerhans cells expressing CD4 antigen in the root sheath. Note the sparse perifollicular infiltrate (alopecia areata, x270)

DISCUSSION

Our study shows a difference in the expression of LC antigens between AA and normal skin. While expression of CD1 and MHC class II antigens by Langerhans cells showed no significant differences, AA was characterized by the occurrence of CD4 positive intraepidermal cells. These cells are virtually lacking in interfollicular and follicular regions of normal skin[13,14].

The antibodies used here stain different LC antigens. Anti-Leu 6 recognizes the antigen CD1. This antigen is found on thymocytes, indeterminate dermal cells and LC[15]. CD1 is the best immunomorphological marker of the LC population[16], the distribution of the antigen is very restricted and all LC containing Birbeck granula express this antigen[17]. The function of the antigen is not known, but relations with endocytotic structures are suggested[18].

MHC class II antigens HLA-DR, -DQ, -DP in normal epidermis are only expressed by LC[19]. Staining of these antigens may recognize activated LC subsets[20]. These antigens are a supposition for an effective antigen-presenting function of LC. We do not know at this time whether differences of the composition of these antigens on the cell surfaces of LC reflect functional differences of these cells.

The expression of the antigen CD4 by LC and monocytoid cells is well documented[13,21,22]. This antigen was originally described as a helper T cell antigen. The expression of this antigen by LC is strictly related to interactions between epidermal cells and infiltrating lymphocytes. LC expressing this antigen are generally found in dermatoses characterized by lymphocytic infiltrates. In other dermatoses these cells are, as in normal skin, rarely found[13,14].

Obviously the expression of this antigen by LC characterizes an activated Langerhans cell subpopulation. The ratio of CD4 and CD1 positive Langerhans cells (Table 3) in alopecia areata is strikingly higher than in normal skin, and is in the same range as in interfollicular epidermis of other dermatoses related to lymphocytic infiltrates[14]. In the hair follicles of AA this ratio seemed to be even higher than in interfollicular epidermis.

Table 3   Ratios of CD4 and CD1 positive Langerhans cells in interfollicular epidermis of different dermatoses and normal skin (see ref. 14)

	CD4/CD1	n
Atopic dermatitis	0.56	18
Alopecia areata	0.28	40
Lupus erythematosus	0.27	11
Parapsoriasis (BROCQ)	0.26	10
Lichen planus	0.25	8
Verruca seborrhoica	0.04	6
Nevus cell nevus	0.02	7
Normal skin	0.02	17

The function of the CD4 antigen on lymphocytic cells is related to the antigen recognition[23,24] and the cell-to-cell contact[25] necessary for effective antigen presentation. We do not know if these functions may be of value for LC expressing the CD4 antigen.

We conclude that the interfollicular and follicular epidermis of patients with AA is different from normal skin not by the number of LC, but by the occurrence of a CD4 expressing Langerhans cell subpopulation. Although the function of this antigen on LC is not known, expression of CD4 by LC may be an indication of the pathogenetic importance of epidermal cell–lymphocyte interactions, and may be a sign of active or reactive involvement of Langerhans cells in this process.

REFERENCES

1. Thies W. Vergleichende histologische Untersuchungen bei Alopecia areata und narbig-atrophisierenden Alopecien. *Arch Klin Exp Dermatol*, **227**, 541–549, 1968
2. Goos M. Zur Histopathologie der Alopecia areata mit besonderer Berücksichtigung ihrer Beziehung zur Dauer, Lokalisation und Progression des Haarausfalles. *Arch Dermatol Forsch*, **240**, 160–172, 1971
3. Messenger AG, Bleehen SS. Expression of HLA-DR by anagen hair follicles in alopecia areata. *J Invest Dermatol*, **85**, 569–572, 1985
4. Peereboom-Wynia JDR, van Joost T, Stolz E, Prins MEF. Markers of immunologic injury in progressive alopecia areata. *J Cutan Pathol*, **13**, 363–369, 1986
5. Perret C, Wiesner-Menzel L, Happle R. Immunohistochemical analysis of T-cell subsets in the peribulbar infiltrates of alopecia areata. *Arch Derm Venereol (Stockh)*, **64**, 26–30, 1984
6. Ranki A, Kianto U, Kanerva L, Tolvanen E, Johansson E. Immunohistochemical and electron microscopic characterization of the cellular infiltrate in alopecia (areata, totalis and universalis). *J Invest Dermatol*, **83**, 7–11, 1984
7. Breathnach AS. The distribution of Langerhans cells within the human hair follicle, and some observations on its staining properties with gold chloride. *J Anat*, **97**, 73–80, 1963
8. Jimbow K, Sato S, Kukita A. Langerhans cells of the normal human pilosebaceous system. *J Invest Dermatol*, **52**, 177–180, 1969
9. Sato S, Kukita A, Jimbow K. Electron microscopic studies of dendritic cells in the human grey and white hair matrix during anagen. *Pigment Cell*, **1**, 20–26, 1973
10. Wiesner-Menzel L, Happle R. Intrabulbar and peribulbar accumulation of dendritic OKT 6-positive cells in alopecia areata. *Arch Dermatol Res*, **276**, 333–334, 1984
11. Happle R, Klein HM, Macher E. Topical immunotherapy changes the composition of the peribulbar infiltrate in alopecia areata. *Arch Dermatol Res*, **278**, 214–218, 1986
12. Hsu SM, Raine L, Franger H. The use of avidin–biotin–peroxidase complex (ABC) in immunoperoxidase techniques. A: A comparison between ABC and unlabeled antibody PAP procedures. *J Histochem Cytochem*, **29**, 577–580, 1981
13. Groh V, Tani M, Harrer A, Wolff K, Stingl G. Leu 3/T4 expression of epidermal Langerhans cells in normal and diseased skin. *J Invest Dermatol*, **86**, 115–120, 1986
14. Niedecken HW, Stefan JA, Bauer R, Kreysel HW. Differential expression of CD1, CD4 and MHC class II antigens on epidermal Langerhans cells. In *Proceedings of the Second Workshop on Langerhans Cells*, (Thivolet J, Schmitt D, eds). In press
15. Takezaki S, Morrison SL, Berger CL, Goldstein G, Chu AC, Edelson RL. Biochemical characterization of a differentiation antigen shared by human epidermal Langerhans cells and cortical thymocytes. *J Clin Immunol*, **2**, 128–134, 1982
16. Harrist TJ, Mühlbauer JE, Murphy GF, Mihm MC, Bahn AK. T6 is superior to Ia (HLA-DR) as a marker for Langerhans cells and indeterminate cells in normal epidermis: a monoclonal antibody study. *J Invest Dermatol*, **80**, 100–103, 1983
17. Murphy GF, Bahn AK, Sato S, Harrist TJ, Mihm MC. Characterization of Langerhans cells by the use of monoclonal antibodies. *Lab Invest*, **45**, 465–468, 1981

18. Hanau D, Fabre M, Schmitt DA, Stampf JL, Garaud JC, Bieber T, Grosshans E, Benezra C, Cazenave JP. Human epidermal Langerhans cells internalize by receptor-mediated endocytosis T6 (CD1, Na 1/34) surface antigen. Birbeck granules are involved in the intracellular traffic of the T6 antigen. *J Invest Dermatol*, **89**, 172–177, 1987

19. Stingl G, Tamaki K, Katz SI. Origin and function of epidermal Langerhans cells. *Immunol Rev*, **53**, 149–174, 1980

20. McKie RM, Turbitt ML. Quantitation of dendritic cells in normal and abnormal human epidermis using monoclonal antibodies directed against Ia and HTA antigens. *J Invest Dermatol*, **81**, 216–220, 1983

21. Stewart SJ, Fugimoto J, Levy R. Human T lymphocytes and monocytes bear the same Leu 3 (T4) antigen. *J Immunol*, **136**, 3773–3778, 1986

22. Wood GS, Warner NL, Warnke RA. Anti-Leu 3/T4 antibodies react with cells of monocyte/macrophage and Langerhans lineage. *J Immunol*, **131**, 212–216, 1983

23. Biddison WE, Rao PE, Talle MA, Goldstein G, Shaw S. Possible involvement of the OKT4 molecule in T cell recognition of class II HLA antigens. Evidence from studies of cytotoxic T lymphocytes specific for SB antigens. *J Exp Med*, **156**, 1065–1076, 1982

24. Meuer SC, Schlossman SF, Reinherz EL. Clonal analysis of human cytotoxic T lymphocytes: T4+ and T8+ effector T cells recognize products of different major histocompatibility complex region. *Proc Natl Acad Sci USA*, **79**, 4395–4399, 1982

25. Marrack P, Endres R, Shimonkewitz R, Ziotnik A, Dianylas D, Fitch F, Kappler J. The major histocompatibility complex-restricted antigen receptor on T cells. II. Role of the L3/T4 product. *J Exp Med*, **158**, 1077–1091, 1983

31
Analysis of T cell, activated T cell and NK cell subsets in peripheral blood lymphocytes from patients with alopecia areata

R Imai, J Miura, K Numata, Y Aikawa, K Takamori and H Ogawa
Department of Dermatology
Juntendo University School of Medicine
Bunkyo-Ku, Tokyo, 113, Japan

ABSTRACT

Forty-one patients with severe alopecia areata (AA) were studied. They were classified into four types according to clinical manifestations (type 1: fixed alopecia universalis or multiple AA, type 2: active alopecia totalis, type 3: active multiple AA and type 4: active multiple AA with anti-thyroid antibodies). T cell, activated T cell and NK cell subsets in the peripheral blood lymphocytes were investigated using a fluorescence activated cell sorter. (1) The percentage of Leu4$^+$ cells in total lymphocytes showed a significant decrease in AA with types 1, 3 and 4 when compared to those of the normal controls. (2) The percentages of Leu3a$^+$-DR$^+$ cells in Leu3a$^+$ cells and of Leu2a$^+$-DR$^+$ cells in Leu2a$^+$ cells were significantly higher in AA with types 1, 3 and 4 than those of the normal controls. (3) The percentages of Leu11$^+$ cells and Leu7$^+$ Leu11$^+$ cells in total lymphocytes were significantly high in AA with type 3. Leu7$^-$ Leu11$^+$ cells were elevated in AA with types 1 and 3. (4) The percentage increase of Leu7$^-$ Leu11$^+$ cells was proportional to the disease activity in AA with type 3. The increase of activated T cell in peripheral blood lymphocytes from AA suggests that immune mechanisms are involved in the pathogenesis of AA. In type 3 AA, NK cell may play an important role in the pathogenesis of AA.

INTRODUCTION

Many hypotheses have been proposed for the pathogenesis of alopecia areata (AA); however, to date they have not been entirely convincing. Recent studies suggested that AA may be caused by the aberrance of cell-mediated immunity[1]. On the other hand, it is unknown whether natural killer (NK) cells play a role in the pathogenesis of AA. In this study we investigated T cell, activated T cell (HLA-DR$^+$ T cell, IL-2R$^+$ T cell) and NK cell subsets in the peripheral blood lymphocytes of AA.

PATIENTS AND METHODS

Patients

Forty-one patients with severe AA were studied. The patients comprised 18 males and 23 females, with an average age of 33. A control group of 16 males and 10 females with an average age of 29 was selected from healthy volunteers.

Patients were classified into four types; type 1: fixed alopecia universalis or multiple AA, type 2: active alopecia totalis, type 3: active multiple AA and type 4: active multiple AA with anti-thyroid antibodies.

Type 1 group consisted of nine patients, four males and five females, with an average age of 26. They were categorized as being in a 'fixed state' as they had not shown any obvious change in the area of AA during the preceding 18 months.

Type 2 group consisted of five patients, one male and four females, with an average age of 36. All patients had experienced an acute onset and had finally developed to alopecia totalis within 1 month.

Type 3 group consisted of 20 patients, 13 males and seven females, with an average age of 34. All patients had multiple (more than 10) patchy areas of AA on their scalp. The hair surrounding each of the areas of AA showed a tendency to fall out easily.

Type 4 group consisted of seven patients, all female, with an average age of 35. They had active MAA and autoantibodies against thyroid constituents in their sera.

Methods

The peripheral blood mononuclear cells (PBMC) were isolated by Ficoll-Hypaque density gradient centrifugation.

Table 1   Monoclonal antibody and target cell

Monoclonal antibody	Target cell
Leu4$^+$	Pan T cell
Leu3a$^+$	Helper/inducer T cell
Leu2a$^+$	Suppressor/cytotoxic T cell
HLA-DR$^+$ -Leu3a$^+$	Activated helper/inducer T cell
HLA-DR$^+$ -Leu2a	Activated suppressor/cytotoxic T cell
IL-2R$^+$ -Leu4$^+$	Activated T cell with IL-2 receptor
Leu7	NK cell
Leu11$_c$	NK cell

Each monoclonal antibody was conjugated with PE (phycoerythrin) or FITC

PBMC were double-stained with phycoerythrin (PE) conjugated monoclonal antibodies (Leu4, Leu7 or HLA-DR) and FITC conjugated monoclonal antibodies (Leu2a, Leu3a, Leu11 or IL-2R) (Table 1) and then analyzed using a fluorescence activated cell sorter (FACStar-I).

RESULTS

Distribution of T cell subsets in the peripheral blood of AA patients

The distribution of T cell subsets in the peripheral blood from AA patients of different clinical types and healthy control subjects was investigated.

The percentage of Leu4$^+$ cells (Pan T cells) in total lymphocytes showed significant decreases in AA with type 1 (60.1 ± 5.13, $p < 0.01$), type 3 (57.9 ± 3.53, $p < 0.001$) and type 4 (56.8 ± 7.90, $p < 0.05$) when compared to those of the normal controls (75.4 ± 1.53).

Activated T cell subsets in each of the T cell subsets

The distribution of activated T cells in each of the T cell subsets was investigated.

The percentages of Leu3a$^+$-DR$^+$ cells (activated helper/inducer T cells) in Leu3a$^+$ cells and Leu2a$^+$-DR$^+$ cells (activated cytotoxic/suppressor T cells) in Leu2a$^+$ cells were significantly higher in AA with types 1, 3 and 4 than that of the normal controls (Figures 1 and 2).

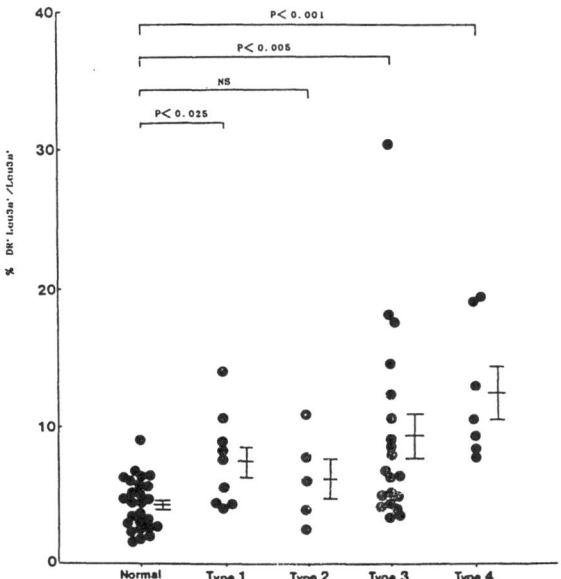

Figure 1 Percentages of activated helper/inducer T cells in Leu3a$^+$ cells in each of the AA types. Brackets represent the mean $\pm$ SE; NS = no signficant differences

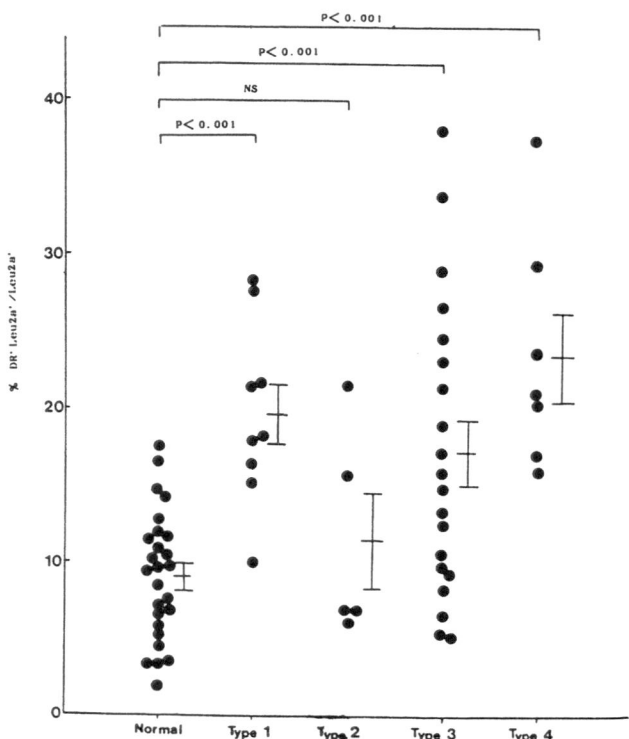

Figure 2 Percentages of activated cytotoxic/suppressor T cells in Leu2a$^+$ cells in each of the AA types. Brackets represent the mean $\pm$ SE; NS = no significant differences

NK cell subsets in total lymphocytes

The distribution of NK cells in total lymphocytes was analyzed using two kinds of monoclonal antibodies against NK cell (Table 1).

The percentages of Leu11$^+$ cells and Leu7$^+$ Leu11$^+$ cells in total lymphocytes showed significant increases in AA with type 3 (19.3 ± 2.94, $p < 0.005/12.1 \pm 2.45, p < 0.025$) when compared to that of the normal controls ($9.91 \pm 1.11/5.75 \pm 0.93$). The percentage of Leu$^-$ Leu11$^+$ cells in total lymphocytes were also strikingly higher in type 1 ($8.30 \pm 1.66, p < 0.025$) and type 3 (7.23 ± 0.87, $p < 0.005$) when compared to that of the normal controls (4.15 ± 0.40).

Correlation of disease activity with the distribution of NK cell subsets in type 3 AA patients

The patients with type 3 AA were divided into three groups based on the extent of the affected area of the scalp, and the respective NK cell subsets subsequently analyzed.

The percentage of Leu⁻Leu11⁺ cells in type 3 was proportional to the extent of the affected area of scalp (normal; 4.15 ± 0.40/mild cases of type 3; 4.84 ± 1.33/medium cases of type 3; 6.70 ± 0.94, $p < 0.025$/serious cases of type 3; 8.70 ± 1.60, $p < 0.01$).

DISCUSSION

The percentage of Pan T cells in total lymphocytes showed significant decreases in acute multiple AA (types 3 and 4). These findings concur with those of D'Ovidio et al.[2]. The significant decrease of Pan T cells was also shown in fixed alopecia universalis and multiple AA (type 1). This suggests that T cells may play a role in the pathogenesis of AA.

The percentages of activated helper/inducer T cells and activated cytotoxic/suppressor T cells were significantly higher in AA with types 1, 3 and 4. This suggests that the activation of T cells is induced in the peripheral blood of AA with types 1, 3 and 4.

It is unknown why the activated T cell increases in peripheral blood; however, as a phenomenon, the increase of activated T cell has been reported in virus diseases such as infectious mononucleosis[3], and in the diseases which were thought to be autoimmune diseases, such as graft-versus-host-disease[4], systemic lupus erythematosus[5], rheumatoid arthritis[5], aplastic anemia[6] and autoimmune thyroid disease[7]. In vitro, considerable increases in the percentages of activated T cells have been found after stimulation with mitogen[8], immunization with tetanus toxoid[9], or during mixed lymphocyte culture reaction[10]. This suggests that activating factor(s) of T cells may exist in above-mentioned diseases, including AA.

Human keratinocytes also express HLA-DR antigen in certain disease states characterized by mononuclear cell infiltrates. Messenger and Bleehen reported that HLA-DR antigens are aberrantly expressed in anagen hair follicle components of AA[11]. The expression of HLA-DR antigens on the anagen hair follicle and the peripheral T cells in AA suggests that immune mechanisms are operating in the pathogenesis of AA.

In this study, each of the subsets of NK cells in AA was also examined. The percentage of Leu⁻Leu11⁺ cells which had the highest cytotoxicity in NK cell subsets[12] was significantly elevated in AA with types 1 and 3. Further, in type 3 we were able to confirm the apparent relationship between disease activity and the percentage of Leu⁻Leu11⁺ cells.

The above suggests that NK cells may also play a role in the pathogenesis of AA.

REFERENCES

1.   Mitchell AJ, Krull EA. Alopecia areata: pathogenesis and treatment. J Am Acad Dermatol, 11, 763–775, 1984

2. D'Ovidio R, Vena GA, Angelini G. Cell-mediated immunity in alopecia areata. *Arch Dermatol Res*, **271**, 265–273, 1981

3. Reinherz EL, O'Brien C, Rosenthal P, Schlossman SF. The cellular basis for viral-induced immunodeficiency: analysis by monoclonal antibodies. *J Immunol*, **125**, 1269–1274, 1980

4. Reinherz EL, Parkman R, Rappeport J, Rosen FS, Schlossman SF. Aberrations of suppressor T cells in human graft-versus-host disease. *N Engl J Med*, **300**, 1061–1068, 1979

5. Yu DTY, Winchester RJ, Fu SM, Gibofsky A, Ko HS, Kunkel HG. Peripheral blood Ia-positive T cells. Increases in certain diseases and after immunization. *J Exp Med*, **151**, 91–100, 1980

6. Zoumbos NC, Gascón P, Djeu JY, Trost SR, Young NS. Circulating activated suppressor T lymphocytes in aplastic anemia. *N Engl J Med*, **312**, 257–265, 1985

7. Chan JYC, Walfish PG. Activated (Ia[+]) T-lymphocytes and their subsets in autoimmune thyroid diseases: analysis by dual laser flow microfluorocytometry. *J Clin Endocrinol Metab*, **62**, 403–409, 1986

8. Ko H-S, Fu SM, Winchester RJ, Yu DTY, Kunkel HG. Ia determinants on stimulated human T lymphocytes. Occurrence on mitogen- and antigen-activated T cells. *J Exp Med*, **150**, 246–255, 1979

9. Yachie A, Miyawaki T, Uwadana N, Ohzeki S, Taniguchi N. Sequential expression of T cell activation (Tac) antigen and Ia determinants on circulating human T cells after immunization with tetanus toxoid. *J Immunol*, **131**, 731–735, 1983

10. Evans RL, Faldetta TJ, Humphreys RE, Pratt DM, Yunis EJ, Schlossman SF. Peripheral human T cells sensitized in mixed leukocyte culture synthesize and express Ia-like antigens. *J Exp Med*, **148**, 1440–1445, 1978

11. Messenger AG, Bleehen SS. Expression of HLA-DR by anagen hair follicles in alopecia areata. *J Invest Dermatol*, **85**, 569–572, 1985

12. Abo T, Miller CA, Balch CM. Characterization of human granular lymphocyte subpopulations expressing HNK-1 (Leu-7) and Leu-11 antigens in the blood and lymphoid tissues from fetuses, neonates and adults. *Eur J Immunol*, **14**, 616–623, 1984

32
Mutagenic evaluation of SADBE in human lymphocytes

E Capelli* and G Orecchia
*Dipartimento di Genetica e Microbiologia
Università di Pavia
Via S. Epifanio, 14
27100 Pavia, Italy
†Clinica Dermatologica
Università di Pavia
Ospedale S. Matteo Pavia, Italy

ABSTRACT

Local treatment with squaric-acid dibutylester (SADBE) is a therapy for alopecia areata[1] and warts[2]. No mutagenic or cell-transforming activities could be shown for SADBE in the Ames test or the BHK cell transforming assay[2]. The aim of the present report is to evaluate the effects of SADBE on cultured human cells. The experiments were carried out on peripheral blood lymphocytes from normal blood donors. Test doses ranged from 0.05 to 500 mg/ml. The cytotoxic effect of the substance was demonstrated by the reduction of survival of PHA-stimulated lymphocytes. Finally the analysis of chromosome preparations obtained from lymphocytes 24 h after treatment with SADBE was performed in the presence and absence of S-9 mix. Treatments with cyclophosphamide and mitomicin C as positive controls were set up. No significant increase in the frequency of aberration was observed, compared to the untreated control, regardless of the presence of S-9 mix.

INTRODUCTION

Squaric acid dibutylester (SADBE) is a potent allergen used for the treatment of severe forms of alopecia areata[1] and of recalcitrant warts[2]. No mutagenic activities could be shown for SADBE in the Salmonella microsome test (Ames test) or in BHK cell transforming assay[3]. The good correlation between carcinogenic and mutagenic activity for a large number of chemical compounds has led to the development of several short-term mutagenicity tests[4]. The evaluation of possible genetic damage cannot be based on a single assay system; a whole battery of tests must be exploited[5,6], including different test organisms: prokaryotes, eukaryotic micro-organisms, and human cells cultured *in vitro*.

To obtain further information on the effects of SADBE we tested the substance on human lymphocytes *in vitro*. Human peripheral blood lymphocytes are a sensitive indicator of both *in vivo*- and *in vitro*-induced chromosomal structural changes[7]. The cytotoxic effect and the induction of chromosome aberration after SADBE treatment *in vitro* were evaluated.

MATERIALS AND METHODS

SADBE ($C_{12}H_{18}O_4$) was dissolved in ethanol at the concentration of 1 g/ml, stored at 4 °C and diluted at the time of use to the concentration required.

Cell cultures

Mononuclear cells obtained from peripheral blood samples of healthy donors by separation with MSL (Eurobio Labs.) were stimulated with 3% phytohemagglutinin (PHA-m, Difco) in complete medium (RPMI 1640 plus 20% of fetal calf serum) at 37 °C.

Toxicity test

A total of 5×10^5 cells were distributed into 24 mm wells (96 well plates) in complete medium with PHA containing SADBE at concentrations ranging from 0.0005% to 5% (0.05–50 mg/ml). The cells were then incubated at 37 °C for 24, 48 and 72 h.

Treatments

The 48 h PHA-stimulated cells, collected by centrifugation, were exposed to SADBE for 2 h in the presence and absence of metabolic activation (S-9 mix). Rat liver microsomes for metabolic activation were prepared from liver homogenates after induction with Aroclor 1254 and the S-9 mixtures were prepared according to the procedure of Ames *et al.*[8]. Treatments with cyclophosphamide (Endoxan, Asta) and Mitomicin C (Kyowa) as positive controls were performed in parallel.

Analysis of chromosome aberrations

After treatment the lymphocytes were resuspended in the 48 h conditioned medium previously stored at 37 °C and the incubation continued for another 24 h, at which time Colcemid (0.025 μg/ml) was added. After 5 h the hypotonic treatment was carried out at 37 °C with KCl 0.56 mol/l for 10 min. The cells were fixed with methyl alcohol–acetic acid solution. The slides were air-dried, stained with Giemsa solution and mounted with DPX (BDH).

RESULTS

A test was performed to obtain a general impression of the cytotoxicity of the tested chemical: the substance was added in different concentrations to the cells, without metabolic activation. Survival of lymphocyte cultures was evaluated at different doses (0.05–50 mg/ml) of SADBE after 24, 48 and 72 h of treatment, by counting the number of cells after trypan blue vital staining.

Figure 1 shows the survival of mononucleated lymphocytes after 24 h treatment with SADBE. The toxic effect of the substance, as demonstrated by the reduction of survival in respect to the untreated cells, increases as the concentration of SADBE increases. After 48 and 72 h culture the cytotoxicity of SADBE is more marked.

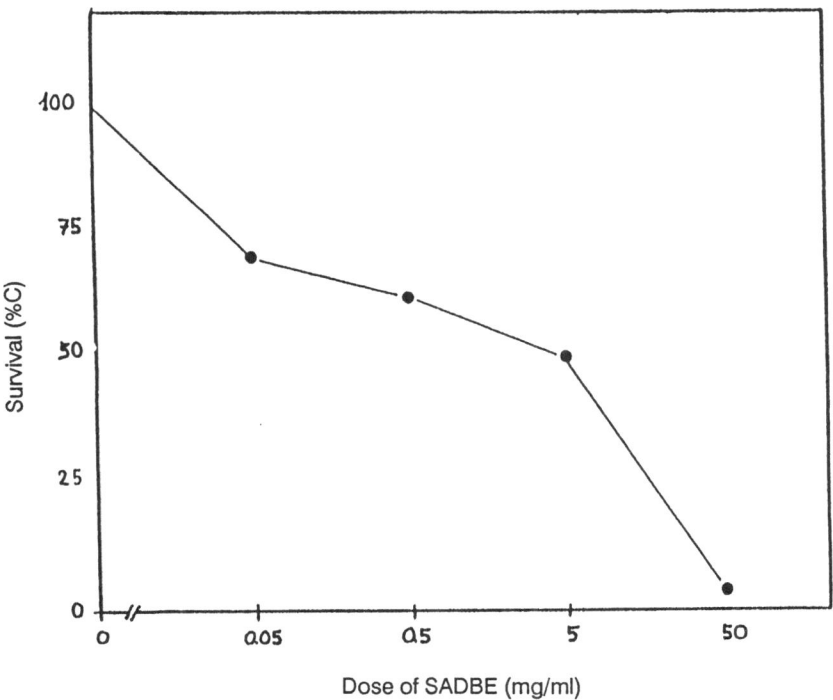

Figure 1   Survival of normal blood lymphocytes after 24 h SADBE treatment

The percentage of mitoses in cells treated for 2 h with SADBE is reported in Figure 2. The percentage of mitoses decreases as the SADBE doses increase (range of doses: 5–500 mg/ml).

The analysis of chromosome aberrations was performed in the presence and in the absence of S-9 on 72 h PHA-stimulated lymphocytes, 24 h after SADBE treatment. The following doses were chosen: 10 mg/ml; 50 mg/ml,

307

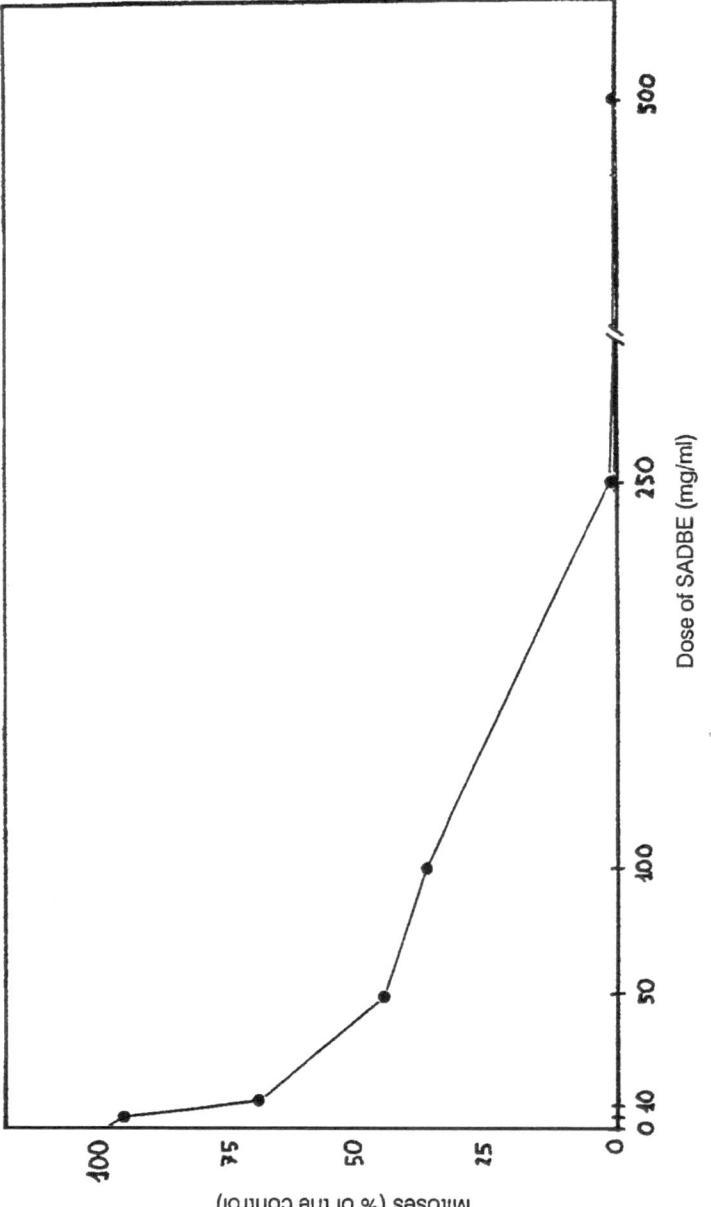

Figure 2 Number of mitoses after 2 h SADBE treatment

and 100 mg/ml, which induced a reduction of mitotic index of 30%, 54% and 62% respectively (Figure 2).

The percentage of mitoses in the samples treated with SADBE was compared to that in the untreated control: the frequency of mitoses decreases as the concentration of SADBE increases. The toxic effect is similar in the presence of microsomes (Figure 3).

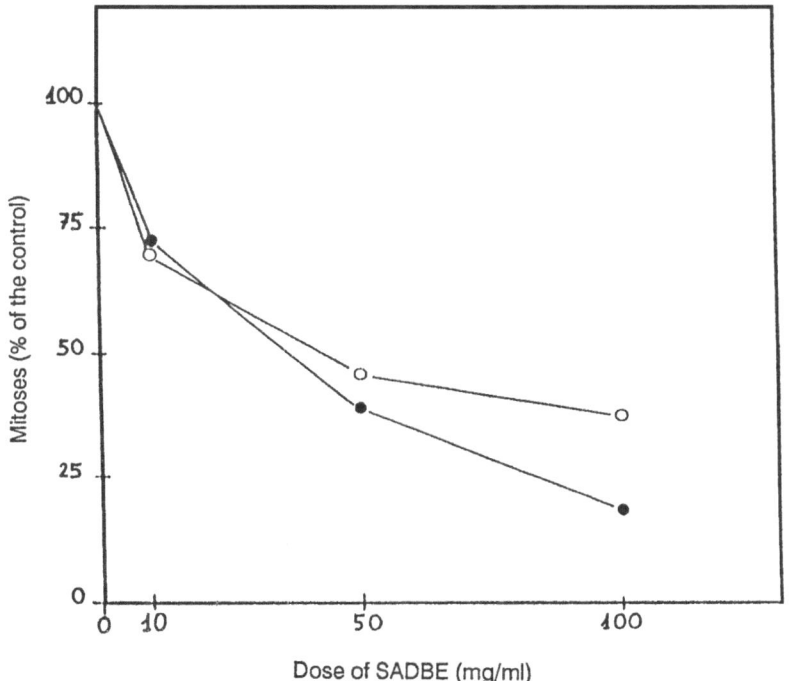

Figure 3 Number of mitoses in cells treated with SADBE in the absence (o–o) and in the presence of (● – ●) of microsomes

The frequency of mitoses showing chromosome aberrations (with and without gaps) was also evaluated. As shown in Table 1, no significant increase in the frequency of aberrations was observed compared to the untreated control, regardless of the presence of S-9. On the contrary, a high frequency of aberrations was detected in the samples obtained from cells treated with mitomicin C in the absence of S-9, and in those cells treated with cyclophosphamide, in the presence of S-9. The aberrant cell frequency in untreated control cells is in the range of the values normally observed, for the same cellular type, in our standard conditions (1–5% for the aberrations including gaps; 0–3% for the aberrations without gaps).

Table 1 **Frequency of chromosome aberrations in lymphocytes after SADBE treatment in the presence and absence of microsomes**

Dose of SADBE (mg/ml)	No of examined mitoses	Percentage of mitoses with aberration			
		− Microsomes		+ Microsomes	
		+ gap	− gap	+ gap	− gap
0	50	4	0	3	1
10	50	2	0	2	0
50	50	0	0	0	0
100	50	2	1	2	0
Dose of cyclophosphamide (µg/ml)					
6	42	10	0	61.0	31.0
Dose of mitomicin C (µg/ml)					
10	50	28	26	ND	ND

CONCLUSIONS

We investigated the potential genotoxic activity of SADBE by determining the induction of chromosomal aberrations in human lymphocytes from normal individuals cultured *in vitro*. The results were compared to those obtained with a direct clastogen (mitomicin C) and with a clastogen requiring metabolic activation (cyclophosphamide).

No significant increase was observed in the frequency of chromosome aberrations in treated cells as compared to the untreated cells regardless of the presence of rat liver microsomes (S-9) for the metabolic activation. A high frequency of aberrations was detected in the samples treated with the positive control cyclophosphamide in the presence of S-9 and with the positive control mitomicin C in the absence of S-9.

Our results, and the reports of other authors[2], concerning SADBE support the idea that this compound does not have mutagenic activity. However, it is still necessary to continue research on SADBE activity in human cells using other mutagenicity tests[9,10] in order to exclude any genotoxic effect.

In conclusion, SADBE must be preferred to DNCB because it is a potent sensitizer having no mutagenic activity[11].

REFERENCES

1.   Giannetti A, Orecchia G. Clinical experience on the treatment of alopecia areata with squaric acid dibutylester. *Dermatologica*, **167**, 280–282, 1983
2.   Strobel R, Röhrborn G. Mutagenic and cell transforming activities of 1-chlor-2, 4-dinitrobenzene (DNCB) and squaric acid dibutylester (SADBE). *Arch Toxicol*, **45**, 307–314, 1980

3. Claudy AL, Roche H. Traitement des verrues multiples et recidivantes par induction d'une hypersensibilité retardée. II Etude critique de l'utilisation du dibutylester de l'acide squarique. *Ann Derm Vénér*, **108**, 765–767, 1981

4. Ashby J, de Serres FJ, Draper M, Ishdate M Jr, Margolin BH, Matter BE, Shelby MD (eds). *Progress in Mutation Research*, Vol. 5: *Evaluation of Short-Term Tests for Carcinogens*. Amsterdam, Oxford, New York: Elsevier, 1985

5. Hollaender (ed.) Cytological methods for detecting chemical mutagens. *Chem Mutagens*, **4**, 1–29, 1973

6. Martin CM, McDermid AC, Garner RC. Testing of known carcinogens and non carcinogens for their ability to induce unscheduled DNA synthesis in HeLa cells. *Cancer Res*, **38**, 2621–2627, 1978

7. Evans HJ, O'Riordan ML. Human peripheral blood lymphocytes for the analysis of chromosome aberration in mutagen tests. *Mutat Res*, **32**, 135–148, 1975

8. Ames BN, McCann J, Yamasaki E. Methods for detecting carcinogens and mutagens with the salmonella (mammalian-microsome mutogenicity test). *Handbook of Mutagenicity Test Procedures* pp. 1–17. Amsterdam, New York, Oxford: Elsevier, 1977

9. Van Zeeland AA. DNA repair. In: *Mutation in Man* (Obe G, ed.), pp. 34–57, Berlin, Heidelberg: Springer Verlag, 1984

10. Fenech M, Morley AA. Measurement of micronuclei in lymphocytes. *Mut Res*, **147**, 29–36, 1985

11. Kratka J, Goerz G, Vizethum W *et al*. Dinitroclorobenzene influence on the cytochrome P-450 system and mutagenic effects. *Arch Dermatol Res*, **226**, 315–318, 1979

33
Treatment of severe alopecia areata by topical applications of cyclosporin A: comparative trial versus placebo in 43 patients

Y de Prost, D Teillac, F Paquez, L Carrugi and
R Touraine
Department of Dermatology
Hôpital Necker, Paris, France

ABSTRACT

Forty-three patients with severe alopecia areata were divided into two groups: group 1 ($n = 22$) treated with once-daily application of 0.5 ml of an oily solution containing 100 mg/ml of cyclosporin A (CyA) to one half of the scalp during 6 months; group 2 ($n = 21$): once-daily application of an oily solution without CyA to one half of the scalp. The development of terminal hairs, generally in the form of small tufts 0.5 to 2 cm in diameter was observed in seven patients in group 1 and not in group 2. No cases of complete hair regrowth were observed. Diffuse vellus hair predominant on the treated side was observed in five patients in group 1 and in three patients in group 2. The local tolerance was good. A few episodes of transient folliculitis (four cases in each group) were noted. The laboratory survey (serum electrolytes, creatinine, uric acid) did not reveal any significant variations and cyclosporin blood levels were always below detectable limits. CyA has never been used topically in man prior to this trial. This comparative trial demonstrated a difference between the two groups, as terminal hairs were observed in seven cases in group 1. This regrowth was mild, of delayed onset and never complete. However, the development of terminal hairs in the treated group suggests a local action of CyA and encourages further therapeutic trials with different concentrations and different vehicles.

The current pathophysiological concepts of alopecia areata involve two immunological mechanisms: autoimmune phenomena and the participation of T cell lymphocytotoxicity, with infiltration of T lymphocytes around the pilosebaceous follicles[1]. The immunosuppressant action of cyclosporin (CyA), especially on the cell-mediated immune response, suggests a possible action in alopecia areata. The development of hypertrichosis during systemic treatment with CyA, although unexplained, also suggests a possible trichogenic effect. CyA has never been applied topically in man. The topical application of 2% CyA in experimental animals decreases delayed hypersensitivity reactions[2].

We studied the therapeutic effect of repeated applications of CyA in patients with severe alopecia areata by means of a comparative trial versus placebo. This study was conducted in 43 patients with severe alopecia areata: 20 cases of universal alopecia, seven cases of total alopecia and 16 cases of patchy alopecia affecting more than 30% of the scalp, present for between 1 and 32 years (mean ≈ 11 years). The patients were divided into two groups: group 1 ($n = 22$): once-daily application of 0.5 ml of an oily solution containing 100 mg/ml of CyA to one half of the scalp; group 2 ($n = 21$): once-daily application of an oily solution without CyA to one half of the scalp for a period of 3 months, followed by the same solution as that used in group 1 for the following 3 months in 12 patients. Serum cyclosporin assays were performed each month during the first months of treatment by means of radioimmunological technique. The lymphocyte sub-populations of the peribulbar infiltrate were studied before and after treatment in 3 patients.

The development of terminal hairs, generally in the form of small tufts 0.5 to 2 cm in diameter, was observed in seven patients in group 1 and none in group 2. These terminal hairs appeared between the second and sixth months of treatment.

No cases of complete hair regrowth were observed. Diffuse down, predominant on the treated side, was observed in five patients in group 1 and diffuse down was observed in three patients in group 2. Only one patient developed terminal hairs after cross-over.

The local tolerance of treatment was good. A few episodes of transient folliculitis (four cases in each group) and occasional transient sensations of pruritus or irritation were noted, but never required withdrawal of treatment. The laboratory survey (serum electrolytes, creatinine, uric acid), performed before and after treatment, did not reveal any significant variations and the serum cyclosporin assays were always below detectable limits. The study of the peribulbar lymphocyte sub-populations in three patients only revealed a modification in the helper/suppressor ratio in one patient, while insufficient infiltrate was obtained in the other two patients. The infiltrate was composed of 90% helper T cells and 5% suppressor T cells before treatment, and the ratio was clearly inverted after treatment in an area of regrowth of terminal hairs (helper 10%, suppressor 75%).

This comparative trial therefore demonstrated a difference between the two groups of patients, as terminal hairs were observed in seven cases in group 1 and never in group 2. This regrowth was mild, of delayed onset and never complete.

CyA has never been used topically in man prior to this trial. The application of 0.5 ml of CyA per day over a period of 6 months was always well tolerated and only caused transient folliculitis and irritation, probably related to the oily nature of the excipient. Serum cyclosporin levels were always below the limits detectable by the method used. The predominance of helper T cells in the peribulbar infiltrate has already been reported in the course of alopecia areata[2]. The inversion of the helper suppressor ratio during regrowth was an interesting finding in one of our patients. However, it does not necessarily directly reflect the action of CyA, but may be a sign of regrowth of terminal hairs.

This comparative trial did not demonstrate any beneficial therapeutic effect in cases of severe alopecia areata. However, the development of terminal hairs in the treated group suggests a local action of CyA in this disease and encourages further therapeutic trials with different concentrations and different vehicles.

REFERENCES

1. Aldridge RD, Thomson AW, Rosslyn Rankin. Inhibition of contact sensitivity reactions to DNFB by topical cyclosporin application in the guinea-pig *Clin Exp Immunol*, **59**, 23–28, 1985
2. Todes Taylor N, Turner R, Wood SG. T cell sub-populations in alopecia areata *J Am Acad Dermatol*, **11**, 216–223, 1984

34
Anatomo-clinical illustration of a hair-follicle nevus

D Tennstedt and JM Lachapelle
Unit and Laboratory of Occupational and Environmental Dermatology
Catholic University of Louvain, 30 Clos Chapelle-aux-Champs
B-1200 Brussels, Belgium

ABSTRACT

A patient, aged 16, sought advice for a tuft of dense eyelashes at the free margin of the right eyelid. The main complaint was the length of the eyelashes, that needed frequent cutting. There was no swelling of the eyelid. When compared to those of the left eyelid, the eyelashes were thinner, longer, more numerous and they were orientated in various directions. The area of skin was removed. Histopathological examination of the specimen revealed the presence of a hair-follicle nevus. The lesion is characterized by the presence of numerous mature hair follicles, containing a hair shaft. The hair bulbs are present at different levels of dermis and are orientated in various directions with regard to epidermis. The hair-follicle nevus is quite infrequent. It was described in 1924 by Fessler, and is illustrated in Civatte's textbook of dermatopathology[1].

INTRODUCTION

The hair-follicle nevus is a very rare hamartoma; a few cases have been reported since the first description by Fessler[2] in 1924. A characteristic lesion has been diagnosed recently at our department.

CASE REPORT

A patient, aged 16, sought advice for a tuft of dense eyelashes at the free margin of the right eyelid. The main complaint was the length of the eyelashes, which needed frequent cutting. There was no swelling of the eyelid. When compared to those of the left eyelid, the eyelashes were thinner, longer, more numerous and they were orientated in various directions (Figure 1). The area of skin was removed. Histopathological examination of the specimen revealed the presence of a hair-follicle nevus (Figure 2). The lesion is characterized by the presence of numerous mature hair follicles, containing a hair

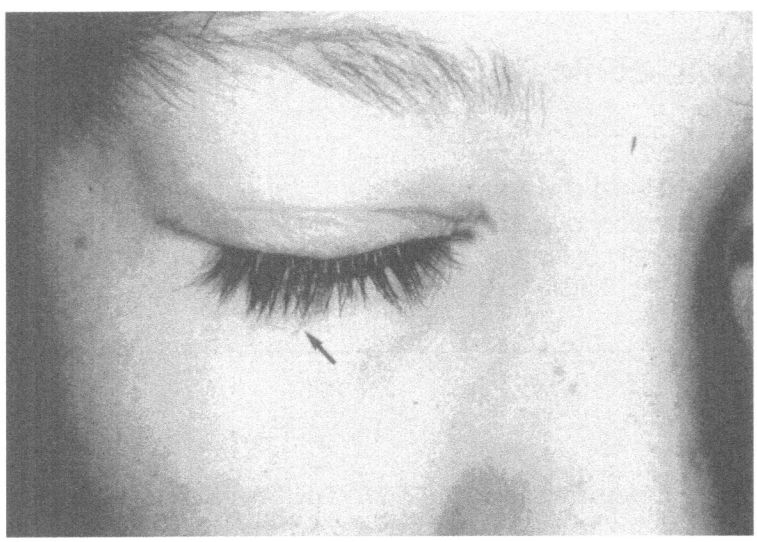

Figure 1 Hair-follicle nevus. The eyelashes are thinner, longer, more numerous and orientated in various directions (see arrow)

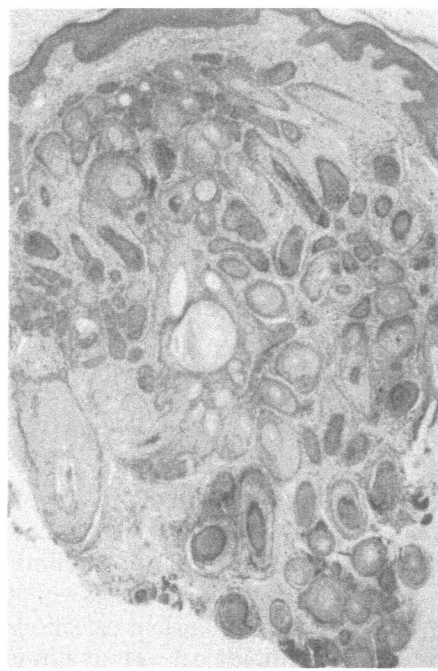

Figure 2 Hair-follicle nevus. A microscopic view of the lesion at low magnification. H and E stain (x 15)

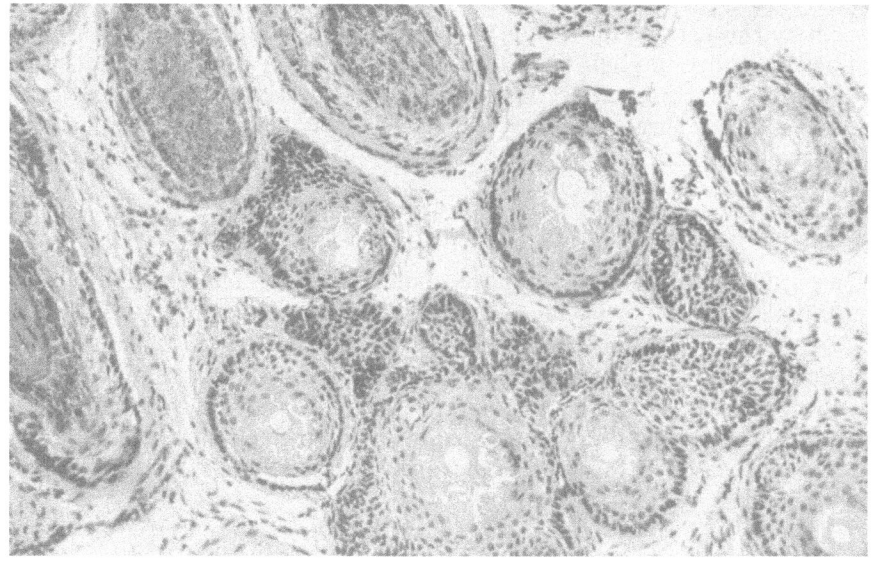

Figure 3   Hair-follicle nevus. The hairs are orientated in various directions. H and E stain (x 70)

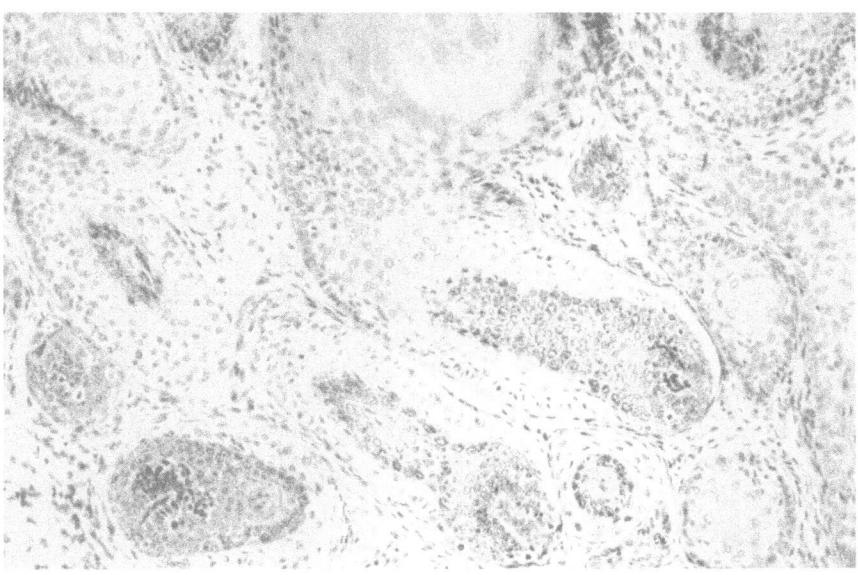

Figure 4   Hair-follicle nevus. The hair bulbs are orientated in various directions. H and E stain (x 100)

shaft (Figure 3). The hair bulbs are located in mid or deep dermis and are orientated in various directions with regard to epidermis (Figure 4). The epidermis above the hair-follicle nevus is not hyperplastic. There is no inflammatory reaction; sebaceous glands are not present. Removal of the lesion by a plastic surgeon was successful. The free margin of the right eyelid is clinically normal.

DISCUSSION

The pure hair-follicle nevus is not frequent. It is characterised by well-differentiated hair follicles. Our observation is quite similar to that illustrated in Civatte's *Textbook of Histopathology* p. 248[3]. In both cases there are no sebaceous glands in the nevus. It is obvious that great variations in the size of hair follicles do exist when we compare histological pictures from various observations: crowding of many tiny mature hair follicles is the essential feature in most cases[3-7]. Some authors mention that small sebaceous glands can be present[4,6].

REFERENCES

1. Civatte J. *Histopathologie Cutanée*. Paris: Flammarion, 1982
2. Fessler A. Angeborene Haargeschwulst. *Arch Dermatol Syphil*, 146, 411–414, 1924
3. Doxanas MT, Green WR, Arentsen JJ, Elsas FJ. Lid lesions of childhood: a histopathological survey at the Wilmer Institute (1923-1974). *J Pediatr Ophthalmol*, 13, 7–39, 1976
4. Grouls V. Hair-follicle nevus or congenital vellus hamartoma. Letter to the Editor. *Am J Dermatopathol*, 7, 304, 1985
5. Pinkus H, Mehregan AH. *A Guide to Dermatohistopathology*, 2nd edn. New York: Appleton, 1976
6. Pippione M, Aloi F, Depaoli MA. Hair-follicle nevus. *Am J Dermatopathol*, 6, 245–247, 1984
7. Weir TW. Hair-follicle nevus. Letter to the Editor. *Am J Dermatopathol*, 7, 304, 1985

35
Headgear induced traumatic alopecia during orthodontic treatment

D Van Neste
Department of Dermatology, Catholic University of Louvain, Brussels, Belgium

ABSTRACT

This short clinical case report illustrates a case of traumatic alopecia appearing during orthodontic therapy. A girl, aged 9 years, presented with a localized alopecia on the vertex. There were obvious signs of microtrauma on the skin surface with moderate erythema and crusting over the area. The alopecia and the irritation developed, while the patient applied a device every night to maintain a constant traction during resting time at the level of the maxillae. The goal of the application of the orthopedic forces was restoration of malocclusion.

The headgear consists of two rims crossing over the vertex. Crossings are fixed with hooks. When traction is applied these hooks are in close contact with the scalp, and friction removes the hair shafts from the area. The hair root status showed 92% anagen, indicating tractional alopecia. Hair regrowth was observed within a few weeks after replacement of the currently used device by a less traumatizing one.

This is a variant of mechanically induced 'iatrogenic' alopecia which is to be added to the list of other forms of traumatic alopecia. Dermatologists and orthodontists should be aware of the existence of this type of alopecia, and the use of harmless devices should be preferred.

INTRODUCTION

The aim of this short clinical case report is to illustrate a poorly known cause of traumatic alopecia appearing during orthodontic therapy. Rarely reported in the medical literature, this condition is worth knowing of and identifying, as specific preventive treatment resolves the problem without any serious defect for the patient.

CASE REPORT

A girl, aged 9 years, presented with a localized alopecia on the vertex. There were obvious signs of microtrauma on the skin surface with moderate erythema and crusting over the area (Figure 1). Alopecia and irritation developed while the patient applied a device every night to maintain a constant traction during resting time at the level of the maxillae. The goal of the application of the orthopedic forces was restoration of malocclusion (Figure 2).

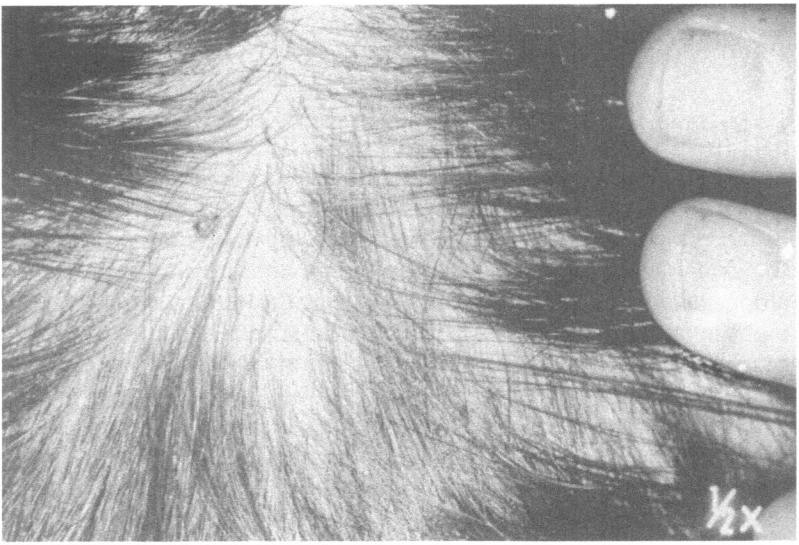

Figure 1   Headgear-induced traumatic alopecia. Microtrauma on the scalp, moderate erythema and crusting over the area of alopecia on the vertex

The headgear consists of two rims crossing over the vertex. Crossings are fixed with hooks (Figure 3). When traction is applied, these hooks are in close contact with the scalp and friction removes the hair shafts from the area. The hair root status showed 92% anagen, indicating tractional alopecia. Hair regrowth was observed within a few weeks after replacement of the currently used device by a less traumatizing one.

DISCUSSION

This case report concerns a patient with a variant of mechanically induced 'iatrogenic' alopecia. Various forms of pressure-induced alopecia have been reported. In most of the cases reported so far, it appeared that the alopecia was due to excessive local pressure with decrease of the skin blood perfusion. Amongst the etiological circumstances reports mainly concern unusually

322

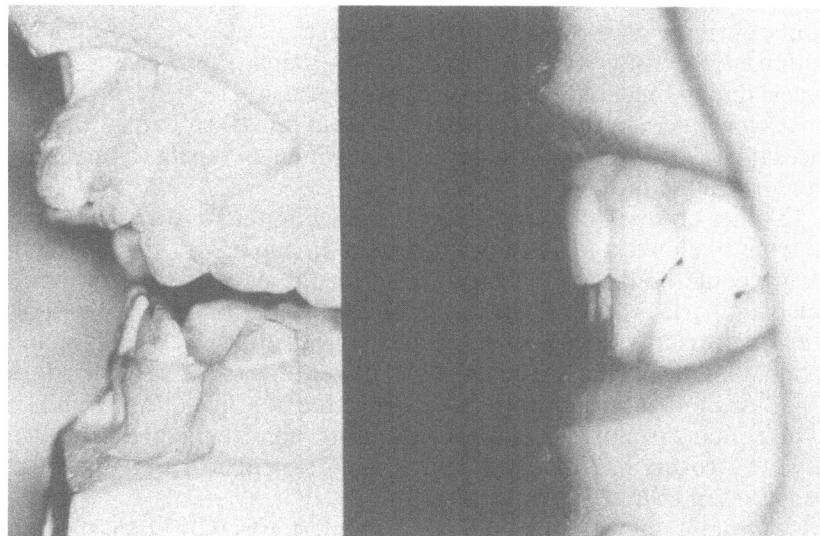

Figure 2 Malocclusion before and after treatment. This illustrates the malocclusion (before treatment), a quite common indication for the application of the orthopedic forces during childhood. The restoration of malocclusion is shown on the right

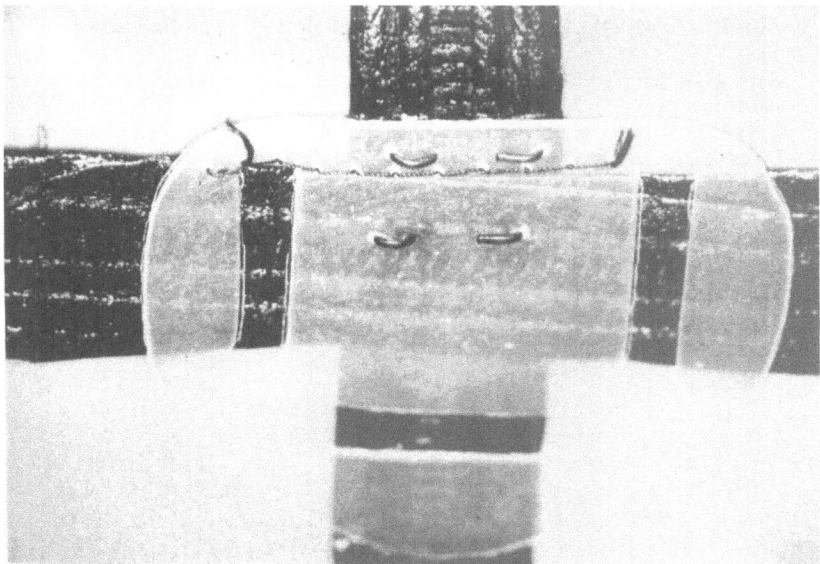

Figure 3 Hooks used for fixing the crossing rims. The headgear consists of two rims crossing over the vertex; crossings are fixed with hooks

323

prolonged periods of intubation (with or without coma), or anesthesia – for example during gynecological[1,2] or open-heart surgery[3]. Depending upon the duration and intensity of the local ischemia, the damage varies from transient alopecia due to functional reduction of skin perfusion to blistering and scar formation with cicatricial alopecia (reviewed in ref. 4). Under such circumstances it is advised to move the head of the patient at regular intervals during the operation or recovery.

In other observations extraoral appliances, better known as 'headgear'. Two types of alopecia must be distinguished. In one report it appeared that pressure could be the trigger mechanism for the development of the first patch of alopecia areata[5]. Even though alopecia areata started at the spot of increased pressure other zones could be involved afterwards. In our patient we think that the patchy hair loss was exclusively due to excessive friction by the hooks removing hairs from the scalp in the absence of any significant pressure-induced alopecia. Indeed, by using non-traumatizing headgear complete recovery was observed. This etiology should be added to the list of other forms of traumatic alopecia[6].

Our intention, with this short clinical report, was to bring to the attention of dermatologists and orthodontists the existence of this type of alopecia, which can easily be prevented by the use of non-traumatizing devices.

REFERENCES

1. Abel RR, Lewis GM. Postoperative (pressure) alopecia. *Arch Dermatol* **81**, 34-42, 1960
2. Berger GS, Peterson B. Pressure alopecia after microsurgical anastomosis. *Am J Obstet Gynecol* (letter), **704**, 1978
3. Lawson NW, Mills NL, Ochsner JL. Occipital alopecia following cardiopulmonary bypass. *J Thorac Cardiovasc Surg*, **71**, 342-347, 1976
4. Wiles JC, Hansen RC. Postoperative (pressure) alopecia. *J Am Acad Dermatol* **12**, 195-198, 1985
5. Zuehlke RL, Bishara S, Price V. Pressure potentiated alopecia areata. *Am J Orthodont*, 437-438, 1981
6. Rook A, Dawber R. *Diseases of the Hair and Scalp*. Oxford: Blackwell, 1982, pp. 121-122

Index

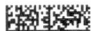